Certification Review for Perianesthesia Nursing

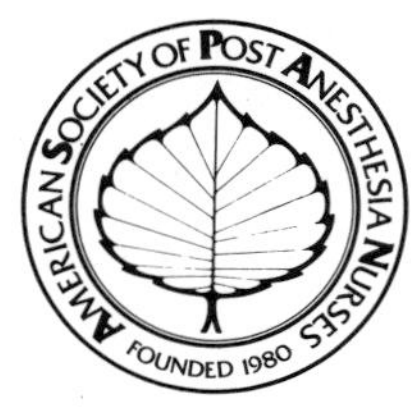

American Society of Post Anesthesia Nurses

Certification Review for Perianesthesia Nursing

Kathy Carlson, RN, MA, BSN, CPAN
Clinical Nurse, Post Anesthesia Care Unit
Abbott-Northwestern Hospital
Minneapolis, Minnesota

Saunders
An Imprint of Elsevier

SAUNDERS

An Imprint of Elsevier

The Curtis Center
Independence Square West
Philadelphia, Pennsylvania 19106

Library of Congress Cataloging-in-Publication Data

Certification review for perianesthesia nursing / Kathy Carlson
[editor]. — 1st ed.
p. cm.
Includes bibliographical references and index.
ISBN 0-7216-4492-9
1. Anesthesiology—Examinations, questions, etc. 2. Post
-anesthesia nursing—Examinations, questions, etc. 3. Nurse
anesthetists. I. Carlson, Kathy.
[DNLM: 1. Anesthesia—nursing—examination questions. 2. Nursing
Process—examination questions. WY 18.2 C418 1996]
RD82.C46 1996
617.9'6'076—dc20
DNLM/DLC 95-36450

NOTICE

Perianesthesia nursing is an ever-changing field. Standard safety precautions must be followed, but as new research and clinical experience broaden our knowledge, changes in treatment and drug therapy become necessary or appropriate. The editors of this work have carefully checked the generic and trade drug names and verified drug dosages to ensure that the dosage information in this work is accurate and in accord with the standards accepted at the time of publication. Readers are advised, however, to check the product information currently provided by the manufacturer of each drug to be administered to be certain that changes have not been made in the recommended dose or in the contraindications for administration. This is of particular importance in regard to new or infrequently used drugs. It is the responsibility of the treating physician, relying on experience and knowledge of the patient, to determine dosages and the best treatment for the patient. The editors cannot be responsible for misuse or misapplication of the material in this work.

THE PUBLISHER

ASPAN: CERTIFICATION REVIEW FOR PERIANESTHESIA NURSING ISBN 0–7216–4492–9

Printed in the United States of America

Last digit is the print number: 9 8 7 6

Contributors

Nurses practicing in perianesthesia settings were invited to collect their best clinical references and to consider clinical topics that every certified perianesthesia nurse must grasp. Questions submitted by the nurses who responded to this call were enfolded into situations that became this book's scenarios and items; issues and concepts raised in the questions expanded into the supporting rationales.

Anonymous

One generous nurse colleague contributed many questions but not her name. Like the prolific poet, I shall call her "Anonymous" and publicly thank her.

Charles N. Aprea, RN, MSN

Nurse Manager, PACU/IV Team, Hospital of Saint Raphael, New Haven, Connecticut

Jolene Carver, RN, BSN, CPAN

Staff Nurse, Iowa Health System, Iowa Lutheran Hospital, Des Moines, Iowa

Donna M. DeFazio-Quinn, RN, MBA, BSN, CPAN, CAPA

Director, Elliot 1-Day Surgery Center, Optima Health, Manchester, New Hampshire

Joyce C. Hadley, RN, BA, CPAN

Clinical Educator, Fairfax Hospital, Falls Church, Virginia

Vallire D. Hooper, RN, MSN, CPAN

Nurse Entrepreneur and Co-founder, Hooper, Keith, & Associates, Augusta, Georgia

Robin M. Kirschner, RNC, MA, BSN, CDE, CPAN

Staff Nurse, St. Francis Medical Center, West Ewa Beach, Hawaii

Kathleen Millican Miller, RN, MSN, CPAN

Perioperative Clinical Nurse Specialist, St. Charles Hospital, Oregon, Ohio

Ellen L. Poole, RN, MS, BSN, CCRN, CPAN, CAPA

Assistant Professor of Nursing, Grand Canyon University Samaritan College of Nursing, Phoenix, Arizona

Jean Sutton, RN, CPAN, CAPA

Staff Nurse, Sacred Heart Medical Center, Spokane, Washington

Joan Vogelsang, RN, EdD, MSN

Staff Nurse, Jewish Hospital Kenwood; Clinical Nurse, University Hospital, Cincinnati, Ohio

Annette S. Williams, RN, BSN, CPAN

Staff Nurse, PACU, Memorial Hospital at Gulfport, Gulfport, Mississippi

Maureen Jo Winter, RN, BS, CPAN

Nurse Clinician, Department of Anesthesia; Unit Manager, Preadmission Service, Monmouth Medical Center, Long Branch, New Jersey

Reviewers

Nancy Burden, RN, BS, CPAN, CAPA
Surgery Team Leader, Morton Plant East Lake Surgery Center, Palm Harbor, Florida

Dolly Ireland, RN, CAPA
William Beaumont Hospital–Troy, Troy, Michigan

Kim Litwack, RN, PhD, CPAN
Associate Professor, University of New Mexico College of Nursing, Albuquerque, New Mexico

Janet L. Ridder, RN, MS, CPAN
Coordinator for Case Management, Hinsdale Hospital, Hinsdale, Illinois

Lois Schick, RN, MBA, MN, BSN, CPAN, CAPA
Saint Joseph Hospital, Denver, Colorado

Cynthia A. Smith, RN, MBA, BSN
Venice Health Park, Venice, Florida

Foreword

ASPAN is pleased to present a new publication entitled *Certification Review for Perianesthesia Nursing.* Kathy Carlson has worked diligently on this project, and we appreciate her efforts.

ASPAN recognizes that PACU nurses are no longer exclusively in the postanesthesia setting. As your professional organization, ASPAN constantly strives to represent nurses in all areas of perianesthesia care. We feel that the title and content of this new publication will address the expanded role of your practice.

As you make preparations to accept the challenge of CPAN or CAPA certification, we hope you will find this resource both beneficial and valuable!

Lois A. Roberts, RN
ASPAN President
1995–1996

Preface

Congratulations! The very act of opening *Certification Review for Perianesthesia Nursing* reflects your interest in professional development. The journey to certification encourages you to excel professionally, and personal excellence is a tandem benefit.

A certification examination asks you to demonstrate your mastery of core knowledge, essential skills, and fundamental principles integral to perianesthesia nursing practice. According to 1990 and 1993 survey responses of your already certified colleagues, earning a certification credential is truly a personally gratifying achievement.

Your primary clinical focus practice determines whether you elect to certify by the CPAN or the CAPA form of the examination. Over 4000 nurses have become certified postanesthesia nurses (CPANs) since 1986. The CPAN credential designates knowledge and skill applied primarily in a *hospital-based, inpatient* setting.

Nurse colleagues who practice primarily in *ambulatory surgery* settings may earn the credential of CAPA, a certified ambulatory postanesthesia nurse. The CAPA examination premiered in November 1994. A nurse who seeks challenge and whose practice balances both the inpatient and ambulatory surgery focus may earn *both* credentials.

The ability to assess, plan, implement, and evaluate the patient condition from presentation through postanesthesia "recovery" requires education and honed skill. *Certification Review for Perianesthesia Nursing* provides each reader with a comprehensive tool to guide a personal learning process, a method to nurture professional growth, a flavor of examination content, and insight into examination development and construction. I believe the questions and concepts presented here can challenge the perianesthesia nurse, certified or not, in *any* setting.

Imagine a patient-focused practice in perianesthesia nursing that extends beyond narrow labels or the territorial, arbitrary limits of a single setting. Break imposed barriers! Apply each bit of knowledge or skill concept globally, whether in a freestanding or hospital-based postanesthesia care unit (PACU), a minimally invasive care setting or critical care unit, a radiology department, mental health unit, and even a physician office. Wherever there is patient care, a perianesthesia nurse weaves the nursing process through the core of essential elements common to these settings: airway management, circulatory support, pharmacologic interactions, education, and attention to positive outcomes for the sedated or anesthetized patient.

Trust yourself. Value your already demonstrated clinical experience. Remember that certification merely validates the knowledge you have already acquired. So, relax. Whether you pass the examination this time or do not, the process of preparing for this goal can only improve your confidence in yourself and your practice. Now *that is* a lofty achievement!

Kathy Carlson
March 1995

Acknowledgments

Out of our questions, we have developed a dialogue of faith in the process that carries us forward.

—Christina Baldwin

The journey of crafting questions for a book was truly a creative adventure. This two-year endeavor tapped my belief in process and my trust that ideas and formats evolve with time. The product weaves together the efforts and energies of many. I particularly appreciate:

- nurses who aspire to grow, to seek knowledge, and to quest for new challenges
- strong women (and men) in ASPAN and ABPANC who mentored me by example and modeled achievement
- ASPAN leaders who dangle challenges before me, test my creativity and trust my determination to succeed
- Charlene Roberts, once my coeditor, whose perspective grounded the book's vision, tone, and style; thanks for sending humor and silent messages of support
- nurse contributors who translated real-life clinical situations into issues and questions that shaped the book
- six respected perianesthesia nurses whose review suggestions became written conversations that encouraged me, inspired content and phrasing adjustments, or brightened my perspective and lightened my heart
- Daniel Ruth, for his persistent encouragement and droll art, and Susan Bielitsky, who shared the wisdom of her experience
- Mary Espenschied of Cracom Corporation and Joan Sinclair at Saunders, who engineered an exceptionally speedy production schedule
- Susan Fetzer, whose regular phone calls sustained my motivation; thanks for postcards, a collaborative history, friendship, and lively conversations
- Jan Rabbers, a true soul connection who also loves questions, stretches my thoughts, and whose world view so complements mine
- my Minneapolis contingent:
  - colleagues in PACU at Abbott-Northwestern Hospital who anchor me, probably without realizing it, through their presence, flexibility, and the constant bond of shared experiences, crises, and laughter over 15 years.
  - thousands of postanesthesia patients who have shared an hour (or four) with me; I've learned to observe closely, ask questions, expect change, and respect intuition.
  - my family, who tolerates my "portable" editing jobs and late night computer hours: *Lee,* for massages, culinary skills, and a quiet love that abides my erratic pace; *Lara,* for her bright smile, bubbling energy, and optimistic young woman-spirit that rejuvenates me; *Brent,* for the impish twinkle in his eye, boyish hugs, and his inquisitive mind and engaging wit; and *Scruffy,* my quiet and everpresent rug-side companion.

Kathy

Contents

Fundamental Concepts

Applied Concepts

Section 4

Section 5

Section 6

Section 7

Section 1

Certification Planning

Information in this section focuses on the process of certification. Concepts include a philosophy of certification, personal discipline and motivation, the perianesthesia role and examination construction and development.

ESSENTIAL CORE CONCEPTS

Preparing for Excellence
Excellence: Personal Development
Excellence: A Professional Intention
Engaging in a Process
Assessment: Knowledge of Candidate and Examination
Assessment of Self
Awareness of Certification Details
Understanding Examination Concepts and Development
Planning and Implementation: Study Strategies
Setting a Pace Toward Certification
Evaluation: Monitoring Achievement
Testing Tidbits
As You Begin . . .

Love the questions.

—Rilke

Life is full of challenging questions. A certification examination just concentrates 200 focused questions into 4 hours! Choosing to respond to these questions involves growth and discovery of your capabilities and of new knowledge.

Welcome the turns and questions along your path. Any growth, including preparing to certify, represents a process that is not necessarily linear, as from point A to point B. Growth more often poses questions and resembles a dance, with steps forward, sideways and back. Perhaps in your past you considered, then dismissed, thoughts of certifying for reasons as diverse as time, lack of knowledge or even fear. Perhaps you needed more tools, an extra ounce of confidence or the comfort of a study circle. Perhaps now a colleague's supportive encouragement, the lure of achievement or your health care facility's merit recognition program entices you. This time, you're ready to accept the challenge.

In the spirit of loving the questions, spend time becoming aware. Reflect on your goals for seeking this new discipline of discovery, consider your personal style of learning, assemble your resources and establish a nurturing web of support. *Here we go!*

PREPARING FOR EXCELLENCE

Why create this guide? Who is the guide's audience?

Excellence: Personal Development

This guide is primarily intended for the perianesthesia nurse who strives toward the certified postanesthesia nurse (CPAN) credential. The certified ambulatory postanesthesia (CAPA) examination candidate, the already certified nurse, and other inquiring readers will also benefit by assimilating the content and practicing the examination style. When creating review questions and rationales, the author assumes most readers have mastered the basic principles that underlie a nursing practice in the perianesthesia specialty and do meet minimum eligibility qualifications to seek certification.

The primary purpose of this resource is to help assess and increase your knowledge of essential perianesthesia concepts. As you prepare for certification, devising sample mini-examinations provides a periodic opportunity to validate your growing grasp of clinical knowledge. Such a "check in" also highlights any troublesome knowledge gaps for detailed review. In addition, this guide expands your repertoire of resources to consult about perianesthesia nursing practice even *after* certification.

The perianesthesia nurse might also creatively apply this resource to:

- augment the collection of references in the facility's library
- challenge critical thinking
- create continuing education ideas
- educate nurse preceptors
- establish a journal club
- expand a personal library
- focus a study group
- identify knowledge gaps
- orient new perianesthesia nurses
- post a unit "question of the week"
- refresh individual clinical knowledge
- stimulate continuing education discussion

Excellence: A Professional Intention

Consumer protection. Seeking certification in a nursing specialty is a voluntary commitment. A nurse who earns a certification credential validates mastery of a core of specialty knowledge. A certification credential does *not* verify practice competence. Through certification, a nongovernmental specialty association also validates that a licensed registered nurse has met a specialty's specific, predetermined standards. Therefore, certification is one method of consumer protection and demonstrates achievement both to oneself and the employer.

Accountability. Development, administration and evaluation of the certification program in the perianesthesia nursing specialty is coordinated through the American Board of Post Anesthesia Nursing Certification (ABPANC). ABPANC is a nonprofit organization incorporated in 1985 with support of the American Society of Post Anesthesia Nurses (ASPAN).The purposes of specialty certification include:

- demonstrating accountability for one's practice to the health care consumer
- promoting quality patient care delivery
- confirming clinical and professional excellence
- validating nursing expertise
- promoting personal satisfaction

ENGAGING IN A PROCESS

Preparing for certification parallels the nursing process. Assessment, planning, intervention and evaluation, the familiar concepts of the nursing process, help the certification candidate to discover the objectives of certification, appreciate methods of constructing examination-level questions and measure growth. Learners circle through these process phases, assessment through evaluation, again and again.

During the *assessment* phase, the certification candidate embarks on a journey of discovery. To *plan* and *intervene* means the candidate does not cram, but creates a confidence-promoting path for study. The candidate "follows through" by enacting the plan and just *doing* it. *Evaluation* is the candidate's soul-search and affirmation that, yes, knowledge is indeed understood and retained. Each reevaluation (reassessment) offers another loop or tangent in a spiral path of learning.

ASSESSMENT: KNOWLEDGE OF CANDIDATE AND EXAMINATION

The assessment phase of the nursing process involves observation and gathering information. Likewise, the assessment phase of the certification process encourages the candidate to gather knowledge about self, the examination and the certification process. This section, therefore, responds to the question *"What do I need to know to certify?"*

Assessment of Self

Understand your motivation. Devise questions to increase your self-awareness about your choice to certify and your commitment to the preparation process. You might reflect in conversation with colleagues or ruminate by writing your thoughts in a journal. Why *do* you seek this credential? What *are* your professional and personal benefits? Who will support and affirm you in this endeavor? How much time can you devote to preparation? Where and when will you sit for the examination? Do you approach testing with an attitude to master a challenge or to face a fear? Do you feel open or resistant?

Determine clinical content you already know. Ponder several clinical topics to appreciate informaton you grasp well and any knowledge deficits. Ask more questions. Will you need 6 weeks or 6 months to prepare? How do you best retain knowledge?

Identify your individual style. The ways individuals process information (learn) and demonstrate knowledge (take tests) vary. Some need a physical learning environment that offers hands-on experience. Others can read a book to understand how to accomplish a task, while still others must see, read and feel to learn. Be aware, too, that test-taking creates very real fear for some people. Do you prefer to study independently, or is a collaborative study group more appealing? Do you relish multiple choice tests or prefer expansive blue book essays?

Awareness of Certification Details

When contemplating certification, be sure you have the *most current edition* of *Post Anesthesia Certification Program: Examination Handbook and Applicatión.* This booklet, available from Professional Examination Service (PES), includes everything you must know to select your examination date and site and to correctly complete your application for either the CPAN or CAPA examination.

Management company. The ABPANC has selected PES to manage, coordinate, and administer the examinations (both the CPAN and CAPA). PES has a long and exemplary history of administering certification examinations. Through its New York office, PES coordinates and administers examinations for other specialty nursing organizations as well, including the critical care registered nurse (CCRN) and certified operating room nurse (CNOR) examinations. PES's expertise is not limited to nursing certification; they also represent such diverse groups as accountants, veterinary medicine practitioners and engineers.

Candidate eligibility. A nurse qualified to apply for certification candidacy must meet two criteria:

1. A currently licensed registered nurse: Licensure must be valid in the United States and be granted based on the N-CLEX examination.
2. Demonstration of a minimum of 1800 hours of postanesthesia or ambulatory postanesthesia nursing practice within the previous consecutive 3 years: Experience must arise from *direct care* of the postanesthesia (for CPAN) or ambulatory postanesthesia (for CAPA) patient through care delivery, leadership, education or research related to perianesthesia care.

The application form requests a copy of your nursing license and verification of your postanesthesia experience.

Examination dates. The certification examinations in postanesthesia nursing are administered twice each year. The first administration is in the spring, usually in April, on the Sunday morning prior to ASPAN's National Conference. The spring examination is administered at the conference site and also in two other strategically selected "hub" locations. The fall administration occurs on the first Saturday in November in at least 40 different locations. Test sites may vary each year, so *be sure* to consult *the most current edition* of *Post Anesthesia Certification Program: Examination Handbook and Application* when planning your test site and date.

Application. *Plan ahead!* Application deadlines for the November examination occur 8 to 10 weeks prior to the examination to allow for processing and securing proctors and examination facilities in multiple cities. Currently, the application deadline for the April administration arrives about 6 weeks prior to examination day, as fewer candidates and only three test sites are involved.

Obtain an application for the certification examinations by writing, telephoning or faxing:

ABPANC Program Director
Professional Examination Service (PES)
475 Riverside Drive
New York, New York 10115
Phone: (212) 870-3248
FAX: (212) 870-3333

Following all instructions to complete the application is critical. All portions of the application *must* be completed and returned by the specified date. No exceptions. The Program Director answers specific questions about the examination application and certification requirements. Direct inquiries about certification-related issues and maintaining your certification to ABPANC's toll-free number:

1-800-6-ABPANC

Understanding Examination Concepts and Development

Development of the certification process for postanesthesia nursing was a daunting undertaking for ABPANC's first Board of Directors. Both PES and ABPANC devoted many months to examination development. The nursing professionals who designed the system were very committed to the excellence of postanesthesia nursing practice and considered certification a serious responsibility.

The underpinnings of the certification examinations are the identified parameters, or *scope,* of postanesthesia or ambulatory surgery practice and the core components, or *domains,* of that role. Essential knowledge and skills, or *task statements,* further define and delineate the perianesthesia roles.

Role delineation. Examination of knowledge in *any* practice area requires that the field's scope, or its boundaries, are clearly specified. This process of determining just what observations, actions, knowledge and skills comprise perianesthesia nursing practice is called *role delineation.*

Role delineation reoccurs every few years to assure an examination's content reflects current practice. The CPAN and CAPA examinations each develop from a separate role delineation. The first statements of postanesthesia nursing's scope arose through collaboration between ABPANC and ASPAN. A cross section of practicing postanesthesia nurses throughout the United States, many of whom were CPANs, amended and revalidated the role delineation in 1991 and again in 1994. The CAPA examination is based on a separate yet similar 1992 role delineation by a different group of nurses whose practice focuses on the ambulatory surgery patient.

Domains. Major categories of responsibility in practice, the domains, are specified and validated. Statements identify the relevant tasks, knowledge and skills required by a competent practitioner to perform the activities of each domain.

Perianesthesia nurses involved in the 1994 delineation of the CPAN role collapsed the five original domains into two. *Direct Care* and *Leadership* are now the fundamental domains of the CPAN examination (Table 1–1). Principles of ethics, research and education are woven through each CPAN's direct patient care and leadership activities and need not be separate domains. The CAPA examination is predicated on three domains: *Direct Care, Education and Leadership* (Table 1–2).

Task, knowledge and skill statements. Each domain of the postanesthesia nursing role delineation requires specific knowledge and skills. A *task* statement identifies a cluster of specific nursing ac-

TABLE 1–1. Domains of the CPAN Role Delineation

Domain I: Direct Care

A. Collect and document pertinent patient data (including but not limited to consultation, record review, interview and physical examination) in order to assess the patient's health status and identify patient problems.
B. Formulate and communicate a nursing diagnosis by analyzing collected data and by collaborating, when appropriate, with the health-care team and the patient's family/significant others, in order to develop a plan of care for each patient.
C. Develop and communicate a plan of care by identifying and prioritizing patient needs and by identifying available resources in order to establish both short and long term goals.
D. Implement and communicate the plan of care by initiating appropriate nursing interventions to assist the patient's return to optimal health status.
E. Evaluate and communicate the results of nursing interventions by ongoing patient assessment and the application of total quality management (TQM) principles or research protocols in order to ensure the quality of patient care.

Domain II: Leadership

A. Contribute to the development, implementation, and evaluation of patient care standards and outcomes by utilizing research and TQM in order to ensure consistent quality care.
B. Collaborate in the management of the patient care environment by utilizing available resources in order to ensure consistent quality care.
C. Promote sharing of knowledge by utilizing available resources in order to advance the practice of post anesthesia nursing.

From *Post Anesthesia Certification Program: Examination Handbook and Application.* Richmond, VA: American Board of Post Anesthesia Nursing Certification, p. 14, 1994.

tions, the recipient of the action and how or why the task is accomplished.

A *knowledge* statement describes information related to a task and how the nurse processes data or incorporates concepts into the patient's care. For example, in the domain of direct care an examination item might validate the nurse's assessment of vital sign parameters and address supportive interventions.

A *skill* statement describes an observable, quantifiable act and the measurable parameters of performance. An examination item might assess the skill or ability to measure vital signs correctly.

Validation study. After each role delineation, PES asks perianesthesia nurses from around the country to confirm, or validate, the domains and scope of practice. Each validator assigns a score, or *weight,* to each domain and its knowledge and skills. Validation focuses on the candidate who meets *the minimum certification eligibility requirements of 1800 hours in practice.*

The assigned weights reflect each validator's evaluationof a domain's relative importance to safe and competent practice in a perianesthesia clinical setting (Tables 1–3 and 1–4). Validators typically assign the greatest weight to the direct care domain. Since the weighted domains form the blueprint, or recipe, that guides construction of the examination, the highest percentage of examination questions also arises from the *direct care* domain.

Examination construction. The actual certification examination is constructed by computer from a large bank of reviewed and validated test questions (items). Both the CPAN and CAPA examinations include 200 multiple choice questions. Based on the weights assigned during role delineation, a specific number of questions are selected from the pool of possible questions (the *item bank*), which is securely housed at PES. The CPAN and CAPA examinations each have a separate bank of items.

Item format. Questions on a certification examination are referred to as items. Each *item* is composed of one stem or premise, three (incorrect) choices or distrac-

Table 1–2. CAPA Role Delineation

Domain I: Direct Care

Collect and document pertinent patient data by interview, consultation, record review, and physical examination in order to assess the patient's health status and identify patient, patient family, and companion needs.

Formulate a nursing diagnosis by analyzing collected data and collaborating with the patient, family or companion, and other health care providers in order to develop a plan of care for each patient.

Develop plan of care by identifying and prioritizing patient needs, especially as related to the impact of anesthesia, the procedure or surgical intervention, and discharge needs, by identifying available resources in order to anticipate and prevent potential complications and to establish goals for discharge readiness.

Implement the plan of care by initiating appropriate nursing interventions to prevent complications and prepare the patient and family/companion for the patient's discharge readiness.

Evaluate the results of nursing interventions by assessment of the patient's response to the implemented plan of care in order to determine the effectiveness of the plan of care or the need to modify it accordingly.

Provide for continuity of care by communicating the patient's health status and response to the plan of care with the patient, the patient's family/companion, and other healthcare providers, in order to provide for optimum recovery.

Domain II: Education

Collect and document pertinent learner characteristics by interview, consultation, record review and physical examination in order to assess educational needs of the patient and family/companion.

Formulate a nursing diagnosis by analyzing collected data and by collaborating with the patient, family/companion and other healthcare providers to develop a teaching plan for each patient and family/companion.

Develop a teaching plan by identifying and prioritizing patient needs in order to individualize patient and family/companion.

Provide education to the patient and the patient's family/companion to prepare the patient both physically and emotionally for the potential impact of anesthesia, the procedure or surgical intervention, and the plan of care in order to assist the patient and family/companion in recognizing and accepting their joint responsibility for the patient's well being.

Provide education to the patient and the patient's family/companion to prepare the patient both physically and emotionally for the consequences of anesthesia, the procedure or surgical intervention, and the plan of care in order to assist the patient and family or companion in recognizing and accepting their joint responsibilities for the patient's pre and post discharge care.

Evaluate the results of the teaching provided by assessing the comprehension of information by the patient and family/companion in order to determine the effectiveness of the teaching or the need to modify it accordingly.

Domain III: Leadership

Participate in the development, implementation, and evaluation of standards and projected outcomes of patient care by utilizing available resources in order to promote the highest quality of patient care.

Utilize available resources within the organization framework to provide for an environment conducive to the highest quality of patient care.

Maintain competence by seeking and sharing information pertinent to ambulatory surgery nursing to promote the highest quality of patient care.

From *Post Anesthesia Certification Program: Examination Handbook and Application.* Richmond, VA: American Board of Post Anesthesia Nursing Certification, pp. 15-16, 1994.

tors, and one correct answer. A brief paragraph or scenario with key points about a patient, a diagram, or an EKG rhythm strip may precede a group of three or four questions. Other items stand alone. Some questions require mere knowledge recall. More sophisticated, higher level questions require the candidate to apply knowledge to a situ-

TABLE 1–3. Role Delineation for the CPAN Examination*

DOMAIN	PERCENT OF EXAMINATION	NUMBER OF ITEMS
Direct Care	80%	160
Leadership	20%	40

*Based on the 1994 CPAN Role Delineation.

TABLE 1–4. Role Delineation for the CAPA Examination*

DOMAIN	PERCENT OF EXAMINATION	NUMBER OF ITEMS
Direct Care	54%	108
Education	24%	48
Leadership	22%	44

*Based on the 1992 CAPA Role Delineation.

ation, or synthesize several pieces of information to determine the correct response.

Item development. The separate item banks for the CPAN and CAPA examinations each consist of hundreds of questions. Questions are written and submitted for consideration by individual CPANs, participants in ABPANC-sponsored workshops, and by members of the ABPANC Board of Directors and its Item Development Committee. Before an item is accepted into the item bank, the question's content, style and distractors are *reviewed,* or critiqued, by at least five practicing perianesthesia nurses. Each item is also *edited* for clarity and accuracy and *referenced* to a source in the current literature. Every item is then *validated* for importance and relevance to practice. Finally, reviewers assign a *level of difficulty* that reflects the kind of knowledge or skill a candidate needs to determine the correct answer.

Level of difficulty. When creating certification level items, the authors strive to develop situations that require the candidate to think, then apply knowledge to resolve the clinical situation. Identifying a correct answer to an examination question often requires more than merely remembering facts.

Each question on the certification examination is assigned a level of difficulty, or a cognitive level. A question that requires ability to recall specific knowledge is a Level I question. A Level II question asks the candidate to relate facts, whereas a Level III question tests the ability to synthesize facts and apply concepts to a situation. Most items require Level II or Level III cognitive skills.

Item bank. Approximately one-third of the questions are rotated, or removed, for each new version of the examination. Each question included in each examination version is statistically evaluated in several different ways to determine its levels of performance. This assessment assures that only the most current and pertinent questions are kept in the item bank. The entire item bank is also routinely reviewed. Questions are edited, rereferenced if the cited reference is more than 5 years old, and reassessed to determine relevance to current practice. Items that no longer meet criteria of accuracy, relevance and clarity are "retired" from the item bank; these never appear on subsequent forms of any certification examination.

Passing point. The passing point for each version of the examination is determined by the ABPANC Board of Directors, using psychometric criteria provided by PES. The current method utilizes the Angoff procedure. Each item on an examination is statistically analyzed to establish the minimum score, or passing point, that a candidate can achieve. A new passing point is established for each new version of the examination.

PLANNING AND IMPLEMENTATION: STUDY STRATEGIES

The *planning* phase of the nursing process involves establishing priorities and designing strategies for nursing intervention. Entering the planning phase for certification means generating a study plan, collecting educational resources and making time.

The *implementation* phase of the nursing process involves the initiative to act and the momentum to proceed with the plan. When applied to planning for certification, implementation involves active review and new learning through reading, practice tests, course participation or discussion with study colleagues.

This section of the resource guide responds to the questions *"How do I use this study guide as one part of my study plan?"* and *"How do I prepare for certification?"*

Setting a Pace Toward Certification

Generate a plan. There is no single "best" way to prepare for certification. Individual study choices might include some combination of ASPAN-sponsored certification review workshops, a discussion group to stimulate critical thinking or sharpen problem-solving skills, and/or a solo (ad)venture reviewing specific resources.

Play with this book's style. Focus your study on specific knowledge gaps in preparation for the "real" test. From the approximately 600 questions in this resource, create brief pretests using the topical index of questions at the end of the book. You probably are already aware of your clinical strengths. Concentrate your study efforts on patient populations, medications, diseases or clinical situations with which you are less familiar. If, for example, you seldom care for an obstetric patient, add care of the pregnant woman to your study plan.

Collect resources. *Abundantly surround yourself with an array of nursing, medical, and pharmacologic literature, both books and journals,* from several disciplines. For diversity, collect critical care, orthopedic, neuroscience, renal, holistic and general surgical nursing texts.

- Use, but do *not* limit yourself to, the "classic" perianesthesia nursing and anesthesia resources!
- Network with other aspiring certification candidates.
- Register for a mind-challenging class.
- Ardently believe that *no single reference,* whether a book, a revered lecturer or a course, *contains all tidbits of information a candidate needs to prepare for certification.*
- Allow the references in the rationales for each question and the annotated bibliography at the end of this guide lead you to other *suggested,* potential resources. Please note that *the references used to create this book are by no means all-inclusive!!*
- Explore the bookshelves of your favorite medical bookstore or library and gather books and journals that appeal to your individual learning style and needs.
- Obtain long-term loans for resources owned by supportive colleagues.
- Refer to the certification preparation materials sponsored by other nursing specialties. Many include sample multiple choice questions and in-depth discussions of useful test-taking approaches.
- Supplement the study materials you've already collected and reinforce your educational objectives by using this resource.

Your *sense of humor,* specific sources of *personal support* and *daily affirmations* are resources too!

- Ask friends and colleagues to support your endeavors toward clinical growth.
- Arrange to contact them when the study is difficult or your discipline wavers.
- Request that they check in with you.
- Locate affirmations that you can repeat regularly. Such positive statements can remind you that your path is worthy and that your progress is steady.

Managing time and energy. *Never "cram" for a certification examination!!* Plan and organize your schedule for study—then stick to it.

- Brief, frequent study periods are often more effective than marathon sessions.
- Set long- and short-term study goals.
- Break the volumes of material to study into small, manageable chunks of information.

Reinforce knowledge. PRACTICE!! REVIEW—then PRACTICE AGAIN!! The style of this book allows the reader to mimic the examination experience—as often as desired.

- Repetition of a concept breeds familiarity while hopefully increasing comfort with one's test-taking skills, item content and the scope and difficulty of the examination.

- Approximately 600 sample questions, each with a referenced rationale, are included in this guide for your review. *Of course none of these questions will actually appear on your examination.*

Create clinical puzzlers. The topic index at the end of this resource leads the reader to specific questions and rationales. *Use the index to locate items with difficult-to-comprehend concepts.* For example, the certification candidate who struggles with distinguishing depolarizing from nondepolarizing muscle relaxants might choose only those questions.

- Answer the questions in the scenarios, understand the accompanying rationales and consult the suggested references for further explanation.
- Seek solutions and information from a myriad of other references as well. Many are identified in this book's annotated bibliography.

Devise multiple tests. RECHALLENGE!! Questions in this resource are cross-referenced by level of difficulty and clinical content.

- Make multiple copies of the answer form.
- Use the questions for personal review or in group discussion to stimulate exchange of ideas and hone problem-solving skills. Remember that several paths might lead you to the same question. For example, you may find one question about succinylcholine referenced in the index under "succinylcholine," "depolarizing muscle relaxants," "hypoxia" and "hypoventilation."
- Access specific concepts or levels of difficulty through the topical index.
- Pattern the "official examination" by choosing a wide range of questions from the domains represented on the examination.
- At the end of your review, challenge yourself by selecting only Level III questions!
- *Devise your own scenarios and questions.* Use these items as a model. You'll challenge your mind—an experience you'll want to tap on a CPAN or CAPA item development team!!

EVALUATION: MONITORING ACHIEVEMENT

The evaluation phase of the nursing process assesses outcomes, determines progress toward goal achievement and amends the plan. When applied to growth and preparing for certification, evaluation provides "stop points" to confirm progress, ferret out the knowledge gaps and places you feel "stuck." Replan, seeking new paths toward understanding. This section responds to the question *"Am I moving along?"*

Ask questions. Reassessment is ongoing and ever evolving. Reconfirm your learning often. Use your ability to answer questions in this guide as one bit of tangible evidence to help you evaluate your certification readiness. How do your answers this week about causes of hypoxia compare with answers you provided last week? Can you verbally contrast metabolic acidosis from respiratory acidosis? How does your explanation of pulmonary artery pressures match with the rationales of related questions?

Check in with yourself. Calmly and repeatedly ask: Do I feel ready? Am I on the right track? Do I know what I need to know? Honestly assess and reassess your growing knowledge and testing skill throughout your planned precertification months. Find and repeat self-affirming messages. Call in your support team.

Examination day: the ultimate evaluation! We cannot prepare indefinitely for life. Eventually, we must commit to the task and "show our stuff." You've planned and replanned for this day. *Now, just do it!!*

TESTING TIDBITS

A written test is currently the most widely recognized method to demonstrate and measure knowledge. Perhaps in the future, a computer-generated examination will adapt a set of questions, and an entire examination, based on each individual's unique responses. Computerized nursing licensure examinations are already available; other testing agencies monitor these attempts closely. Meanwhile, paper and pencil tests with computerized scoring remain the norm.

A flair for testing. Ability to pour out your mastery of concepts through a multiple choice test is a developed skill. Successful test-takers develop strategies to approach questions (Table 1–5). You've practiced and repracticed sample questions from this and other study resources. You apply the new knowledge you've gained through your disciplined study each day in your perianesthesia practice. Now, transfer your critical thinking skills from your practice setting to this examination setting.

TABLE 1–5. Test-taking Strategies

Before the examination:
- Assess and reassess self-knowledge
- Believe you are prepared
- Assemble and bring the REQUIRED MATERIALS
- Arrive at the test site ON TIME
- Practice relaxation!

During the examination:
- Read carefully!
  - Directions
  - Questions
- Approach each question critically
- Answer only what the question asks
  - DO NOT "read in"
  - Consider usual situations, not exceptions
- There is only *one* correct answer
- Identify KEY WORDS
  - Negative words: *except, not, least*
  - Similar emphasis in stem and distractor
  - Absolutes: all, none
  - Qualifiers: usually, most
- Identify essential information
  - What does the question ask?
  - Turn each possible answer (distractor) into a question and determine whether it is true
  - Mark ideas, similar words in the test book
  - Observe patterns, relationships
- CAREFULLY mark the answer form
  - Watch numbering!
  - Blacken your correct response by the corresponding number
  - Recheck every few questions
- Guess without penalty!

Remember that *the goal of a certification examination is to discern the clinically knowledgeable practitioner.* Though there are no "trick questions," the correct answer may not be immediately obvious. One question's distractors may seem equally plausible to a candidate who lacks sufficient knowledge. The certified nurse has the knowledge, integrated understanding or reasoning ability to identify some critical difference that makes one choice stand out as correct and the others as incorrect.

During the test experience, you may find a scenario with clinical information that precedes several questions. Read the scenarios *carefully* to discriminate information required to answer a question from any unnecessary or distracting data. Each scenario and its cluster of related questions, will be clearly and boldly identified on the examination.

Use only the information provided in the question. *DO NOT "read in"* or imagine that a question asks for more information than it states. Exactly what does the question ask? Does more than one answer seem possible? What key words or special knowledge distinguishes the correct answer from its possible, but absolutely incorrect, distractors? Does the question ask you to identify the only possible solution, or must you select the single *in*correct choice?

Self-care. Be kind to yourself. After you have achieved your review goals, build in time to relax!

- Call in your support team for affirming wishes.
- Reread positive affirmations with messages that inspire your confidence and strength.
- The night before the examination, try to eat a balanced meal, pursue a relaxing activity and be sure to find enough time to sleep. A relaxed candidate who takes the examination after a good night's sleep enhances the chances of passing far more than the candidate who crams for the test until the early morning hours.

Believe you can do this! On the morning of the examination, repeat more affirming messages. Anticipate and minimize unncessary stress.

- Leave your books and notes at home!!
- Pace yourself to allow enough time to arrive at the test site *early*.
- Arrive with your REQUIRED MATERIALS: pencil, admission card and PHOTO IDENTIFICATION.
- Arrive rested, confident, and ON TIME!

Celebrate your success! You already know this information—and apply it each day in practice. You've done your best to prepare for the examination. You're confident and glowing. Now, just *do* it. Best wishes!!

AS YOU BEGIN. . .

This resource was developed in a way similar to the construction of a certification examination:

- Nursing practice presents an infinite number of situations. Only a few were actually captured as items—this time.
- These scenarios and items were contributed by certified ASPAN members, were newly created by the author or were irrevocably altered items retired from ABPANC's item bank.
- Each item, rationale and answer was stringently reviewed by a panel of six expert perianesthesia nurses who commented on accuracy, relevance, clarity and level of difficulty.
- Scenarios and items that apply similar nursing knowledge and skills were placed together in one section. For example, assessment of microcirculation and nerve function follows an orthopedic, neurologic *and* neurovascular procedure.
- Scenarios consider preanesthesia, postanesthesia and ambulatory surgery concepts. Whether a woman plans to return home after a laparoscopy or is admitted to the hospital after hysterectomy, the nurse assesses this patient for intraabdominal bleeding.
- Scenarios that portray concepts such as educational priorities, pain management, ethics, acid-base balance or research are considered in several sections. These aspects of practice are woven through direct care and leadership concepts related to any procedure or anesthesia technique.
- References selected to verify the concepts in the items and scenarios are not the *only* relevant sources; books and journals that you choose will also verify concepts.
- Many scenarios and rationales are lengthy and span several items. The purpose is to illustrate perianesthesia practice and to explain nursing priorities. Examination items are generally more brief.

With positive thoughts, enjoy and have fun!!

Section 2

Professional Issues Applied to Perianesthesia Nursing Practice

Scenarios and items in this section reflect the dimensions of professional nursing practice in the perianesthesia environment. These issues tap only a few of the myriad situations encountered by the nurse in clinical practice and are important because:

- professional growth and delivery of high-level patient care asks each nurse to stretch beyond the limits of traditional, delegated functions.
- each nurse weaves clinical research, ethical dilemmas, legal concerns and education concepts through daily clinical practice.

ESSENTIAL CORE CONCEPTS	AFFILIATED CORE CURRICULUM CHAPTERS
Perianesthesia Nursing	
Establishing Priorities	
Nursing Process	Chapter 2
Scope of Practice	
Standards of Practice (ASPAN)	Chapter 2
Professional Practice and Clinical Intersections	
Applied Clinical Research	Chapter 3
Research Process	
Participating in Data Collection	
Critiquing Research Design	
Linking Research With Practice	
Educational Principles	Chapter 6
Adult Learning Theory	
Patient Education	
Assessing Readiness	
Discharge Information	
Ethical Dilemmas in Clinical Practice	Chapter 5
Principles of Ethics	
Perianesthesia Issues	

SET I

Items 2.1-2.30

NOTE: Consider scenario and item 2.1 together.

Three clinical registered nurses working in Phase I PACU anticipate five patient admissions during the next 90 minutes and collaboratively plan nursing care assignments. Patients already in PACU include a sedated 13 year old boy whose oral airway was just removed and now has an SpO_2 of 98% and respiratory rate of 15 breaths per minute, and an awake 9 year old girl who is accompanied by her mother. The staff intends to provide safe nursing care that aligns with staffing recommendations in ASPAN's *Standards of Perianesthesia Nursing Practice.* One suggested assignment option is to have one nurse care for both children and to admit one adult woman after her cardioversion ends in 5 minutes.

2.1 After reviewing ASPAN's recommended patient classification guidelines, the staff determines that this assignment option is:

a. appropriate if a medical aide admits the new woman
b. inappropriate; only two patients per nurse in Phase I
c. inappropriate; the 13 year old boy requires 1:1 care
d. appropriate as suggested and an easy assignment

2.2. Conditions most associated with increased risk of nosocomial infection include all of the following *except:*

a. broad-spectrum antibiotics
b. applied asepsis principles
c. multiple invasive catheters
d. concurrent multisystem illnesses

NOTE: Consider scenario and item 2.3 together.

The PACU's competency-based continuing education program reviews ASPAN's recommendations for necessary equipment and supplies to respond to a malignant hyperthermia (MH) crisis. Evaluation and successful completion of the competency include gathering *initial* supplies for a mock MH situation in PACU.

2.3. The nurse obtains the most appropriate supplies including dantrolene sodium and:

a. bag-valve-mask unit with oxygen, iced crystalloid, and sodium bicarbonate
b. succinylcholine, ventilator and renal-dose dopamine
c. chilled gastric lavage, lidocaine, and pressure monitoring equipment
d. phenylephrine, cooling blanket, and midazolam

NOTE: Consider scenario and items 2.4-2.8 together.

A PACU nurse observes that patients who develop postanesthesia shaking and complain of pain typically stop shaking after receiving meperidine 25 mg for analgesic purposes. This nurse chooses to examine whether meperidine suppresses shaking.

2.4. The nurse conducts a review of the literature to:

a. establish the chemical configuraton of meperidine
b. clearly and concisely state the research problem
c. determine side effects of meperidine
d. relate the identified problem to previous research

2.5. The nurse-researcher develops a theoretical framework for this study to:

a. guide the study and provide a context for findings
b. describe meperidine's physiologic effect on shaking
c. define parameters for the study sample and setting
d. declare the problem statement and study methods

2.6. To best examine whether meperidine suppresses postanesthesia shaking, the researcher designs a:

a. longitudinal data collection tool
b. postoperative patient survey
c. factorial construct analysis
d. nonexperimental descriptive study

2.7. The most appropriate data analysis procedure for this research is:

a. stepwise regression
b. descriptive statistics
c. analysis of variance
d. meta-analysis

2.8. The research hypothesis for this study:

a. is synonymous with the purpose statement
b. rises from collected data
c. states the relationship among study variables
d. is unnecessary with descriptive designs

2.9. A student nurse is assigned to work with an expert PACU nurse. During delivery of nursing care, the PACU nurse "thinks aloud." This process demonstrates a teaching strategy that primarily:

a. decreases student anxiety in clinical settings
b. improves a student's decision-making skills
c. confuses the student with multiple options
d. increases the student's technical skill

NOTE: Consider scenario and item 2.10 together.

During a postoperative transfusion of banked packed red blood cells through an electrically operated blood warmer, Mr. F's temperature increases to 39° C. The nurse observes the color of blood entering Mr. F is bright red; the blood tubing feels hot. The transfusion is immediately discontinued and returned to the blood bank, where the blood temperature registers 42° C. An "overtemperature" alarm failed to signal increasing blood temperature before cell hemolysis.

2.10. The clinical nurse's responsibility includes:

a. determining whether long-term patient harm occurred
b. reporting the incident directly to the manufacturer
c. informing facility managers of the malfunction
d. returning the equipment for quick biomedical repair

NOTE: Consider scenario and items 2.11-2.12. together.

Mr. M is nonresponsive and has an oral airway when admitted to PACU after an emergency appendectomy. Initial nursing assessment indicates shallow, rhythmic, diaphragmatic breathing, flaccid, relaxed muscles and absent eyelid reflexes.

2.11. At this moment, the nurse's plan of care focuses on Mr. M's *most immediate* risk, which is potential for:

a. corneal abrasion
b. emergence delirium
c. silent regurgitation
d. respiratory alkalosis

2.12. As Mr. M's anesthetic depth changes to more resemble Stage II, nursing priorities shift and the nurse's greatest priority for Mr. M becomes:

a. managing restlessness
b. reorientation to time
c. preliminary discharge education
d. support of diaphragmatic breathing

2.13. For each functioning operating room, ASPAN's standards recommend that the Phase I inpatient PACU provide patient privacy, isolation as needed and:

a. a minimum of 4 feet between stretchers
b. space for one bed and one recliner per operating suite
c. one handwashing sink per two patient cubicles
d. separation of general anesthesia patients from regional anesthesia patients

NOTE: Consider scenario and items 2.14-2.15 together.

The orthopedist orders 5 mg midazolam and 25 mg meperidine intravenously for Mr. G's conscious sedation, then requests sterile gloves, an antibiotic and steroid medications, which are located in the preanesthesia unit.

2.14. In this situation, the PACU nurse's primary responsibility is to:

a. administer medications as ordered, then obtain supplies
b. locate an anesthesia-certified colleague to administer medications
c. collaborate with the surgeon to adjust and individualize these doses
d. obtain the supplies while the orthopedist medicates Mr. G and begins the procedure

2.15. The PACU nurse reminds the orthopedist that Mr. G takes phenelzine (Nardil) each day for depression. Last dose was 9 PM last evening. One medication to avoid is:

a. streptomycin
b. midazolam
c. ketorolac
d. meperidine

2.16. Privacy, informed consent, confidentiality of communications, and continuity of care are expectations mandated by the:

a. Joint Commission on Accreditation of Healthcare Organizations (JCAHO)
b. Patient Self-Determination Act
c. Patient's Bill of Rights
d. American Nurses Association Standards of Nursing Practice

NOTE: Consider scenario and items 2.17-2.18 together.

A researcher designs a quasiexperimental study to determine if permitting visitors in the PACU affects the anxiety of postoperative patients. Since one study group will receive visitors and the second will not, a PACU normally closed to visitors is selected as the study site.

2.17. While instructing prospective data collectors, the researcher discovers the study PACU actually does permit visitation. Based on this knowledge, the researcher determines this PACU cannot be a study site because the design:

a. lacks a logical purpose and external validity
b. denies standard PACU care to nonvisited patients
c. conflicts with a patient's legal right to privacy
d. prevents proving a cause-effect relationship between variables

2.18. The researcher selects another study site, a PACU that denies visitation in any circumstance. When considering the researcher's proposal to conduct the study, this facility's Institutional Review Board assures that the proposed research:

a. studies a significant clinical problem with measurable variables
b. assures the target population is randomly assigned, diverse and anonymous
c. obtains the subject's informed consent to perform parametric tests and generalize hypotheses
d. protects the patient's privacy, confidentiality, and freedom from harm

2.19. According to ASPAN's *Standards of Perianesthesia Nursing Practice*, observation of a preanesthesia patient should best occur:

a. apart from any Phase I postanesthesia patient
b. anywhere there is available space
c. in Phase I PACU when no critical care patients are there
d. among Phase I patients who received epidural steroids

2.20. ASPAN's *Standards of Perianesthesia Nursing Practice* recommends that renewal of the PACU nurse's cardiopulmonary resuscitation (CPR) credential occur:

a. annually
b. every 2 years
c. every 3 years
d. prior to JCAHO visitation

2.21. A critical element of the postanesthesia nurse's educational growth is willingness to:

a. work alone to provide care and education for four patients in Phase II PACU
b. demonstrate selected PACU competencies each year
c. delegate mandibular support to the medical aide
d. attend one educational seminar, then adapt content to orient a colleague

NOTE: Consider items 2.22-2.23 together.

2.22. Mr. I has methicillin-resistant *Staphylococcus aureus* (MRSA). To provide safe nursing care following today's nephrectomy, the PACU nurse's *most appropriate* action is to:

a. concurrently care for Ms. D, who will soon transfer to Phase II PACU for discharge
b. provide strict isolation to protect Mr. I, who has minimal immunity and low resistance from MRSA
c. wear a gown, gloves, and mask, then segregate Mr. I to prevent colonizing PACU staff and patients
d. admit Mr. I among other PACU patients and don sterile gloves and a surgical mask to change wet dressings

2.23. The antibiotic of choice to treat a patient with methicillin-resistant staphylococcus aureus (MRSA) is:

a. oxacillin
b. cefoxitin
c. imipenem
d. vancomycin

NOTE: Consider scenario and item 2.24 together.

When presenting the structure and function of the PACU to a nurse-orientee, the preceptor describes available equipment as recommended in ASPAN's *Standards of Perianesthesia Nursing Practice.*

2.24. In addition to a pulse oximeter, necessary equipment for *each* patient in Phase I includes a/an:

a. portable end-tidal CO_2 monitor
b. active rewarming system
c. cardiac monitor
d. pulmonary artery pressure transducers

NOTE: Consider scenario and items 2.25-2.26 together.

A 14 year old girl, Carrie, fractured several fingers in her left hand while playing baseball. Following surgical repair with general anesthesia, she is drowsy but arousable and has both hemodynamic and neurovascular stability after 15 minutes in PACU. The nurse observes complete heart block and consults with the anesthesiologist, who disagrees with the nurse's interpretation, leaves no orders and departs.

2.25. The *most appropriate* nursing action is to document events and:

a. inform the surgeon of the complete heart block
b. recontact the anesthesiologist only if symptoms develop
c. obtain a 12-lead EKG, interpret, then administer atropine sulfate
d. advise the parents and transfer Carrie to coronary care

NOTE: The scenario continues.

Carrie is scheduled for ambulatory surgery discharge when appropriately awake. She remains hemodynamically and surgically stable, though a 12-lead EKG confirms complete heart block.

2.26. The PACU nurse prepares Carrie and parents for anticipated discharge to:

a. home with telephone follow-up and Holter monitor
b. inpatient telemetry unit for cardiac evaluation
c. home with orthopedic instructions and cardiology referral
d. cardiac unit for immediate transvenous pacemaker

NOTE: Consider scenario and item 2.27 together.

The PACU nurse reviews literature describing visitation by family members in PACU for the unit's monthly Journal Club meeting. After critiquing several studies that report anxiety reduction among visited patients, he supports incorporating study recommendations into unit practice.

2.27. When preparing his Journal Club presentation, this nurse carefully phrases research conclusions as:

a. proof that visited patients have shorter PACU stays
b. decisive evidence that refutes skepticism of peers
c. a technique to encourage family bonding
d. information to support a PACU policy for visitation

NOTE: Consider scenario and item 2.28 together.

After general anesthesia and a 5 hour procedure to treat documented ovarian cancer, a newly admitted 45 year old woman requests to see her husband.

2.28. When considering this request, the PACU nurse recalls clincal research that suggests the presence of family members generally:

a. reduces patient and family anxiety
b. detracts from establishing nurse-patient mutuality
c. invades privacy of other anesthetized patients
d. disrupts nursing activity and attention

NOTE: Consider items 2.29-2.30 together.

2.29. The staff nurse chairperson prepares the agenda for the monthly meeting of the PACU collaborative governance council. Ideally, the agenda:

a. details all identified problems in PACU
b. identifies leader preferences about an item
c. suggests resolutions for identified issues
d. presents the sequence of topics for discussion

2.30. The meeting coordinator appoints a recorder to document meeting activity. The purpose of this documentation is to:

a. quote individual remarks
b. summarize major points
c. detail controversial issues
d. present all discussion

SET II

Items 2.31-2.44

NOTE: Consider scenario and items 2.31-2.32 together.

A PACU nurse is named in a malpractice lawsuit 6 months after a patient alleges she developed a back wound infection on the day of L3-L4 hemilaminectomy and microdiscectomy. The complaint states that the PACU was busy and that her nurse care provider improperly changed her bleeding back wound dressing after caring for another patient with hepatitis and then failed to inform the neurosurgeon of bleeding.

2.31. To demonstrate negligence, this patient must prove:
- a. legal duty
- b. harmful intent
- c. undesirable outcome
- d. damaging conduct

2.32. Criteria used to measure this nurse's clinical performance may include showing that her nursing care aligned with accepted community practice and demonstrating:
- a. that a nurse is only accountable to the unit manager
- b. compliance with standards of perianesthesia nursing
- c. lack of proximate cause during wound assessment
- d. that her skills equal the performance of a certified colleague

2.33. The clinical nurse manager creates an empowering environment when encouraging PACU nursing staff members to:
- a. consult with the manager prior to revising a patient's plan of care
- b. present each committee decision for administrative approval
- c. collaborate with a multidisciplinary team to enact a research protocol
- d. invite the anesthesiologist to redesign the PACU's educational objectives

2.34. In an inservice conducted for nurses who will assist in data collection for a research project, a graduate student explains the study's procedures and tools. This inservice is necessary to improve the study's:
- a. interrater reliability
- b. construct validity
- c. internal consistency
- d. content analysis

NOTE: Consider scenario and items 2.35-2.36 together.

Following general anesthesia for a diagnostic bronchoscopy, a coughing and restless 38 year old man is admitted to PACU Phase I. Eighteen months ago, lab tests confirmed he had antibodies to the human immunodeficiency virus (HIV). The nurses' goal is to demonstrate attention to efficient care delivery, adequate infection control, optimum staff safety and positive patient outcomes.

2.35. The staff quite appropriately assigns this man's care to:
- a. an HIV-negative PACU registered nurse who uses needle precautions
- b. two PACU nurses who deliver his postanesthesia care in the OR
- c. two HIV-positive hospital staff members who use universal precautions in PACU
- d. a PACU nurse who covers her moist skin eruptions with gloves and who concurrently cares for another drowsy patient

2.36. Transmission of HIV is *least* likely to occur when the nurse is:

a. obtaining an arterial sample of serum electrolytes
b. suctioning the oropharynx for endotracheal extubation
c. discontinuing an infiltrated intravenous catheter
d. assisting with insertion of spinal anesthetic

NOTE: Consider scenario and item 2.37 together.

A 95 year old resident of a long-term care facility with a "do not resuscitate or intubate" (DNR/DNI) advance directive fell and broke her hip. The physician orders a "no-CPR" status for the duration of the hospitalization. Her family signs a consent for surgical repair.

2.37. With regard to the advance directive in PACU, ethical guidelines as interpreted by the American Heart Association recommend:

a. perioperative continuation of the DNR/DNI directive
b. automatic revocation until return to long-term care
c. focused review of intent for perianesthetic period
d. suspension of the DNI directive and retention of the DNR portion

NOTE: Consider scenario and item 2.38 together.

The surgical services business manager chooses to orient interested medical-surgical staff nurses for weekend and on-call positions in Phase I of the hospital-based PACU. The professional practice arm of the PACU's collaborative governance structure craft a proposal that recommends that only nurses with critical care experience be placed in these positions.

2.38. The proposal cites ASPAN's *Standards of Perianesthesia Nursing Practice,* which recommends that a Phase I PACU nurse demonstrate competence in:

a. identifying heart block and stating indications for beta blockers
b. adjusting pacemaker parameters and administering intracardiac epinephrine
c. interpreting electroencephalogram patterns and managing phenytoin protocols
d. cardioversion techniques, intubation skill and central venous cannulation

2.39. After emptying a wound drain, the nurse spills a graduate containing 100 ml of bloody fluid onto the floor. The nurse advises personnel who clean this spill to wear protective gloves, dispose of cleaning materials in a biohazard waste bag, and use a solution of:

a. scalding water and detergent
b. double strength 80% methyl alcohol
c. 1:10 dilution of sodium hypochlorite
d. 35% povidone-iodine

NOTE: Consider scenario and item 2.40 together.

The collaborative governance council of a combined inpatient and ambulatory PACU is responsible for demonstrating quality improvement. Two staff nurses are selecting quality indicators for consideration by the council.

2.40. An example of a perioperative quality improvement (QI) indicator relevant to the Joint Commission on Accreditation of Healthcare Organizations (JCAHO) Agenda for Change is:

a. reporting numbers of newly inserted pacemakers
b. monitoring a nurse's PACU documentation for completeness
c. listing occurrence of perioperative normothermia
d. correlating PACU hypoxemia in ASA III patients with distance from OR

2.41. The nurse's advocacy role to promote patient well-being is predicated on the ethical principle of:

a. beneficence
b. autonomy
c. fealty
d. justice

NOTE: Consider scenario and item 2.42 together.

A preoperative nurse meets a patient for a preoperative interview. Surgery is scheduled in 2 hours. She quickly discovers the patient speaks little English, yet he appears to understand some information. The nurse is uncertain that the patient truly comprehends surgical events. An operative consent is unsigned, as the surgeon normally waits until just before surgery to obtain consent.

2.42. This nurse's *most appropriate* intervention is to:

a. proceed with assessment as consent is implied by arrival for surgery
b. delay surgical preparations and await the surgeon's arrival
c. locate an interpreter to translate medical events
d. explain the surgical procedure with photographs and hand-drawn pictures

NOTE: Consider scenario and item 2.43 together.

At 12:30 PM in the Phase I PACU, patients include a 38 year old drowsy woman who arrived 30 minutes ago after an elective postpartum tubal ligation with general anesthesia and a 7 year old boy whose oral airway was removed 5 minutes ago after a tonsillectomy. His mother is at his side. One nurse is at lunch in the PACU conference room and another wants to transfer an intubated patient to the intensive care unit, leaving one expert nurse and an experienced medical assistant in PACU.

2.43. A prudent nursing decision in this situation, based on ASPAN's *Standards of Perianesthesia Nursing Practice,* is to:

a. locate a second licensed nurse to stay in PACU during the transfer period
b. assign the medical aide to observe the woman and admit a sedated postendoscopy patient
c. delegate transfer responsibility to the medical aide and anesthesia personnel
d. assure no patients will be admitted from OR and transfer as planned

NOTE: Consider scenario and item 2.44 together.

The PACU nurse administers small doses of intravenous midazolam and assesses Ms. O while the orthopedic surgeon realigns Ms. O's hip dislocation. Ms. O winces and is not relaxed when realignment requires increasingly more pressure and manipulation. The orthopedist asks the nurse to administer methohexital 50 mg.

2.44. A legally appropriate response is for the PACU nurse to ask the physician to delay further manipulation and:

a. observe Ms. O while the nurse obtains methohexital
b. ask an anesthesia provider to administer methohexital
c. quickly review the state's Nurse Practice Act
d. attach a pulse oximeter and cardiac and blood pressure monitors

SET I

Answer Key

2.1. b
2.2. b
2.3. a
2.4. d
2.5. a
2.6. d
2.7. b
2.8. c
2.9. b
2.10. c
2.11. c
2.12. a
2.13. a
2.14. c
2.15. d
2.16. c
2.17. b
2.18. d
2.19. a
2.20. b
2.21. b
2.22. c
2.23. d
2.24. c
2.25. a
2.26. b
2.27. d
2.28. a
2.29. d
2.30. b

SET I

Rationales and References

2.1. Correct Answer: **b**

In this situation, one nurse can be appropriately assigned to provide care for the children in their current stages of recovery, but accepting responsibility for a third patient would not be wise. ASPAN's *Standards of Perianesthesia Nursing Practice* specifies that one nurse in Phase I PACU may provide care for "two conscious stable, 11 years of age and under." One registered nurse, never a medical aide, admits, assesses and creates a plan of care for a new PACU patient. One other licensed staff member must also be *present.*

American Society of Post Anesthesia Nurses (ASPAN): Standards of Perianesthesia Nursing Practice, *Resource 9. Thorofare, NJ, ASPAN, p. 47, 1995.*

2.2. Correct Answer: **b**

Health care providers who follow principles of asepsis and universal precautions reduce the spread of nosocomial, or hospital-acquired, infections. Handwashing and attention to cleanliness limit microorganism numbers. Coexisting illnesses, many care providers, prolonged hospitalization and multiple invasive procedures are conditions most associated with increased risk of nosocomial infection. Indwelling catheters, including monitoring lines and urinary catheters, introduce exogenous infection. Broad-spectrum antibiotics alter the patient's normal body flora, creating imbalance and allowing microorganisms, including antibiotic-resistant strains, to colonize and rapidly proliferate.

Long, M & Miller, MD: Infection Control in Basic Nursing: Theory and Practice, *3rd ed (Potter, PA & Perry, AG, Eds). Philadelphia, Saunders, p. 612, 1994.*

2.3. Correct Answer: **a**

Initial treatment of malignant hyperthermia crisis requires many vials of dantrolene sodium, cold IV saline for infusion, cooling blankets, sodium bicarbonate, mannitol, and 100% oxygen for possible delivery with positive pressure. The patient may or may not be intubated. IV lidocaine and succinylcholine are considered possible triggers of malignant hyperthermia and are not given to any patient with suspected MH.

American Society of Post Anesthesia Nurses (ASPAN): Standards of Perianesthesia Nursing Practice, *Resource 5. Thorofare, NJ, ASPAN, p. 37, 1995; Litwack, K:* Post Anesthesia Care Nursing, *2nd ed. St. Louis, Mosby, pp. 472-475, 1995.*

2.4. Correct Answer: **d**

A preliminary research step, the review of the literature, helps the researcher to identify, select and critically analyze the range of existing information in the published literature about the study topic. This literature review helps clarify known and unknown aspects of a topic and guides the researcher to form a research problem. In this scenario, meperidine is not the study focus; a literature review is *not* a problem statement for a particular study.

Polit, DF & Hungler, BP: Nursing Research: Principles and Methods, *4th ed, Philadelphia, Lippincott, pp. 87-110, 1991; Miller, BK: The Literature Review in* Nursing Research: Methods, Critical Appraisal, and Utilization, *3rd ed (LoBiondo-Wood, G & Haber, J, Eds). St. Louis, Mosby, pp. 111-115, 1994.*

2.5. Correct Answer: **a**

A theoretical framework provides a context to guide a study, a rationale for predictions posed in a research problem, an organized structure to link study results with findings of previous research and to relate variables. This framework is a context on which to ground concepts and research findings or observations and also to examine relationships for meaningful, generalizable results. Grounding the scientific research approach in a theoretical framework also tests the theory and may suggest theory modifications or adaptations.

Polit, DF & Hungler, BP: Nursing Research: Principles and Methods, *4th ed. Philadelphia, Lippincott, pp. 113-132, 1991; Summers, S: Nursing Research in* ASPAN's Core Curriculum for Post Anesthesia Nursing Practice, *3rd ed (Litwack, K, Ed). Philadelphia, Saunders, pp. 17-18, 1994.*

2.6. Correct Answer: **d**

The researcher chooses a descriptive design to focus on describing the phenomenon of postanesthesia shaking and to summarize the status of this phenomenon. Longitudinal designs collect the same data over two or more points in time; surveys collect information about people's past, present or future actions; factorial study designs manipulate more than one variable.

Polit, DF & Hungler, BP: Nursing Research: Principles and Methods, *4th ed. Philadelphia, Lippincott, pp. 175-188, 1991; LoBiondo-Wood, G & Haber, J:* Nursing Research: Methods, Critical Appraisal, and Utilization, *3rd ed. St. Louis, Mosby, pp. 231-235, 1994.*

2.7. Correct Answer: **b**

A researcher uses descriptive statistics to summarize and describe the study's observations and measurements. These statistics give meaning to the collected data (numbers) and characteristics of the study sample. The researcher might describe the sample by central tendency (mode, mean or median scores), by variability (range, standard deviation) or by strength of correlation among study variables.

Polit, DF & Hungler, BP: Nursing Research: Principles and Methods, *4th ed. Philadelphia, Lippincott, pp. 206-427, 1991; Bello, A: Descriptive Data Analysis: in* Nursing Research: Methods, Critical Appraisal, and Utilization, *3rd ed (LoBiondo-Wood, G & Haber, J, Eds). St. Louis, Mosby, pp. 385-403, 1994.*

2.8. Correct Answer: **c**

When stating a research hypothesis, the researcher assumes, then declares, how two or more study variables will relate. Thus, the hypothesis is stated in advance of data collection and specifies study variables, names the study population and predicts outcomes. A hypothesis is a clearly expressed statement to tie the theoretical framework with the literature review and problem statement.

Polit, DF & Hungler, BP: Nursing Research: Principles and Methods, *4th ed. Philadelphia, Lippincott, pp. 206-427, 1991; Summers, S: Nursing Research in* ASPAN's Core Curriculum for Post Anesthesia Nursing Practice, *3rd ed (Litwack, K, Ed). Philadelphia, Saunders, pp. 17-18, 1994.*

2.9. Correct Answer: **b**

When an expert nurse "thinks aloud," the student hears the rationale behind specific nursing actions. Narratives reveal a nurse's judgment and reflect the skills embedded in patient assessment and nurse decision making. Sharing these assists the student's learning process and helps nurses highlight essential elements of practice.

Corcoran, S, Narayan, S & Moreland, H: "Thinking Aloud" as a Strategy to Improve Clinical Decision Making. Heart and Lung *17(5): 465-568, 1988; Bowers Feldman, ME: Uncovering Clinical Knowledge and Caring Practices.* Post Anesth Nurs *8(3): 159-162, 1993; Benner, P: From Novice to Expert: Excellence and Power in* Clinical Nursing Practice. *Menlo Park, CA, Addison Wesley, 1984.*

2.10. Correct Answer: **c**

Any patient complication related to medical device use must be reported to the Food and Drug Administration (FDA) and the manufacturer. The staff nurse need not directly inform these agencies but must set the facility protocol in motion so mandatory reporting is completed within 10 days of an incident. In 1990, a federal law, The Safe Medical Devices Act (SMDA), was enacted to protect consumers from product-related illness, injury or death. The law requires the health care worker in hospitals, ambulatory facilites and nursing homes to report device malfunctions.

Allen A: Medical Device Reporting: A New Challenge for Perioperative Nurses. Post Anesth Nurs *7(5): 352-353, 1992; News Notes:* Post Anesth Nurs *7(5): 135, 1992.*

2.11. Correct Answer: **c**

The immediate nursing priority for Mr. M's current postanesthesia care is astute observation to prevent pulmonary aspiration of silent emesis. Emergency surgery and his current unconsciousness and anesthesia depth (resembling Stage III, the level of surgical anesthesia) increase Mr. M's aspiration risk. He is totally unaware and unmoving, has blunted reflex responses, probably uses his abdominal and diaphragmatic muscles to breathe, has little intercostal muscle movement and may require jaw support. When Mr. M metabolizes anesthetic medications, risk for corneal abrasion increases and will become a priority concern as he groggily reawakens and moves. Now, the nurse positions herself near Mr. M's head and MUST remain continuously attentive.

Drain, C: The Post Anesthesia Care Unit: A Critical Care Approach to Post Anesthesia Nursing, *3rd ed. Philadelphia, Saunders, pp. 190-192, 1994; Burden, N:* Ambulatory Surgical Nursing. *Philadelphia, Saunders, pp. 253-266, 1993.*

2.12. Correct Answer: **a**

Increased potential for disoriented activity and restless (emergence delirium), active vomiting and airway irritability with laryngospasm most resemble the classic Stage II of anesthesia, the stage of delirium. He now may behave with restless abandon—confused, agitated, trying to get off the stretcher and looking disoriented. Nursing priorities now shift to protect the semiconscious Mr. M from injury. Stage II is mercifully brief, particularly when short-acting general anesthetics are used.

Drain, C: The Post Anesthesia Care Unit: A Critical Care Approach to Post Anesthesia Nursing, *3rd ed. Philadelphia, Saunders, pp. 190-192, 1994.*

2.13. Correct Answer: **a**

According to ASPAN's *Standards of Perianesthesia Nursing Practice* and based on guidelines of the American Institute of Architects, a Phase I inpatient PACU provides a "minimum of 80 square feet for each patient bed" and "clearance of at least 4 feet" between beds and from any wall.

American Society of Post Anesthesia Nurses (ASPAN): Standards of Perianesthesia Nursing Practice, *Resource 5. Thorofare, NJ, ASPAN, p. 36, 1995.*

2.14. Correct Answer: **c**

This nurse must recognize the need for dose reduction in an elderly, small or debilitated patient, then collaborate with the physician to adjust Mr. G's dose. In addition, the nurse assigned to Mr. G's care must *establish priorities:* continuously monitoring his response during conscious sedation and emergency intervention are the nurse's *only* responsibilities. Obtaining supplies, not patient observation, must be delegated. Even though he is a healthy man, a 5 mg dose of midazolam likely will oversedate an elderly man like Mr. G; his ability to independently maintain his patent airway, a requirement of conscious sedation, could also be eliminated. Meperidine augments these effects.

(Collaborative Statement): The Role of the Registered Nurse in the Management of Patients Receiving IV Conscious Sedation for Short-Term Therapeutic, Diagnostic, or Surgical Procedures in Standards of Perianesthesia Nursing Practice, *Resource 14. Thorofare, NJ, ASPAN, pp. 54-55, 1995. Burden, N:* Ambulatory Surgical Nursing. *Philadelphia, Saunders, pp. 139-149, 1993.*

2.15. Correct Answer: **d**

Meperidine and antidepressant monoamine oxidase inhibitors (MAOI) like phenelzine (Nardil) don't mix. The combination could produce profound hypertension. MAOIs promote storage of epinephrine, which meperidine releases. In some patients, this catecholamine surge can produce wildly fluctuating blood pressures with agitation and headache. Appreciating the potential consequences of combining meperidine with an MAOI medication and then questioning the physician's order are nursing responsibilities related to drug administration.

Burden, N: Ambulatory Surgical Nursing. *Philadelphia, Saunders, pp. 199, 273 & 278, 1993; Morgan, GE & Mikhail, MS:* Clinical Anesthesiology. *Norwalk, CT, Appleton & Lange, p. 449, 1992.*

2.16. Correct Answer: **c**

Respect, privacy, informed consent and confidentiality are

among the tenets of a Patient's Bill of Rights. The American Hospital Association presented this Patient's Bill of Rights to "contribute to more effective patient care" and recognize the legal and supportive roles of the physician and hospital in assuring patient satisfaction.

American Hospital Association: A Patient's Bill of Rights in Standards of Perianesthesia Nursing Practice, *Resource 1. Thorofare, NJ, ASPAN, pp. 22-23, 1995.*

2.17. Correct Answer: **b**

Protection of human rights means research cannot deny a patient the normal or standard care offered in that facility. Denying visitors to one-half of the participants at this study is, therefore, unethical in a PACU in which allowing visitors is part of standard care. This study's quasiexperimental design does not prove true cause and effect relationships; rather, the researcher compares differences in group outcomes.

Polit, DF & Hungler, BP: Nursing Research: Principles and Methods, *4th ed. Philadelphia, Lippincott, pp. 30-38. 1991; Massey, VH:* Nursing Research: A Study and Learning Tool. *Springhouse, PA, Springhouse Corp, pp. 50-55, 1991.*

2.18. Correct Answer: **d**

The primary purpose of an Institutional Review Board (IRB), or human subjects committee, is to protect human rights. Research that passes IRB scrutiny satisfies *ethical* requirements of informed consent, protects a subject's privacy, anonymity and confidentiality and provides reasonable freedom from harm. An IRB considers methodology but only in relation to protection of human rights. The National Research Act of 1974 requires facilities that conduct health or behavioral research using human subjects to follow the Code of Federal Regulations.

Polit, DF & Hungler, BP: Nursing Research: Principles and Methods, *4th ed. Philadelphia, Lippincott, pp. 40 & 646. 1991; Jackson, BS: Legal and Ethical Issues in* Nursing Research: Methods, Critical Appraisal and Utilization, *3rd ed (LoBiondo-Wood, G & Haber, J, Eds). St. Louis, Mosby, pp. 330-333, 1994.*

2.19. Correct Answer: **a**

A preoperative patient may have increased anxiety after observing the blunted motor and sensory functions of a postanesthesia patient. In a patient-focused system, the nurse's *priority* is to minimize the preanesthesia patient's potential for anxiety. Therefore, in Phase I PACU "preoperative patients are not present when patients are recovering from anesthesia." Situations that increase anxiety fail to achieve this standard. Each facility must identify and evaluate an appropriate space for preanesthesia and postanesthesia patients to assure a "safe, comfortable and therapeutic environment" apart from "environmental risk factors."

American Society of Post Anesthesia Nurses (ASPAN): Standards of Perianesthesia Nursing Practice, *Standard II. Thorofare, NJ, ASPAN, pp. 9-10, 1995.*

2.20. Correct Answer: **b**

Renewal of the CPR credential occurs every 2 years; a review of CPR-related content and practice of technique is an annual event. The ASPAN standard recommends Advanced Cardiac Life Support (ACLS) competency because "perianesthesia nursing practice involves autonomous decision-making and implementation of interventions in a crisis situation."

American Society of Post Anesthesia Nurses (ASPAN): Standards of Perianesthesia Nursing Practice, *Standards II & X. Thorofare, NJ, ASPAN, pp. 9 & 19, 1995.*

2.21. Correct Answer: **b**

Standards state each PACU develops a written plan for orientation and ongoing education to improve competency of nurses and support staff. Critical elements for achievement include annual demonstration of required competencies. Working alone with any postanesthesia patient or delegating a nursing function like jaw support do not comply with established standards.

American Society of Post Anesthesia Nurses (ASPAN): Standards of Perianesthesia Nursing Practice, *Resources 9, 15 & 17. Thorofare, NJ, ASPAN, pp. 47, 56 & 61-71, 1995.*

2.22. Correct Answer: **c**

To prevent colonization of other patients and health care workers and rampant spread of infection, a patient with methicillin-resistant staphylococcus aureus (MRSA) organisms must be isolated. In addition, handwashing, wearing gloves, mask and gown, and careful contact with the patient are important for anyone in the MRSA patient's presence. MRSA organisms are virulent gram-positive bacteria. MRSA-related nosocomial pneumonias and bacteremia infections of epidemic proportions ravage hospitals in increasing numbers.

McCraney, S & Rapp, RP: Antibiotic Agents in Critical Care. Crit Care Nurs Clin North Am *5(2): 319-320, 1993; Long, M & Miller, MD: Infection Control in* Basic Nursing: Theory and Practice, *3rd ed (Potter, PA & Perry, AG, Eds). Philadelphia, Saunders, pp. 620-623, 1994.*

2.23. Correct Answer: **d**

Vancomycin is the medication of choice to treat MRSA. Methicillin-resistant strains of staphylococci are not susceptible to penicillinase-resistant antibiotics, the usual antibiotic choice for staphylococcal infections. Most staphylococci produce the enzyme penicillinase; these infections are treated with narrow-spectrum, penicillinase-resistant antibiotics. These include methicillin, nafcillin, amd oxacillin.

McCraney, S & Rapp, RP: Antibiotic Agents in Critical Care. Crit Care Nurs Clin North Am *5(2): 319-320, 1993; Ma, MY: Antibacterial Agents in* Clinical Pharmacology and Nursing, *2nd ed (Baer, CL & Williams, BR, Eds). Springhouse, PA, Springhouse Corp, pp. 1038-1040, 1992.*

2.24. Correct Answer: **c**

ASPAN standards recommend an available cardiac monitor and pulse oximeter for each patient. In addition, a minimum of one ventilator is available in the PACU, with other ventilators accessible as needed. ASPAN standards recommend that the PACU be supplied with equipment to rewarm patients, though the type of rewarming system is not specified.

American Society of Post Anesthesia Nurses (ASPAN): Standards of Perianesthesia Nursing Practice,

Resource 5. Thorofare, NJ, ASPAN, pp. 35-38, 1995.

2.25. Correct Answer: **a**

The nurse has a legal and ethical responsibility to this patient to determine if the rhythm is truly complete heart block. The nurse should document observations, any related sequelae, interventions and patient responses, people informed and the reponse. Negligence surrounds failure to follow professional standards and facility protocols or to *report changes* in the patient's condition. Reporting includes the appropriate physicians, the designated PACU manager and perhaps even hospital managers. Carrie is asymptomatic—now. Observation without treatment may be appropriate for awhile, but true complete heart block cannot be ignored. This is a serious arrhythmia that can deteriorate to asystole.

American Society of Post Anesthesia Nurses (ASPAN): Standards of Perianesthesia Nursing Practice, *Standards VI & VII. Thorofare, NJ, ASPAN, pp. 15-16, 1995; Thelan, LS, Davie, JK, Urden, LD, et al:* Critical Care Nursing: Diagnosis and Management. *St. Louis, Mosby, p. 224, 1994; Litwack, K:* Post Anesthesia Care Nursing, *2nd ed. St. Louis, Mosby, pp. 44-55, 1995.*

2.26. Correct Answer: **b**

Hospital admission for further observation is appropriate—and necessary for Carrie's safety. Complete heart block has the potential to create life-threatening complications. The health care team has no information to determine whether this complete heart block is a new development or an undiagnosed congenital problem that requires investigation.

Burden, N: Ambulatory Surgical Nursing. *Philadelphia, Saunders, pp. 367-368, 1993; Thelan, LS, Davie, JK, Urden, LD, et al:* Critical Care Nursing: Diagnosis and Management. *St. Louis, Mosby, p. 224, 1994.*

2.27. Correct Answer: **d**

Research supports, or fails to support, a research position or hypothesis. Research conclusively *proves* nothing. Using research to support a policy change is appropriate, though this critic should describe a variety of studies to present a balanced and well-supported position. Researcher (or research consumer) bias or judgments might mean a study's conclusions are interpreted in ways that stretch beyond information provided in the study. For example, permitting visitation does not *cause* shorter PACU stays but may be one supportive factor in anxiety reduction so the result is earlier discharge.

Poole, EL: The Effects of Postanesthesia Care Unit Visits on Anxiety of Surgical Patients. Post Anesth Nurs *8(6): 386-394, 1993; LoBiondo-Wood, G:* Nursing Research: Methods, Critical Appraisal, and Utilization, *3rd ed. St. Louis, Mosby, pp. 424–437, 1994.*

2.28. Correct Answer: **a**

Postanesthesia, critical care and coronary care literature consistently indicate that the presence of family members or significant others decreases situational anxiety. Both patients and family members consistently report positive aspects of visitation. PACU-focused studies found other patients do not report privacy violation.

Poole, EL: The Effects of Postanesthesia Care Unit Visits on Anxiety of Surgical Patients. Post Anesth Nurs *8(6): 386-394, 1993; Vogelsang, J: Nurses' Assumptions About Patients' Perceived Needs in the PACU.* Crit Care Nurs *6: 44-54, 1986; Noonan, AT, Anderson, P, Newlon, P, et al: Family-centered Nursing in the Postanesthеisa Care Unit: The Evaluation of Practice.* Post Anesth Nurs *6: 13–16, 1991.*

2.29. Correct Answer: **d**

An agenda merely announces the meeting's issues, indicates the order for presentation and provides structure for a productive meeting. Advance awareness of the topics planned for discussion enables committee members to prepare for the meeting. Indicating the sequence of topics sets the stage for a positive working environment; an agenda might start with a topic that encourages concensus. Likewise, the meeting might close with another unifying topic to promote a group's feeling of accomplishment and productivity.

Schegel, JF: Board Primer. Leadership, 1994, p. L-47.

2.30. Correct Answer: **b**

Major points of a meeting discussion should be summarized rather than detailed. Specific individuals need no identification in the minutes, except to document a formal motion. Minutes should be simply written in a short form. This allows easy review by committee members or other interested readers.

Schegel, JF: Board Primer. Leadership, 1994, p. L-48.

SET II

Answer Key

2.31. d
2.32. b
2.33. c
2.34. a
2.35. a
2.36. b
2.37. c
2.38. a
2.39. c
2.40. d
2.41. a
2.42. c
2.43. a
2.44. b

SET II

Rationales and References

2.31. Correct Answer: **d**

A charge of negligence means the patient (plaintiff) must *prove* that damage (the wound infection) actually occurred as a direct result of the accused nurse's actions (changing the dressing after caring for a patient with an infection). Even undesirable outcomes must be directly linked to a specific alleged action. Negligence commonly includes failure to inform the physician of condition changes, failure to monitor condition and failure to accurately document observed events and physician notification. The nurse has a legal responsibility (duty) to provide safe patient care without the intention to harm.

Litwack, K: Post Anesthesia Care Nursing, *2nd ed. St. Louis, Mosby, pp. 42-56, 1995; Calloway, SD: Legal Issues in Post Anesthesia Care Nursing in* ASPAN's Core Curriculum for Post Anesthesia Nursing Practice, *3rd ed (Litwack, K, Ed). Philadelphia, Sau(lers, pp. 26-29, 1994.*

2.32. Correct Answer: **b**

Standards of care (whether established by state or federal law, nursing and specialty organization or accrediting agencies) are legal measures to determine the acceptability of a nurse's professional actions. Nurses must meet the same standard of acceptable care whether certified or not. Expert witnesses may attest to whether this nurse acted responsibly to provide nursing care as another "ordinary, prudent nurse would have performed in the same or similar manner" and in a similar circumstance. The plaintiff who brings the lawsuit, not the nurse-defendant, must prove both proximate cause and damage.

Calloway, SD: Legal Issues in Post Anesthesia Care Nursing in ASPAN's Core Curriculum for Post Anesthesia Nursing Practice, *3rd ed (Litwack, K, Ed). Philadelphia, Saunders, pp. 26-29, 1994; Litwack, K: Post Anesthesia Care Nursing, 2nd ed. St. Louis, Mosby, pp. 42-56, 1995.*

2.33. Correct Answer: **c**

Drawing ideas from the PACU staff, encouraging collaboration among health care team members and incorporating multiple ideas to create a unit plan or project are empowering acts. Empowerment is defined as a "true opportunity for employees throughout the company to create the future together." Among this item's examples, involvement with a multidisciplinary group holds greater potential for creativity, enrichment, diverse solutions—and empowerment—than when requesting permission, approval or conceding a project.

Prim, RG: Communication: Coping with the Unspoken Dance, Nurs Manag *24(3): 33–35, 1993; Duck, JD: Managing Change: The Art of Balancing.* Harv Bus Rev, *Nov-Dec 1993. p. 118; Muller-Smith, PA: PACU Management in* ASPAN's Core Curriculum for Post Anesthesia Nursing Practice, *3rd ed (Litwack, K, Ed). Philadelphia, Saunders, pp. 39-41, 1994.*

2.34. Correct Answer: **a**

Research consistency requires each data collector (rater) consider each subject with identical tools and criteria. Observational research methods are vulnerable to human error. Researchers educate observers to maximize accuracy and reliability of data and to minimize bias, then evaluate the observers in a practice session and compare their answers for agreement.

Polit, DF & Hungler, BP: Nursing Research: Principles and Methods, *4th ed. Philadelphia, Lippincott, pp. 331 & 372, 1991; Summers, S: Nursing Research in* ASPAN's Core Curriculum for Post Anesthesia Nursing Practice, *3rd ed (Litwack, K, Ed). Philadelphia, Saunders, pp. 19-22, 1994.*

2.35. Correct Answer: **a**

Risk of occupational exposure to this patient's HIV is low. Principles of universal precautions and ASPAN standards are applied in this situation to assure positive outcomes for staff and patient. This patient can receive care in PACU and does not need to be isolat in the OR. Universal precautions and protective barriers are necessary when contacting *any* patient, not merely the patient with a specific disease. The caregiver's HIV status need not affect patient assignment decisions, though a nurse with open, weeping skin lesions should not care for this patient. ASPAN standards recommend that one registered nurse, not any "staff member," care for no more than one patient during admission to PACU, or two drowsy, anesthetized patients in Phase I PACU.

Sommargren, CE: Environmental Hazards in AACN's Clinical Reference for Critical-Care Nursing *(Kinney, MR, Packa, DR & Dunbar, SB, Eds). St. Louis, Mosby, pp. 99-100, 1993; Burden, N:* Ambulatory Surgical Nursing. *Philadelphia, Saunders, pp. 411-414 & 701-702, 1993; Morgan, GE & Mikhail, MS:* Clinical Anesthesiology. *Norwalk, CT, Appleton & Lange, p. 659, 1992.*

2.36. Correct Answer: **b**

Discontinuing an airway and suctions presents low risk of HIV transmission. Saliva, sputum and nasal secretions typically contain little or no blood. Contact with cerebrospinal fluid and blood may increase exposure risk, though incidence of HIV transmission to health care workers remains less than 1%. Following principles of universal precautions is a recommended standard of practice whenever the nurse anticipates contact with potentially infectious body secretions.

Sommargren, CE: Environmental Hazards in AACN's Clinical Reference for Critical-Care Nursing *(Kinney, MR, Packa, DR & Dunbar, SB, Eds). St. Louis, Mosby, pp. 99-100, 1993; Burden, N:* Ambulatory Surgical Nursing. *Philadelphia, Saunders, pp. 411-414, 1993.*

2.37. Correct Answer: **c**

A specific "no-CPR" request is only one portion of an advance directive. The American Heart Association recommends that no-CPR or DNR/DNI orders be reviewed with the surgical patient and family by the attending physician and anesthesiologist. Discussion focuses on the desired response by the health care team for specific perioperative potential events. Based on this discussion, the orders may be continued or suspended. Individual health care facilities often establish specific protocols to consider DNR/DNI orders for the perianesthesia period; situational concerns can be directed to a facility's ethics committee.

Litwack, K: Post Anesthesia Care Nursing, *2nd ed. St. Louis, Mosby, pp. 57-65, 1995; Golanowski, M: Do Not Resuscitate: Informed Consent in the Operating Room and Postanesthesia Care Unit.* Post Anesth Nurs *10(1): 9-11, 1995; American Heart Association: Ethical Considerations in Resuscitation.* JAMA *268(16): 2282-2287, 1992.*

2.38. Correct Answer: **a**

The PACU is considered a critical care area. ASPAN standards recommend that the registered nurse practicing in a perianesthesia area achieve competencies related to airway management, circulatory support, comfort and thermoregulation. In addition, ASPAN standards recommend ACLS certification or demonstration of equivalent competence. Content in a recommended competency-based education program and ACLS-equivalent program include critical care concepts like arrhythmia identification, pharmacologic interventions and defibrillation or cardioversion techniques. Appropriate documentation includes written tests, algorithm knowledge and return demonstration.

American Society of Post Anesthesia Nurses (ASPAN): Standards of Perianesthesia Nursing Practice, *Standard X and Resource 17. Thorofare, NJ, ASPAN, pp. 19 & 61-71, 1995; Muller-Smith, PA: PACU Management in* ASPAN's Core Curriculum for Post Anesthesia Nursing Practice, *3rd ed (Litwack, K, Ed). Philadelphia, Saunders, pp. 39-41, 1994.*

2.39. Correct Answer: **c**

Specific dilutions of sodium hypochlorite (bleach) inactivate both blood-borne hepatitis B virus and HIV within 10 minutes. Any body substance is presumed to be potentially infectious. Principles endorsed by the Centers for Disease Control and Prevention (CDC) regarding universal precautions direct handling of body secretions, including cleaning spills. Optimal solutions for disinfection are not specified in these principles, though detergents must be registered as hospital-grade disinfectants for cleaning use.

Pfaff, SJ: Infection Prevention and Control in Ambulatory Surgical Nursing *(Burden, N, Ed). Philadelphia, Saunders, pp. 633-640, 1993.*

2.40. Correct Answer: **d**

"Modern" QI requires action and changing practice to continuously improve patient outcomes, not merely record numbers. QI indicators are patient-focused descriptions of an event, outcome or pattern of care for a specific subgroup of patients. JCAHO guidelines advocate patient-focused evaluations that target high-volume, high-risk or problem-prone patient care issues. For example, ASA III patients or orthopedic patients might represent a unique subgroup of the perioperative population. Hypoxemia is one relevant, patient-focused PACU issue. If correlation indicates patients enter PACU with hypoxia after long transports from the OR, outcome improvement involves a new action, perhaps transporting patients with oxygen, and ongoing monitoring.

Joint Commission on Accreditation of Health care Organizations (JCAHO): Accreditation Manual for Hospitals. *Oak Brook Terrace, Ill, JCAHO, pp. 1-12, 1994; Buss, HE: Continuous Quality Improvement: Adaptation of the 10-Step Model With Postanesthesia Care Unit Application.* Post Anesth Nurs *8(4): 238-248, 1993; Ventura, MR, Rizzo, J & Lenz, S: Quality Indicators: Control Maintains—Propriety Improves.* Nurs Manag *24(1): 46-50.*

2.41. Correct answer: **a**

The ethical principle of beneficence obligates a health care provider to act in ways to provide more benefit than harm or burden. Whether positive benefit occurs is established from the patient's perspective.

American Society of Post Anesthesia Nurses (ASPAN): Standards of Perianesthesia Nursing Practice, *Standard I. Thorofare, NJ, p. 8, 1995; American Nurses Association:* Code for Nurses with Interpretive Statements. *Washington, DC, American Nurses Association, 1995; Rushton, CH & Reigle, J: Ethical Issues in Critical Care in* AACN's Clinical Reference for Critical-Care Nursing, *3rd ed (Kinney, MR, Packa, DR & Dunbar, SB, Eds). Philadelphia, Saunders, pp. 12-14, 1993.*

2.42. Correct Answer: **c**

Ethical and legal principles mandate that the patient *comprehend* information to achieve informed consent. Thus the nurse must act to assure information is conveyed in a way the patient can understand. An interpreter can translate information to the patient's language and confirm that information is also understood. Responsibility for informing a patient about operative events rests with the surgeon (physician), though a nurse can facilitate the process by obtaining diagrams, booklets or interpreters that remove language barriers and increase potential for mutual understanding.

Burden, N: Ambulatory Surgical Nursing. *Philadelphia, Saunders, pp. 610-611, 1993; Rushton, CH & Reigle, J: Ethical Issues in Critical Care in* AACN's Clinical Reference for Critical-Care Nursing *(Kinney, MR, Packa, DR & Dunbar, SB, Eds). St. Louis, Mosby, pp. 16-18, 1993.*

2.43. Correct Answer: **a**

The nurse must either locate a second nurse, call the lunching nurse back to PACU or defer the transfer to ICU. *Standards of Perianesthesia Nursing Practice* developed and promoted by ASPAN recommends that two licensed nurses be present *whenever any patient* is in Phase I PACU. Though sending the medical aide to ICU assures two nurses remain in PACU, it is potentially unsafe for the patient being transferred.

American Society of Post Anesthesia Nurses (ASPAN): Standards of Perianesthesia Nursing Practice, *Resource 9. Thorofare, NJ, ASPAN, p. 47, 1995.*

2.44. Correct Answer: **b**

Methohexital is classified as an anesthetic medication for intravenous induction; therefore, administration is usually beyond the scope of practice of the nonanesthetist RN. Any nurse who assists with conscious sedation should review and understand in advance which medications can be given with a physician's order. Institutional policy, standards of care and that state's nurse practice act specify this information. The nurse managing care must then demonstrate competence in care of patients receiving IV conscious sedation, including monitoring of blood pressure, heart rate and oxygen saturation.

(Collaborative Statement): The Role of the Registered Nurse in the Management of Patients Receiving IV Conscious Sedation in ASPAN's Standards of Perianesthesia Nursing Practice, *Resource 14. Thorofare, NJ, ASPAN, pp. 54-55, 1995; Burden, N:* Ambulatory Surgical Nursing. *Philadelphia, Saunders, pp. 241-247, 1993.*

Section 3

Perianesthesia Considerations Across the Life Span

Scenarios and items in this section focus on *pediatric, obstetric* and *geriatric* patient populations. These concepts are considered together because:

- significant anatomic and/or physiologic differences or changes distinguish these patients from the "classic" adult patient.
- nursing assessment, intervention, education and psychosocial support for the perianesthesia patient consider these unique variables to deliver safe care.

ESSENTIAL CORE CONCEPTS	AFFILIATED CORE CURRICULUM CHAPTERS
Nursing Process	**Chapters 2, 7, 8 & 24**
Assessment	
Planning and Implementation	
Evaluation	
The Pediatric Patient	**Chapter 8**
Anatomy: Child vs. Adult	
Developmental Concepts	
Education	
Family Dynamics	
Psychosocial	
Physiologic "Normals"	
Perianesthesia Issues:	
Airway Compromises	
Anesthetic Specifics for Children	
Operative Specifics for Children	
Prematurity	
Specific Patient Care Concerns	
Awakening, Restlessness and Emesis	
Pain Management: Drugs and Alternatives	
Thermal Balance	
Parent Education	

The Obstetric Patient **Chapter 24**

Physiology of Pregnancy
  Expected Organ Systemic Changes
  Managing Organ Pathophysiology
Pregnancy-Associated Disorders
  Assessing Preterm Labor
  Hemorrhagic Emergencies
  Hypertension: Eclampsia and Seizures
  Placentas: Hypovolemia and Embolism
  Postpartum/Postcesarean Observation
Perianesthesia Specifics
  Anesthetic Options
  Pharmacologic Intervention
  Observation of Mother and Fetus After Surgery

The Geriatric Patient **Chapter 7**

Physiology of Aging
  Age-related Organ Dysfunction
  Pharmacologic Responses
    Anesthetic Options
    Prescribed Medications
Perianesthesia Specifics
  Barriers: Special Needs
  Education Considerations
  Risk Factors and Disease
  Ventilation, Temperature, Fluids and Comfort

SET I

Items 3.1-3.30

3.1. A 9 year old girl with a long history of otitis media will have a right tympanic membrane graft today. A characteristic that makes nitrous oxide a poor anesthetic choice for this child is its potential to:

a. diffuse rapidly into hepatic tissue
b. irritate tissue at the glottis
c. expand air-filled compartments
d. trigger emergence delirium

3.2. Soft, low-pitched respiratory sounds over most of an infant's lung surface during inspiration indicate:

a. hyaline membrane disease
b. vesicular breathing without disease
c. obstructive pulmonary disease
d. restrictive pulmonary disease

3.3. Factors that prolong an 85 year old woman's clinical response to a 3 mg dose of IV morphine sulfate include:

a. decreased serum albumin and total body water
b. vasoconstriction and higher sensitivity to carbon dioxide
c. increased volume of distribution and protein binding
d. morphine's lipid-soluble structure and inotropic effects

3.4. Ten year old Trevor has cerebral palsy and is scheduled for extraction of two infected teeth. An advantage of propofol to induce his anesthesia is its:

a. neuroleptic effect
b. painless injection
c. high analgesic quality
d. prompt redistribution

3.5. Following inhalation anesthesia, clinical signs that indicate a 3 month old infant's extubation readiness include all of the following *except:*

a. pink skin and regular diaphragmatic breathing
b. deep, regular ventilations at 28 breaths per minute
c. eye opening and coughing on the endotracheal tube
d. prolonged expiration and heart rate 92 beats/minute

3.6. Following aorta to femoral artery bypass with in situ graft, the PACU nurse best promotes a 79 year old woman's vascular patency by:

a. reporting the new, loud bruit near her knee
b. preventing fluid volume deficit
c. assuring a high Fowler's position
d. maintaining slight hypercarbia

NOTE: Consider scenario and items 3.7-3.9 together.

A 22 year old woman, $8\frac{1}{2}$ months pregnant, had general anesthesia and emergency cesarean section for abruptio placentae and is now in PACU. She developed sudden, severe abdominal pain of 1 hour's duration and was admitted to Labor and Delivery prior to surgery. Her baby did not survive.

3.7. This patient has increased potential for pulmonary aspiration because:

a. general anesthesia increases lower esophageal sphincter tone
b. gastric acidity varies widely during pregnancy
c. pregnancy delays gastric emptying
d. uterine contractions stimulate the chemoreceptor zone

3.8. This obstetric patient now is more likely to develop:

a. HELLP syndrome
b. noncardiogenic pulmonary edema
c. neuromuscular irritability
d. disseminated intravascular coagulopathy

3.9. The most appropriate nursing interventions to address this patient's psychosocial, grief and emotional needs include:

a. support, empathy, and a nonjudgmental style
b. sedation with an amnesic sedative
c. ignoring patient inquiries about the baby
d. focusing attention on physiologic parameters

NOTE: Consider scenario and items 3.10-3.15 together.

Sydney, a $2\frac{1}{2}$ year old boy, is admitted to PACU after a complex 10-hour procedure involving interdental wires and significant oropharyngeal reconstruction to correct craniosynostosis, a craniofacial anomaly. Breathing is spontaneous and regular at 22 breaths per minute through a nasotracheal tube with humidified oxygen delivered by T-piece at $FiO_2 = 0.6$. Oxygen saturation, measured with pulse oximeter, is greater than 97%. Pupils are equal and react to light. He opens his eyes to a painful stimulus.

3.10. The PACU nurse observes right-sided facial droop and immediately:

a. lowers the head of the bed
b. notifies the surgeon
c. turns the child to his left side
d. consults the medical history

3.11. After 3 hours in PACU, the anesthesiologist extubates Sydney according to established criteria. Fifteen minutes later Sydney begins to vomit. The nurse's most appropriate intervention is prompt:

a. prone repositioning and vigorous chest vibration
b. jaw band severing, then oropharyngeal suction
c. nasal reintubation and bronchial lavage
d. intravenous ondansetron, then gentle oral suction

NOTE: The scenario continues.

Thirty minutes after resolution of the vomiting episode this patient receives oxygen at FiO_2 of 0.6 L/min by humidified face tent. Sydney's heart rate increases to 150 beats per minute, and oxygen saturation slowly decreases to 92%. Breath sounds are audible bilaterally and without wheezes or crackles.

3.12. The nurse does hear stridorous sounds and immediately:

a. reintubates orally, then reapplies dental bands
b. lavages oropharynx with racemic epinephrine and suctions
c. repositons the head, then continues misted oxygen
d. stimulates deep breathing and hyperextends the head

3.13. Despite these interventions, the child's airway remains obstructed. He is swiftly returned to the OR for tracheostomy. When planning nursing care after this second surgery, the PACU nurse plans sterile, atraumatic suction technique and:

a. anticipates copious bloody secretions
b. selects suction catheters sized at 75% of tracheostomy tube diameter
c. intends to maintain a tracheostomy cuff inflation pressure of 35 mmHg
d. prepares to increase FiO_2 prior to suctioning.

3.14. Suctioning irritates the child's trachea and he coughs out his new airway. Airway patency is best supported by immediately:

a. suctioning the meatus
b. reinserting the tracheostomy tube

c. suctioning the oropharynx
d. providing oxygen with bag-valve-mask apparatus

3.15. The nurse tactilely assesses the tracheostomy site to detect:
a. subcutaneous emphysema
b. neck vein distention
c. tracheoesophageal fistula
d. unsuctioned secretions

NOTE: Consider items 3.16-3.17 together.

3.16. Age-related physiologic changes that alter a medication's pharmacokinetics in an 89 year old man include all of the following *except* his:
a. larger residual lung volume
b. increased aldosterone secretion
c. prolonged circulation time
d. greater number of lipid storage sites

3.17. For this patient, the likely pharmacodynamic outcomes related to thiopental administration include:
a. hyperventilation
b. rapid return to consciousness
c. intraoperative temperature rise
d. orthostatic hypotension

3.18. Forty-five minutes after Cesarean section, the PACU nurse palpates a woman's uterus and expects:
a. posterior displacement and soft tissue
b. nodular tissue and three saturated perineal pads
c. firm fundus located near the umbilicus
d. left tenderness and a continuous trickle of blood

3.19. Compared with the adult airway, the child's airway has a:
a. narrower cricoid and higher glottis
b. smaller tongue and nares
c. minimal curve between vocal cords and epiglottis
d. broader cricoid and narrower glottis

NOTE: Consider scenario and items 3.20-3.21 together.

An apprehensive and diaphoretic 88 year old man with history of chronic obstructive pulmonary disease (COPD) and hypertension expectorates frothy sputum. Respirations are 40 breaths per minute with suprasternal retractions; the PACU nurse hears crackles and scattered expiratory wheezes throughout the lung fields and notes an S_3 heart sound. The cardiac monitor shows sinus tachycardia at 152 beats per minute. The patient received 2500 ml crystalloid during a 2 hour Austin Moore hip prosthesis with isoflurane and fentanyl anesthesia.

3.20. The patient's symptoms are most likely due to:
a. increased pulmonary hydrostatic pressure
b. decreased rate of glomerulofiltration
c. increased interstitial clearance
d. decreased alveolar excursion

3.21. For this patient, one nursing intervention with both physiologic and comfort outcomes is to:
a. place patient in side-lying position
b. administer morphine sulfate in 2 mg doses
c. suction trachea and oropharynx every 10 minutes
d. elevate legs on two pillows

3.22. To set 7 year old Chelsea's left comminuted tibial fracture, the anesthesia provider placed a bupivacaine spinal anesthetic. To illustrate the sequential onset of spinal blockade, the preanesthesia nurse explains that Chelsea will most likely notice:
a. pain relief, then inability to wiggle her toes
b. her leg feels heavy before her pain is relieved
c. she cannot bend her knee, then a numb knee
d. absent right thigh motion before left hip numbness

3.23. The child *most* at risk to develop postextubation laryngeal edema with inspiratory stridor is a:

a. 4 month old premature infant
b. 12 month old term toddler
c. 9 year old preteen boy
d. 3 year old preschool girl

3.24. A healthy, 5 months pregnant woman had emergency surgery to repair and cast a tibial fracture. The PACU nurse anticipates pregnancy-related physiologic alterations are reflected in arterial blood gas with:

a. pCO_2 increased, pO_2 decreased, pH decreased
b. pCO_2 normal, pO_2 decreased, pH increased
c. pCO_2 decreased, pO_2 increased, pH normal
d. pCO_2 decreased, pO_2 normal, pH decreased

3.25. Factors that increase the potential for postextubation laryngeal edema in children include all of the following *except:*

a. coughing while intubated
b. Down syndrome
c. preoperative asthma
d. surgery in prone position

3.26. When compared with inhaled gases, propofol affects anesthetic outcomes for pediatric patients by:

a. reducing airway obstruction and nausea
b. increasing pain relief and decreasing emesis
c. reducing airway obstruction and increasing emesis
d. increasing both airway obstruction and pain relief

NOTE: Consider items 3.27-3.28 together.

3.27. A woman who is 22 weeks pregnant dozes calmly in PACU after a cervical cerclage to "repair" an incompetent cervix. Blood pressure is 128/60, heart rate is 98 beats per minute in sinus rhythm, respiratory rate is 24 breaths per minute and SpO_2 = 97%. The normal physiologic increase in aldosterone associated with her pregnancy promotes:

a. glucose reduction
b. water excretion
c. sodium retention
d. hemoglobin elevation

3.28. The nurse is *most concerned* when postoperative observations indicate:

a. consistent fetal heart rate of 148 beats per minute
b. increased intrauterine activity reported by patient
c. absent uterine sensations in side-lying position
d. patient and fetal heart rate synchrony during sleep

3.29. Following cleft palate repair, 9 month old Sadie cries loudly and flails her arms. Nursing interventions include parental visitation, ice on her sutures and:

a. 4 oz of apple juice
b. secure arm restraint
c. gentle oral suction
d. acetaminophen suppository

NOTE: Consider scenario and item 3.30 together.

A 64 year old postoperative patient with chronic obstructive pulmonary disease (COPD) develops wheezing, nonproductive cough and severe dyspnea. His speech is interrupted to breathe. The nurse observes diaphoresis, heart rate of 130 beats per minute, and respiratory rate of 36 breaths per minute. Oxygen saturation measured by a pulse oximeter is 88%.

3.30. The most appropriate *immediate* intervention to resolve this patient's respiratory crisis promotes:

a. oxygenation, by delivering humidified oxygen per catheter
b. airway relaxation, by aerosolizing bronchospastic mediators
c. secretion mobilization, by postural drainage and stir-up activity
d. bronchodilation, by inhaling anticholinergic medications

SET II

Items: 3.31-3.52

NOTE: Consider items 3.31-3.32 together.

3.31. An infant born 2 months prematurely is now 4 months old and today he had surgery to correct congenital right club foot. The PACU nurse expects to observe a respiratory pattern characterized by:

a. episodic apnea
b. stridor with retraction
c. alternating bradypnea and tachypnea
d. barking cough

3.32. The management of this infant's care will likely include close nursing observation and:

a. intubation and mechanical ventilation for 5 hours
b. pulse oximeter in PACU for 10 hours
c. overnight hospitalization and apnea monitor
d. discharge to home if no apnea occurs in 4 hours

NOTE: Consider scenario and items 3.33-3.34 together.

Following Cesarean section delivery of her first child, who has Down's syndrome, an 18 year old woman complains of epigastric pain and headache. She is drowsy, resting in PACU and responsive. Her deep tendon and plantar reflexes are brisk. By her choice, significant family members are with her. Her blood pressure has been 158-168/100-110 since hospital admission 12 hours ago; prehospital BP measures were stable near 120/72. Her heart rate is 98 beats per minute.

3.33. Today's most appropriate priority to maximize positive outcomes for this woman is:

a. anxiety reduction through today's grief support group
b. pain management with increased rate of epidural morphine infusion
c. preload reduction with nitroglycerin infusion titrated to effect
d. neuromuscular suppression through magnesium sulfate therapy

NOTE: The scenario continues.

Laboratory analysis confirms slight proteinuria and glucosuria; hemoglobin is 10.3 mg/dl and potassium is 4.2 mEq/L; urine volume is 25 ml/hour. Pharmacologic intervention is initiated. Within 1 hour the PACU nurse observes first degree atrioventricular (AV) block on EKG, SaO_2 is 94% with abdominal breathing, and slight movement to patellar stimulation.

3.34. The PACU nurse reassures the patient, documents observations, informs the physician and prepares to:

a. administer hypertonic sodium chloride and midazolam
b. discontinue the magnesium sulfate infusion
c. add a rapid fluid challenge to vasodilator therapy
d. begin a double strength magnesium sulfate drip

3.35. The preanesthesia nurse expects a healthy 4 month old infant's resting heart rate to be:

a. 70-90 beats per minute
b. 100-110 beats per minute
c. 130-140 beats per minute
d. 160-180 beats per minute

3.36. The PACU nurse estimates that the endotracheal tube required to reintubate his average-sized 6 year old male patient is size:

a. 2.5 mm
b. 4.0 mm
c. 5.5 mm
d. 7.0 mm

3.37. A drowsy 7 year old child is admitted to PACU following tonsillectomy and has no evident oral secretions. Estimated intraoperative blood loss was 30 ml. BP is 90/56, heart rate 108 beats per minute and respiratory rate is 26 breaths per minute. Appropriate nursing intervention is to:

a. observe and regularly reassess apical heart rate
b. provide analgesia to decrease pain-related hyperventilation.
c. administer 100 ml fluid challenge for hypotension
d. infuse propranolol 1.0 mg to reduce tachycardia

3.38. The patient most likely to have an acquired deficiency of pseudocholinesterase is a:

a. child with diabetes mellitus
b. 55 year old man with 3 day old appendix perforation
c. teen with malignant hyperthermia
d. 78 year old woman with hemoglobin loss

3.39. Ideally, an infant's congenital cleft lip is repaired before age 3 months for the benefit of the infant's natural:

a. circulating maternal antibodies
b. low bleeding potential
c. lack of detachment anxiety
d. strong sucking reflex

3.40. The PACU nurse is *least concerned* when a 15 year old's endotracheal tube cuff:

a. remains uninflated after transport from the OR
b. allows speech; cuff pressure measures 9 cm H_2O
c. has an intracuff pressure measure of 25 cm H_2O
d. has a flexible, low-volume design

NOTE: Consider items 3.41-3.42 together.

3.41. A 75 year old man had bilateral knee arthroplasties this morning. One intraoperative dose of epidural morphine sulfate (Duramorph) was instilled between his L3-L4 vertebrae. Morphine sulfate will affect opiate receptors at his:

a. synovial fluid within 1 hour
b. temporal blood-brain barrier in 12 hours
c. dorsal horn and C nerve fibers
d. L3-L4 spinal dermatomes only

3.42. This man states severe pain when the PACU nurse initiates his continuous epidural infusion of morphine sulfate (Duramorph) with bupivacaine. As the epidural dose increases, the nurse assesses him for a bupivacaine-related:

a. allergic response from pseudocholinesterase hydrolysis
b. inability to dorsiflex and plantarflex his feet
c. urinary incontinence from bladder relaxation
d. lack of analgesic effect due to age and anatomy

NOTE: Consider scenario and items 3.43-3.44 together.

Prior to a planned 90 minute outpatient orthopedic procedure, a 10 year old diabetic girl's presurgical blood glucose is 96 mg/dl. She is currently alert and talking, and her vital signs are stable.

3.43. After consultation with the anesthesiologist and pediatrician, the PACU nurse's plan of care will include:

a. cancellation of surgery and infusion of dextrose 50%
b. continued surgical preparation with usual AM dose of short-acting insulin.
c. delay of surgery while cause of infection is sought
d. preparation for surgery and 50% of usual AM dose of intermediate-acting insulin

NOTE: The scenario continues.

This child received a preoperative dose of intermediate-acting insulin 3 hours ago. In PACU, her glucometer-measured glucose is 165 mg/dl. She is drowsy and moves extremities to touch stimulus; respirations are adequate; skin is warm and dry.

3.44. When planning postoperative management of glucose-insulin balance, the PACU nurse considers that:
a. insulin's action will peak within 6-8 hours
b. glucose measure probably reflects impending ketogenesis
c. preoperative insulin is no longer effective
d. Somogyi effect will occur within 1 hour

3.45. A perioperative activity *most appropriate* to a 4 year old's psychosocial development is:
a. using distraction techniques during mask induction of halothane anesthesia
b. watching a film of a school-aged child in the preadmission testing area
c. discussing the child's fear of needles and demonstrating IV therapy equipment
d. providing oral suction equipment for the child to manipulate and use on a doll.

3.46. The patient at greatest risk for hyperosmolar nonketotic syndrome (HNKS):
a. is younger than 28 years
b. dehydrates due to diabetes insipidus
c. produces no endogenous insulin
d. uses oral antihyperglycemic medication

NOTE: Consider scenario and items 3.47-3.48 together.

After carotid endarterectomy, a 74 year old woman will remain in PACU overnight and then transfer to a nursing unit. During the late evening, approximately 12 hours postoperatively, she complains of severe right-sided headache.

3.47. After determining that this woman has no neurologic changes, the PACU nurse appropriately:
a. raises the head of the bed
b. administers ordered intramuscular heparin 2000 u
c. increases intravenous fluid rate to 175 ml/hour
d. encourages her to hyperventilate

3.48. Before offering oral fluids to this woman, the PACU nurse assures integrity of cranial nerves:
a. I and III
b. VI and VII
c. X and XII
d. II and V

3.49. The patient at greatest risk for postoperative discomfort or injury related to position during hemorrhoidectomy and repair of a rectal-vaginal fistula is:
a. a healthy, lactating new mother
b. a 96 kg woman who had a total knee arthroplasty 2 years ago
c. a 60 kg woman with unrepaired carpal tunnel syndrome
d. an elderly woman with preexisting lumbar pain

NOTE: Consider scenario and items 3.50-3.51 together.

Following insertion of a multilumen central venous catheter by sedation with monitored anesthesia care (MAC), 92 year old Mr. Y is admitted to Phase I PACU. Nursing home documentation outlines a discussion 6 months ago between the physician, Mr. Y, and his family about do not resuscitate (DNR) status. The physician included a DNR order in Mr. Y's hospital admission record. When planning Mr. Y's care, the nurse considers the potential for lethal cardiac arrhythmias in PACU.

3.50. Anticipating this situation, the nurse most appropriately plans to:

a. defibrillate until Mr. Y is unmedicated and again legally competent to reconfirm his DNR status
b. negate the DNR status for 36 hours postprocedure
c. obtain a surgeon order for a slow, medication-only resuscitation
d. reconfirm and document physician and family resuscitation expectations

3.51. Following the insertion of a multilumen central venous catheter, Mr. Y has increased statistical risk of:

a. pulmonary artery rupture
b. intrapleural hemorrhage
c. nosocomial septicemia
d. medication precipitation

3.52. The child *most likely* to deal with developmental issues of trust is a:

a. crawling, smiling 10 month old
b. curious 18 month old toddler
c. crying 5 year old kindergartner
d. creative 9 year old prodigy

Set I

Answer Key

3.1.	c
3.2.	b
3.3.	a
3.4.	d
3.5.	d
3.6.	b
3.7.	c
3.8.	d
3.9.	a
3.10.	d
3.11.	b
3.12.	c
3.13.	d
3.14.	b
3.15.	a
3.16.	b
3.17.	d
3.18.	c
3.19.	a
3.20.	a
3.21.	b
3.22.	a
3.23.	d
3.24.	c
3.25.	c
3.26.	a
3.27.	c
3.28.	d
3.29.	d
3.30.	d

SET I

Rationales and References

3.1. Correct Answer: **c**

Patients having tympanic procedures do not receive nitrous oxide. Nitrous oxide easily diffuses into air-containing body spaces and expands the space. After tympanic surgery, an expanded middle ear compartment can produce severe pain and rupture the graft. Patients with pneumothorax, air embolism, bowel obstruction or intracranial air also have risk if these air-filled compartments expand. Nitrous oxide is considered nonirritating and nontoxic; unlike halothane, nitrous oxide is not associated with hepatitis.

Burden, N: Ambulatory Surgical Nursing. *Philadelphia, Saunders, pp. 70-71, 1993; Munson, ES: Complications of Nitrous Oxide Anesthesia for Ear Surgery.* Anesth Clin North Am *11(3): 559-572, 1993.*

3.2. Correct Answer: **b**

Vesicular sounds represent normal breathing and are auscultated throughout the lung field. These sounds are soft and low pitched, prolonged during inspiration and nearly silent during expiration. The inspiratory phase is heard longer and more loudly than the expiratory phase.

Stiesmeyer, JK: A Four-Step Approach to Pulmonary Assessment. Am J Nurs *93(8): 22-28, 1993; Taylor, C, Lillis, C & Le Mone, P:* Fundamentals of Nursing: The Art and Science of Nursing, *2nd ed. Philadelphia, Lippincott, pp. 447-449, 1993.*

3.3. Correct Answer: **a**

The aging process gradually decreases albumin and available protein to bind with drugs. Total body water also decreases and a drug's plasma *concentration* increases. Geriatric patients also have decreases in cardiac output, slowed circulation time, delays in renal metabolism, and decreased blood vessel tone. These all alter morphine's pharmacokinetics, or its concentration, at a mu receptor site. Morphine has little direct heart rate (chronotropic), rhythm, or contractile force (inotropic) effect, but does increase the likelihood of positional or orthostatic hypotension from vasodilation and peripheral blood pooling.

Litwack, K: ASPAN's Core Curriculum for Post Anesthesia Nursing Practice, *3rd ed. Philadelphia, Saunders, pp. 52-56, 1994; Drain, C:* The Post Anesthesia Care Unit: A Critical Care Approach to Post Anesthesia Nursing, *3rd ed. Philadelphia, Saunders, pp. 216-217 & 544-548, 1994.*

3.4. Correct Answer: **d**

Trevor's surgery will probably be brief; a short-acting sedative achieves one anesthetic goal for a pediatric patient—quick and nontraumatizing induction. Propofol, an intravenous sedative/hypnotic, acts rapidly and clears quickly, allowing early wakefulness, few side effects, and early discharge time. Propofol has no analgesic properties, it is not a neuroleptic medication, and injection may be painful. Inhalation agents, typically halothane, have historically been considered the superior choices for induction in part to avoid the trauma of injection.

Hannallah, RS: Induction Dose of Propofol in Unpremedicated Children. Semin Anesth *XI(1, Suppl 1): 48-49, 1992; Martin, TM: Nicolson, SC & Bargas, MS: Propofol Anesthesia Reduces Emesis and Airway Obstruction in Pediatric Outpatients.* Anesth Analg *76: 144-148, 1993.*

3.5. Correct Answer: **d**

A prolonged expiratory phase and heart rate less than 100 beats per minute indicate an infant in physiologic distress. This baby should not be extubated. Bradycardia often precedes cardiac arrest. Forced exhalation indicates obstruction. Specific criteria that herald extubation readiness are controversial; some guidelines include wakefulness, attempts to self-extubate, regular diaphragmatic breathing, presence of swallowing reflex, and physiologic stability.

American Heart Association: Textbook of Advanced Cardiac Life Support *(Cummins, RO, Ed). Dallas, American Heart Association, pp. 1.60-1.68, 1994; Roberts, CC & Okula, SN: The Pediatric Patient in* ASPAN's Core Curriculum for Post Anesthesia Nursing Practice, *3rd ed (Litwack, K, Ed). Philadelphia, Saunders, pp. 65-66, 1994.*

3.6. Correct Answer: **b**

Hypotensive episodes related to fluid volume deficit will only decrease perfusion to this elderly woman's leg. Graft occlusion, venostasis, ischemia or thrombosis may result; severe pain often indicates circulatory compromise, particularly to small, distal vessels. She already has age-related vascular disease, a likely result of either atheroschlerosis or diabetic vasculopathy. Colloid or crystalloid infusion and perhaps vasopressors maintain adequate blood pressure. Sitting flexes a grafted extremity and compresses or occludes blood flow. A bruit over the graft site and bounding peripheral pulses indicate adequate blood flow through the graft; document these normal and undisturbing findings without further intervention.

Sanders, JB: Peripheral Arterial Disease in Critical Care Nursing, *2nd ed (Vazquez, M, Lazear, SE & Larson, EL, Eds). Philadelphia, Saunders, pp. 260-265, 1992; Christensen, TW: Recovery of the Vascular Surgery Patient in* Manual of Post Anesthesia Care *(Jacobsen, WK, Ed). Philadelphia, Saunders, p. 79, 1992.*

3.7. Correct Answer: **c**

Normal gastrointestinal physiology changes during pregnancy. Delayed gastric emptying, decreased lower esophageal sphincter tone and increased gastric acidity and volume result. Uterine enlargement displaces the stomach and intestines, also increasing gastric pressure. All combine to create a "functional hiatal hernia" and increase risk of aspiration. Clinically, pulmonary aspiration has 10-25% mortality. In addition, timing of emergency surgery prevents the usual NPO status with elimination of gastric contents.

Litwack, K: Post Anesthesia Care Nursing, *2nd ed. St. Louis, Mosby, pp. 375-379, 1995; Cheek, TG & Gutsche, BB: Maternal Physiologic Alterations During Pregnancy in* Anesthesia for Obstet-

rics, 3rd ed (Shnider, SM & Levinson, G, Eds). Baltimore, Williams & Wilkins, pp. 3-15, 1993.

3.8. Correct Answer: **d**

Massive bleeding from abruptio placentae prompts release of tissue thromboplastin and begins the events that lead to disseminated intravascular coagulopathy (DIC). Incidence of DIC after abruptio placentae with fetal death approaches 30%. Other potential causes of DIC include eclampsia, retained dead fetus and amniotic fluid embolus. The normal sequence of coagulation events is disrupted in DIC. Shock, infection or obstetric complications stimulate circulation of excessive thrombin, overwhelming antithrombin. This activates a "sequence of hematological events producing hypercoagulability, retraction, and depletion of circulating clotting factors," which is DIC.

Mayer, DC: Hemorrhagic Obstetric Emergencies. Semin Anesth XI(1): 32-42, 1992; Poole, J: HELLP Syndrome and Coagulopathies of Pregnancy. Crit Care Nurs Clin North Am *5(3): 475-487, 1993; Tribett, D: Hematological Disorders in* AACN's Clinical Reference for Critical-Care Nursing, *3rd ed (Kinney, MR, Packa, DR & Dunbar, SB, Eds). St. Louis, Mosby, pp. 998-1001, 1994.*

3.9. Correct Answer: **a**

A supportive, empathetic and nonjudgmental attitude by the nurse, while attending to the patient's physiologic necessities, allows the patient to vent her anger, grief and concerns about the loss of her baby.

Litwack, K: Post Anesthesia Care Nursing, *2nd ed. St. Louis, Mosby, p. 386, 1995; Burden, N:* Ambulatory Surgical Nursing. *Philadelphia, Saunders, p. 516, 1993.*

3.10. Correct Answer: **d**

Before assuming new nerve damage, consult the patient's preoperative records. While the symptoms *may* indicate new neurologic damage or increased intracranial pressure, many children who require corrective facial surgery have significant preoperative craniofacial anomalies and nerve deficits. Extensive facial edema, especially about the eyes, can be expected and may alter assessment of facial function. While any preoperative deficit should be relayed by the anesthesia team or operating room nurse during report, the PACU nurse should also think of the possibility of preexisting neurologic deficit.

Brucker, JM & Laurent, JP: Pediatric Craniofacial Reconstruction: An Overview of Perioperative Management. J Neurosci Nurs *20(3): 159-168, 1988; Palmisano, BW:* Anesthesia for Plastic Surgery in Pediatric Anesthesia, *3rd ed (Gregory, GA, Ed). New York, Churchill-Livingstone, pp. 711-724; 1994. Newfield, P & Hamid, RKA: Pediatric Neuroanesthesia.* Semin Anesth *XI(4): 332, 1992.*

3.11. Correct Answer: **b**

The first priority is to asssure a patent airway. Severing wires and rubber bands allows quick access to the mouth to remove secretions. While preparing to cut the dental bands, initial response may be to turn the patient to one side, allow some secretions to drain and apply gentle oral suction inside the mouth. Administering an antiemetic delays suction to remove vomitus; chest physiotherapy techniques like percussion and vibration are used to free retained pulmonary secretions; intubation (by the anesthesiologist, not the nurse) may be necessary but is not a first response.

Newfield, P & Hamid, RKA: Pediatric Neuroanesthesia. Semin Anesth *XI(4): 332, 1992; Mussler, CA: Post Anesthesia Care of the Plastic Surgical Patient in* The Post Anesthesia Care Unit: A Critical Care Approach to Post Anesthesia Nursing, *3rd ed (Drain, C, Ed). Philadelphia, Saunders, p. 496, 1994; Brucker, JM & Laurent, JP: Pediatric Craniofacial Reconstruction: An Overview of Perioperative Management.* J Neurosci Nurs *20(3): 159-168, 1988.*

3.12. Correct Answer: **c**

Symptoms indicate partial airway obstruction. Airway edema within and around the airway are likely after this surgery, making airway patency a potential difficulty. Cool, humidified oxygen and close monitoring help to maintain airway patency and reduce swelling. If needed, the physician, not the nurse, would likely reintubate this patient, perhaps with fiberoptic bronchoscope guidance. Hyperextending the airway of a young child may further occlude the airway or disrupt surgical incisions. Racemic epinephrine is effective for bronchial constriction when inhaled, not lavaged.

Neelakanta, G: Pediatric Airway Anatomy and the Difficult Airway. Semin Anesth. *XI(3): 220-228, 1992; Brett, CM, Zwass, MS & France, NK: Eyes, Ears, Nose, Throat and Dental Surgery in* Pediatric Anesthesia, *3rd ed (Gregory, GA, Ed). New York, Churchill-Livingstone, pp. 690-692, 1994.*

3.13. Correct Answer: **d**

Assuring airway patency and maintaining cleanliness of the respiratory tract after loss of natural anatomic protection are major considerations after tracheostomy. Briefly hyperoxygenate and hyperinflate lungs prior to applying suction, then return to ordered parameters thereafter. Report significant volumes of bloody secretions; suction catheter should not exceed 50% of the tracheal tube size; tracheal wall circulation is obliterated at cuff pressures greater than 30 mmHg—and cuffed tubes are generally not used for children under 10 years to prevent tissue trauma.

Marks, L, Gurwin, A & Farrar, S: Post Anesthesia Care of the Ear, Nose, Throat, Neck and Maxillofacial Surgical Patient in The Post Anesthesia Care Unit: A Critical Care Approach to Post Anesthesia Nursing, *3rd ed (Drain, C, Ed). Phildelphia, Saunders, pp. 334-338, 1994; Brett, CM, Zwass, MS & France, NK: Eyes, Ears, Nose, Throat and Dental Surgery in* Pediatric Anesthesia, *3rd ed (Gregory, GA, Ed). New York, Churchill-Livingstone, pp. 670-671, 1994.*

3.14. Correct Answer: **b**

Protecting the airway is the PACU nurse's primary concern. Instruction and practice in proper technique to replace tracheostomy tubes is important, and if the tube cannot be easily reinserted, the stoma must be held open until resecured by the surgeon. Oxygenation by face mask is futile in a patient with tracheostomy; unnecessary suction reduces available oxygen, and when applied at the meatus, suction may instigate spasm.

Brett, CM, Zwass, MS & France, NK: Eyes, Ears, Nose, Throat and Dental Surgery in Pediatric Anesthesia, *3rd ed (Gregory, GA, Ed). New York, Churchill-Livingstone, pp. 670-671, 1994; Marks, L, Gurwin, A & Farrar, S: Post Anesthesia Care of the Ear, Nose, Throat, Neck and Maxillofacial Surgical Patient in* The Post Anesthesia Care Unit: A Critical Care Approach to Post Anesthesia Nursing, *3rd ed (Drain, C, Ed). Philadelphia, Saunders, pp. 334-338, 1994.*

3.15. Correct Answer: **a**

After tracheostomy, an overly large incision or partially obstructed tube can allow air entry to subcutaneous tissues. This potential requires observation, particularly for children, whose smaller airway size cannot withstand even small obstructions without compromise.

Marks, L, Gurwin, A & Farrar, S: Post Anesthesia Care of the Ear, Nose, Throat, Neck and Maxillofacial Surgical Patient in The Post Anesthesia Care Unit: A Critical Care Approach to Post Anesthesia Nursing, *3rd ed (Drain, C, Ed). Philadelphia, Saunders, pp. 334-338, 1994.*

3.16. Correct Answer: **b**

Aging decreases aldosterone secretion. *Pharmacokinetic* properties are factors that affect a medication's concentration at the site of action. Ways a drug is absorbed, distributed, biotransformed and excreted determine its pharmacokinetics. For example, aging decreases renal, hepatic and cardiovascular function; one related pharmacokinetic effect is increased circulation time. Aging also increases the number of lipid storage sites because the fat percentage of body weight increases; residual lung capacity increases with age, while other respiratory capacities decrease.

Litwack, K: Post Anesthesia Care Nursing, *2nd ed. St. Louis, Mosby, pp. 316-322, 1995; Britt, TL: Elderly Patients in* Critical Care Nursing *(Clochesy, JM, Breu, C, Cardin, S, et al, Eds). Philadelphia, Saunders, pp. 1351-1369, 1992.*

3.17. Correct Answer: **d**

This patient is old, and position-related (orthostatic) hypotension is likely. Age decreases the ability to respond to shifts in position and blood flow. A medications's *pharmacodynamics* refer to the *response* (physiologic action) it produces at a receptor site. Pharmacodynamics and pharmacokinetics are both altered by aging. Thiopental (Pentothal Sodium) is a barbiturate and respiratory depressant used to induce and maintain unconsciousness during surgery. Circulatory depression associated with aging can be expected to extend thiopental's "normal" metabolic rate of 10% each hour. This effect would delay consciousness and suppress respirations. Aging, not thiopental, more likely promotes hypothermia than hyperthermia.

Litwack, K: Post Anesthesia Care Nursing, *2nd ed. St. Louis, Mosby, pp. 316-322, 1995; Drain, C:* The Post Anesthesia Care Unit: A Critical Care Approach to Post Anesthesia Nursing, *3rd ed. Philadelphia, Saunders, pp 205-206 & 544-548, 1994; Britt, TL: Elderly Patients in* Critical Care Nursing *(Clochesy, et al, Eds). Philadelphia, Saunders, pp. 1351-1369, 1992.*

3.18. Correct Answer: **c**

After delivery, the nonpregnant uterus feels firm, indicating contraction, and is positioned near the woman's umbilicus. Significant postdelivery bleeding can be life-threatening. Red lochia, or vaginal drainage, is expected; frank blood of more than 100 ml (one perineal pad) is not. Inform the physician whenever a soft, boggy uterus does not become firm with massage to the fundus or when bleeding persists.

Litwack, K: Practical Points in the Care of the Obstetric Surgical Patient. J Post Anesth Nurs *5(3): 182-185, 1990; Poole, JH & White, D: The Obstetric Surgical Patient in* ASPAN's Core Curriculum for Post Anesthesia Nursing Practice, *3rd ed (Litwack, K, Ed). Philadelphia, Saunders, p. 501, 1994.*

3.19. Correct Answer: **a**

The child's airway is short, funnel shaped, broader at the larynx and narrow near the cricoid ring (vocal cords). The tongue is also proportionately larger, while nares are smaller than the adult's. Glottis and vocal cords are positioned higher than in the adult. These anatomic differences may mean easy airway obstruction. The tongue easily falls back to obstruct the upper airway; the narrowed glottis may precipitate postextubation edema.

Miller-Browne, DK & Britt-Lightkep, D: The Special Needs of Pediatric Patients in Ambulatory Surgical Nursing *(Burden, N, Ed). Philadelphia, Saunders, pp. 418-439, 1994; Roberts, CC & Okula, SN: The Pediatric Patient in* ASPAN's Core Curriculum for Post Anesthesia Nursing Practice, *3rd ed (Litwack, K, Ed). Philadelphia, Saunders, p. 63, 1994.*

3.20. Correct Answer: **a**

This man's symptoms indicate pulmonary edema, which is characterized by frothy, blood-tinged sputum. Increased hydrostatic pressures push pulmonary capillary fluid across interstitial spaces and into alveoli. Elderly age and a relatively large intravenous fluid volume administered over a brief time period contributed to produce the apparent pulmonary edema. An S_3 heart sound occurs with congestion.

Morgan, GE & Mikhail, SM: Clinical Anesthesiology. *Norwalk, CT, Appleton & Lange, pp. 707-709, 1992; Burden, N:* Ambulatory Surgical Nursing. *Philadelphia, Saunders, pp. 136-138, 1993.*

3.21. Correct Answer: **b**

Morphine decreases respiratory effort, anxiety and venous return and is the first-choice medication to treat pulmonary edema. With multiple doses, observe respiratory response for depression of rate and depth.

Burden, N: Ambulatory Surgical Nursing. *Philadelphia, Saunders, pp. 136-137, 1993; Pillion, JM: Care of the Cardiac Patient in* Comprehensive Cardiac Care, *7th ed (Kinney, MR, et al, Ed). St. Louis, Mosby, pp. 289-290, 1991.*

3.22. Correct Answer: **a**

Chelsea's spinal blockade should progress in a sequence that begins with sympathetic block (loss of vascular tone) and progresses to sensory block (loss of pain, then touch sensation). The ability to move below the level of block follows sensory loss. Inability to detect pressure and no sense of extremity position follow motor loss. Chelsea's position during placement of the block may affect distribution of intraspinal medication, so the drug may have greater effect on her left (operative) side. If so, she should notice left-sided numbness before she loses right-sided movement. Chelsea can expect the block to resolve in reverse sequence.

Burden, N: Ambulatory Surgical Nursing. *Philadelphia, Saunders, p. 309, 1993; Litwack, K:* Post Anesthesia Care Nursing, *2nd ed. St. Louis, Mosby, pp. 172-178, 1995.*

3.23. Correct Answer: **d**

The 2 to 5 year old child more commonly develops postextubation laryngeal edema (postintubation croup). Surgical trauma, extended or difficult intubation and coughing while still intubated can cause this form of airway obstruction. Premature infants rarely develop croup.

Roberts, CC & Okula, SN: The Pediatric Patient in ASPAN's Core Curriculum for Post Anesthesia Nursing Practice, *3rd ed (Litwack, K, Ed). Philadelphia, Saunders, p. 67, 1994; Hall, SC: Perioperative Pediatric Care in* Post Anesthesia Care *(Vender, JS & Speiss, BD, Eds). Saunders, Philadelphia, pp. 256-268, 1992.*

3.24. Correct Answer: **c**

Pregnancy produces expected, gradual physiologic changes. Oxygen consumption increases as much as 20% and minute ventilation by 50%. Functional reserve capacity (FRC) decreases by as much as 20%. pCO_2 decreases by up to 30%, although any pH change is compensated by metabolic change in serum bicarbonate.

Morgan, GE & Mikhail, SM: Clinical Anesthesiology. *Norwalk, CT, Appleton & Lange, pp. 600-601, 1992; Poole, JH & White, D: The Obstetric Surgical Patient in* ASPAN's Core Curriculum for Post Anesthesia Nursing Practice, *3rd ed (Litwack, K, Ed). Philadelphia, Saunders, pp. 473-476, 1994.*

3.25. Correct Answer: **c**

Asthma is a reactive lower airway spasm of bronchi. Postextubation edema and croup involve nonthoracic, upper airway structures. Even small amounts of swelling around the narrowest portion of the child's airway near the cricoid cartilage interferes with airway patency. A congenitally narrow larynx, as in Down syndrome, traumatic or prolonged (more than 1 hour) intubation, resisting the endotracheal tube and nonsupine surgical position increase the likelihood of upper airway edema.

Litwack, K: Post Anesthesia Care Nursing, *2nd ed. St. Louis, Mosby, pp. 333-335 & 342-343, 1994; Cote, CJ & Todres, ID: The Pediatric Airway in* A Practice of Anesthesia for Infants and Children, *2nd ed. Philadelphia, Saunders, pp. 62-66, 1993.*

3.26. Correct Answer: **a**

Incidence of propofol-induced airway obstruction in PACU is low. Propofol seems to have "built-in" antiemetic properties—incidence of postoperative nausea and vomiting is lower among patients who receive propofol anesthetics. Propofol's sedative and hypnotic actions occur rapidly (less than 1 minute) after infusion begins and dissipate quickly. The patient wakens with few residual effects, even though propofol is considered a "relatively modest inhibitor" of the metabolism of other drugs. Halothane and other inhaled gases delay the metabolism and clearance of many medications, thereby continuing their effects. Unpleasant odor and higher incidence of laryngospasm (5%) with isoflurane and seizures (7%) with enflurane make these less popular inhalation anesthetic choices than halothane.

Wood, M: Comparison of the Effect of Intravenous Propofol Anesthesia With Inhalational Anesthesia on Propranolol Drug Distribution and Metabolism. Semin Anesth *XI(1, Suppl 1): 48-49, 1992; Martin, TM, Nicolson, SC & Bargas, MS: Propofol Anesthesia Reduces Emesis and Airway Obstruction in Pediatric Outpatients.* Anesth Analg *76:144-148, 1993.*

3.27. Correct Answer: **c**

Pregnancy increases aldosterone secretion, which encourages the kidneys to reabsorb sodium in exchange for potassium. Water passively follows the movement of sodium, so fluid volume increases as serum sodium increases. Plasma volume increases up to 50% during pregnancy, alters (usually decreases) effective medication dose requirements and produces "physiologic" or dilutional anemia.

Poole, JH & White, D: The Obstetric Surgical Patient in ASPAN's Core Curriculum for Post Anesthesia Nursing Practice, *3rd ed (Litwack, K, Ed). Philadelphia, Saunders, pp. 473-476, 1994; Morgan, GE & Mikhail, MS:* Clinical Anesthesiology. *Norwalk, CT, Appleton & Lange, p. 516, 1992.*

3.28. Correct Answer: **d**

This patient is sleeping and her heart rate is less than 100 beats/minute; this slow fetal heart rate or rapid accelerations then periods of rate deceleration signal fetal distress. The mother should be repositioned to the far left side, receive oxygen and perhaps additional fluid volume to promote maximum uterine and fetal blood flow. Healthy fetal heart tones range between 120-160 beats per minute. Intrauterine activity indicates a busy fetus; a silent uterus (no contractions) indicates no preterm labor. Continuous monitoring of fetal heart rate and to detect any uterine contractions is advised in PACU whenever a pregnant patient has surgery.

Litwack, K: Post Anesthesia Nursing, *2nd ed. St. Louis, Mosby, pp. 379-384, 1995; Levinson, G & Shnider, SM: Anesthesia for Surgery During Pregnancy in* Anesthesia for Obstetrics, *3rd ed. Baltimore, Williams & Wilkins, pp. 272-276, 1993.*

3.29. Correct Answer: **d**

Crying often indicates pain and should be treated, usually with acetaminophen rather than narcotics. Prolonged crying can disrupt hemostasis and cause severe bleeding from vascular mouth tissues. Sadie's loud cry indicates an adequate airway, though monitoring patency and oxygenation are ongoing observations. Oral suction should be performed as indicated by inspection or repeated swallowing. Intravenous, not oral, fluids are provided until bleeding is unlikely.

Saleh, KL: Practical Points in the Care of the Patient Post-Cleft Lip and Palate Repair. Post Anesth Nurs *8(1): 35-37, 1993; Mussler, CA: Post Anesthesia Care of the Plastic Surgical Patient in* The

Post Anesthesia Care Unit: A Critical Care Approach to Post Anesthesia Nursing *(Drain, C, Ed). Philadelphia, Saunders, pp. 496-497, 1994.*

3.30. Correct Answer: **d**

Anticholinergic medications can be delivered by aerosol inhalation and are "considered the first-line drug of choice" to treat patients with COPD, a common presurgical condition in the geriatric population. Anticholinergic (parasympatholytic) medications inhibit reflexive bronchoconstriction "monitored" by the vagus nerve. Therefore, the larger bronchial smooth muscle relaxes and dilates. A parasympatholytic-like ipratropium bromide (Atrovent) with a beta-2 sympathomimetic-like albuterol (Proventil) bronchodilator may be combined to dilate the COPD patient's upper and lower bronchial airways.

Marley, R: Postoperative Administration of Aerosolized Medications: Part I—The Basics. Post Anesth Nurs *9(5): 285-296, 1994.*

Set II

Answer Key

3.31. a
3.32. c
3.33. d
3.34. b
3.35. c
3.36. c
3.37. a
3.38. d
3.39. a
3.40. c
3.41. c
3.42. b
3.43. d
3.44. a
3.45. d
3.46. d
3.47. a
3.48. c
3.49. b
3.50. d
3.51. c
3.52. a

SET II

Rationales and References

3.31. Correct Answer: **a**

The incidence of episodic apnea occurs in up to 37% of infants between 32 and 55 weeks postconceptual age. Apnea is a likely event for up to 12 hours postoperatively and increases the perianesthetic risk for premature infants. This child was born at 28 weeks gestation and is now 16 weeks old; therefore he is 44 weeks postconceptual age.

Roberts, JD, Todres, ID & Cote, CJ: Neonatal Emergencies in A Practice of Anesthesia for Infants and Children, *2nd ed (Cote, CJ, et al Eds). Philadelphia, Saunders, pp. 225-228; Gregory, GA:* Pediatric Anesthesia, *3rd ed. New York, Churchill Livingstone, p. 368, 1994.*

3.32. Correct Answer: **c**

Preterm infants less than 6 months old are typically admitted to the hospital with apnea monitors for overnight nursing assessment. Apnea lasting longer than 20 seconds is life threatening, but a history of apnea does not predict that postoperative apnea will occur. Controversy surrounds identifying the premature infant who is truly at risk todevelop apneic episodes.

Litwack, K: Post Anesthesia Care Nursing, *2nd ed. St. Louis, Mosby, pp. 342-343, 1994; Gregory, GA:* Pediatric Anesthesia, *3rd ed. New York, Churchill Livingstone, p. 368, 1994; Hall, SC: Perioperative Pediatric Care in* Post Anesthesia Care *(Vender, JS & Speiss, BD, Eds). Saunders, Philadelphia, 1992, p. 265.*

3.33. Correct Answer: **d**

Priorities for this young woman's care focus on seizure prevention and blood pressure reduction; magnesium sulfate suppresses neuromuscular irritability, and a vasodilator like nitroprusside decreases afterload. Symptoms suggest preeclampsia; even though she has delivered her baby, this woman's risk continues for up to 24 hours. A first pregnancy, young age, and an infant with chromosomal abnormalities increase her preeclampsia risk. Pregnancy-induced hypertension, or gestational hypertension, may develop without the proteinuria and edema that characterize preeclampsia. Other preeclampsia symptoms include hyperreflexia, headache and epigastric pain.

Gahart, BL: Intravenous Medications, *10th ed. St. Louis, Mosby, pp. 433-435, 1994; Gutsche, BB & Cheek, TG: Anesthetic Complications in Preeclampsia-Eclampsia in* Anesthesia for Obstetrics, *3rd ed (Shnider, SM & Levinson, G, Eds). Baltimore, Williams & Wilkins, pp. 309-318, 1993; Gelfand, RE: Obstetric Patients in the PACU and ICU in* Post Anesthesia Care *(Vender, JS & Speiss, BD, Eds). Philadelphia, Saunders, pp. 356-358, 1992.*

3.34. Correct Answer: **b**

Magnesium sulfate successfully reduced neuromuscular irritability and the immediate risk of seizure. Unfortunately, smooth, skeletal and cardiac muscle functions were suppressed as well.

The infusion must now be discontinued or the rated significantly reduced. Reflex suppression, hypoventilation and cardiac depression indicate a serum magesium level well beyond the therapeutic range of 4-8 mg/dl. The focus of nursing assessment now must be preventing hypoventilation and cardiac decompensation until serum magnesium returns to normal. The physician mayrequest calcium chloride to reverse a very elevated Mg^{+}.

Gahart, BL: Intravenous Medications, *10th ed. St. Louis, Mosby, pp. 433-435, 1994; Poole, SH & White, D: The Obstetric Surgical Patient in* ASPAN's Core Curriculum for Post Anesthesia Nursing Practice, *3rd ed (Litwack, K, Ed). Philadelphia, Saunders, pp. 470-484 & 507, 1994.*

3.35. Correct Answer: **c**

Heart rate decreases as a child develops. The heart rate of a 3 to 12 month old child can be expected to be approximately 130-140 beats per minute, though the rate can range widely from approximately 110-180 beats per minute. A 1 month old infant's heart rate is approximately 160 beats per minute, while a 4 year old's is 100 beats per minute.

American Heart Association: Textbook of Advanced Cardiac Life Support *(Cummins, RO, Ed). Dallas, American Heart Association, p. 1.65, 1994; Miller-Browne, DK & Britt-Lightkep, D: The Special Needs of Pediatric Patients in* Ambulatory Surgical Nursing *(Burden, N, Ed). Philadelphia, Saunders, pp. 418-439, 1994.*

3.36. Correct Answer: **c**

The following formula is based on a child's age and can be used to *roughly* estimate an appropriate endotracheal tube (ETT) size:

$$\frac{16 + \text{child's age}}{4} = \text{approximate ETT size}$$

For this child the estimated ETT size is

$$16 + \text{age } 6 = \frac{22}{4} = 5.5 \text{ mm.}$$

Children of similar age vary greatly in size, so each child's airway and clinical situation must be individually considered. Multiple tube sizes must be available in the PACU.

Roberts, CC & Okula, NS: The Pediatric Patient in ASPAN's Core Curriculum for Post Anesthesia Nursing Practice, *3rd ed (Litwack, K, Ed). Philadelphia, Saunders, pp. 65-68. 1994; Miller-Browne, DK & Britt-Lightkep, D: The Special Needs of Pediatric Patients in* Ambulatory Surgical Nursing *(Burden, N, Ed). Philadelphia, Saunders, pp. 427-429, 1993.*

3.37. Correct Answer: **a**

This child's vital signs are within age-appropriate limits; astute nursing observation is appropriate at this point. A 7 year old's blood pressure is normally 92/62, heart rate 95 beats/minute and respiratory rate 22-28 breaths per minute. Auscultating an apical pulse is the accepted standard because a child's radial pulse is not always palpable.

Roberts, CC & Okula, NS: The Pediatric Patient in ASPAN's Core Curriculum for Post Anesthesia Nursing Practice, *3rd ed (Litwack, K, Ed). Philadelphia, Saunders, pp. 70-71, 1994; Miller-Browne, DK & Britt-Lightkep, D: The Special Needs of Pediatric Patients in* Ambulatory Surgical Nursing

(Burden, N, Ed). Philadelphia, Saunders, pp. 418-439, 1994.

3.38. Correct Answer: **d**

Geriatric age, severe anemia, poor nutrition, pregnancy, hypothermia, malignancy and some medications, including propranolol and echothiophate iodide eye drops, are among conditions that decrease *production* of pseudocholinesterase. Such acquired reductions occur more commonly than the genetically predetermined variation in enzyme activity.

Schweinefus, R & Schick, L: Succinylcholine: "Good Guy, Bad Guy." Post Anesth Nurs *6(6): 410-419, 1991; Drain, C:* The Post Anesthesia Care Unit: A Critical Care Approach to Post Anesthesia Nursing. *Philadelphia, Saunders, pp. 234-236, 1994.*

3.39. Correct Answer: **a**

Maternal antibodies support the infant's immature immune system to minimize potential for infection. The child's hemoglobin is also high at this age. Bleeding is a primary postoperative concern after cleft lip repair. Efforts to reduce crying from pain or separation from the primary caregiver minimize the potential for bleeding.

Saleh, KL: Practical Points in the Care of the Patient Post-Cleft Lip and Palate Repair. Post Anesth Nurs *8(1): 35-37, 1993; Mussler, CA: Post Anesthesia Care of the Plastic Surgical Patient in* The Post Anesthesia Care Unit: A Critical Care Approach to Post Anesthesia Nursing *(Drain, C, Ed). Philadelphia, Saunders, pp. 496-497, 1994.*

3.40. Correct Answer: **c**

This adolescent's endotracheal tube cuff should be inflated to seal the trachea, prevent air loss, protect the lungs from aspiration and exert low tracheal pressure. Pressure from endotracheal cuff inflation can exceed the trachea's capillary filling pressure of 27-29 cm H_2O and can damage tracheal tissue. A recommended cuff pressure ranges between 15-25 cm H_2O (NOTE: pressure values expressed as *mm Hg* differ from cm H_2O values). A high-volume cuff exerts the least pressure. Cuffs are intentionally not inflated only when a child is under age 8.

Alspach, JG: AACN's Core Review for Critical Care Nursing, *2nd ed. Philadelphia, Saunders, pp. 16 & 47, 1991; Drain, C:* The Post Anesthesia Care Unit: A Critical Care Approach to Post Anesthesia Nursing. *Philadelphia, Saunders, pp. 308-309, 1994; Fisher, DM: Anesthesia Equipment for Pediatrics in* Pediatric Anesthesia, *3rd ed (Gregory, GA, Ed). New York, Churchill Livingston, pp. 214-216, 1994.*

3.41. Correct Answer: **c**

The dorsal horn of the spinal cord receives pain messages along C nerve roots and transmits them to the brain. Opiates affect receptors in the brain and spinal cord. Morphine sulfate's (Duramorph's) *site* of action does not vary with patient age, though this aging man may have a different *pharmacodynamic* response than a younger patient. A hydrophilic medication like Duramorph (preservative-free morphine) does not remain localized when delivered epidurally but distributes through the cerebrospinal fluid across several dermatomes. After injection, the morphine gradually migrates toward the brain stem by rostral spread and can depress respiratory effort for up to 24 hours.

Willens, JS: Giving Fentanyl for Pain Outside the OR. Am J Nurs *94(2): 24-28, 1994; Wild, L & Coyne, C: The Basics and Beyond: Epidural Analgesia.* Am J Nurs *92(4): 26-36, 1992.*

3.42. Correct Answer: **b**

Sudden motor weakness may indicate catheter migration into the subarachnoid space, local anesthetic blockade and a spinal anesthetic. Adding bupivacaine (Marcaine) to an epidural solution also increases the potential for some sensory deficit and signs of sympathetic block, such as hypotension. Medication spread through the CSF may occur more quickly in an elderly patient, though adding bupivacaine to an epidural infusion may mean the patient uses less narcotic. Bupivacaine is classified as an amide local anesthetic, which is usually not an allergen.

Wild, L & Coyne, C: The Basics and Beyond: Epidural Analgesia. Am J Nurs *92(4): 26-36, 1992; Drain, C:* The Post Anesthesia Care Unit: A Critical Care Approach to Post Anesthesia Nursing, *3rd ed. Philadelphia, Saunders, pp. 246-249, 1994.*

3.43. Correct Answer: **d**

Surgical plans can continue with attention to glucose-insulin balance and prevention of hypoglycemia and ketosis. One approach to glucose management is to provide a slow glucose infusion and up to one-half of the child's usual AM dose of intermediate-acting insulin to prevent hyperglycemia. Short-acting regular insulin is avoided preoperatively. Serum glucose is monitored at 30-60 minute intervals intraoperatively.

Kirschner, RM: Diabetes in Pediatric Ambulatory Surgical Patients. J Post Anesth Nurs *8: 322-326, 1993; Steward, DJ:* Manual of Pediatric Anesthesia, *3rd ed. New York, Churchill-Livingstone, pp. 124-126, 1990.*

3.44. Correct Answer: **a**

Onset of an intermediate-acting insulin's effect is expected within 2 hours; peak action occurs 6-12 hours later—most likely during the postoperative period. Effect can persist 24 hours later. Therefore regular postoperative monitoring of serum glucose is important to observe trends toward hypoglycemia or whether additional short-acting insulin is needed to prevent extreme hyperglycemia.

Kirschner, RM: Diabetes in Pediatric Ambulatory Surgical Patients. J Post Anesth Nurs *8: 322-326, 1993; Kestel F: Are You Up To Date On Diabetes Medications?* Am J Nurs *94: 48-52, 1994.*

3.45. Correct Answer: **d**

Gear teaching to social play, acting, drawing and touching equipment. The 3 to 6 year old preschooler is curious, literal, imaginative and likes to explore. Emotional development at this age focuses on what Erik Erikson calls a stage of initiative vs. guilt. However, fear caused by separation from the primary care giver may still be an issue. A video may be a helpful adjunct, especially if the character is familiar or of a similar age. Distraction is best used for a toddler and discussion for the older school-aged child.

Frederick, C & Reining, KM: Essential Components of Growth and Development. J Post Anesth Nurs *10(1): 12-17, 1995; Litwack, K:* Post Anesthesia Care Nursing, *2nd ed. St. Louis, Mosby, pp. 336-338, 1995.*

3.46. Correct Answer: **d**

The elderly patient with non-insulin-dependent Type II diabetes mellitus is more likely to develop hyperosmolar nonketotic syndrome (HNKS). Pronounced glucose elevations with dehydration depletes cerebral water, prompting seizures and eventual impaired renal function.

Jones: TL: From Diabetic Ketoacidosis to Hyperglycemic Hyperosmolar Nonketotic Syndrome. Crit Care Nurs Clin North Am *6(4): 712-719, 1994; Loriaux, TC & Drass, JA: Endocrine and Diabetic Disorders in* AACN's Clinical Reference For Critical-Care Nursing *(Kinney, MR, Packa, DR & Dunbar, SB, Eds). St. Louis, Mosby, pp. 942-958, 1993.*

3.47. Correct Answer: **a**

An upright position often relieves the vascular headache that may develop 1-2 days after surgical relief of high-grade (>75%) carotid artery stenosis. Cerebral blood flow markedly increases, causing hyperperfusion and paralyzed autoregulation. Symptoms of hyperperfusion include vascular headache on the surgical side, cerebral hemorrhage and seizure. Hyperperfusion syndrome is more likely among elderly patients or patients with chronic cerebral hypoperfusion or abnormal prothrombin time.

Fode, NC: Carotid Endarterectomy: Nursing Care and Controversies. J Neurosci Nurs *22(1): 25-30, 1990.*

3.48. Correct Answer: **c**

Cranial nerves X (vagus) and XII (hypoglossal) are primarily responsible for adequate chewing and swallowing. Intraoperative damage increases the risk of postoperative aspiration. Compression or trauma to these nerve fibers results in difficult swallowing, loss of gag reflex and deviation of tongue alignment.

Kristt, AM: The Peripheral Vascular Surgical Patient in ASPAN's Core Curriculum for Post Anesthesia Nursing Practice, *3rd ed (Litwack, K, Ed). Philadelphia, Saunders, pp. 294-296, 1994; Johnson, SM & Anderson, B: Carotid Endarterectomy: A Review.* Crit Care Clin North Am *3(3): 499-505, 1991.*

3.49. Correct Answer: **b**

Patients with obesity and preexisting knee conditions like arthritis or total knee arthroplasty have greatest risk of postoperative joint pain, damage or displacement after hemorrhoidectomy. The kneeling position, a variation of the prone and jackknife positions, is used for rectal surgery. The patient's knees bear most of the body weight; despite padding on the surgical frame, skin and joint trauma occurs. Eye injury, ear compression and brachial plexus stretch may also occur.

Litwack, K: Post Anesthesia Care Nursing, *2nd ed. St. Louis, Mosby, pp. 488-490, 1995 Walsh, J: Postop Effects of OR Positioning.* RN *56(2): 50-58, 1993.*

3.50. Correct Answer: **d**

This nurse must now inquire about physician, patient and family expectations regarding extent of resuscitation; in addition this nurse should be aware of facility protocols regarding DNR status during the intraoperative period. The perianesthetic period is currently an ethical "gray zone" with regard to a patient's wishes specified in an advance directive. Ideally, conversations occur prior to surgery and mutual understanding among the physician, patient and family are clearly documented. Despite a patient's DNR status, interventions to restore chemical, fluid and thermal physiologic balance and to reverse cardiac and respiratory depression specifically related to anesthetic medications occur in PACU.

Troug, RD: Do Not Resuscitate Orders in the Operating Room: Where Have We Been, Where Are We Going? Semin Anesth *12(3): 178-186, 1993; American Heart Association:* Textbook of Advanced Cardiac Life Support *(Cummins, RO, Ed). Dallas, American Heart Association, pp. 15-2 to 15-6, 1994.*

3.51. Correct Answer: **c**

Rate of nosocomial infections in the bloodstream is higher with central venous catheters than with other types of vascular access devices. Approximately 80-90% of septicemias occur with centrally inserted catheters. Thin skin of elderly patients easily colonizes with bacteria. In addition, elderly patients are immunosuppressed compared to younger patients; Mr. Y, therefore, is "uniquely susceptible" to sepsis, which may contribute to his mortality. Attention to principles of asepsis during dressing changes and when accessing this central catheter for blood sampling or fluid or medication administration are critical to Mr. Y's health.

Stengle, J & Dries, D: Sepsis in the Elderly. Crit Care Nurs Clin North Am *6(2): 421-427, 1994; Smith, RN, Leyerle, BJ & Shabot, MM: Instrumentation in* AACN's Clinical Reference for Critical-Care Nursing *(Kinney, MR, Packa, DR & Dunbar, SB, Eds). St. Louis, Mosby, pp. 90-91, 1993.*

3.52. Correct Answer: **a**

Trust that basic needs of food and comfort will be met is a major issue of psychologic development for the infant. Anxiety about separation from known nurturing adults stresses this infant. According to Erik Erikson's stages of psychologic development, this trust vs. mistrust psychosocial stage continues until approximately age 1 year.

Frederick, C & Reining, KM: Essential Components of Growth and Development. J Post Anesth Nurs *10(1): 12-17, 1995; Litwack, K:* Post Anesthesia Care Nursing, *2nd ed. St. Louis, Mosby, pp. 336-338, 1995.*

Section 4

Pharmacologic Considerations

Scenarios and items in this section focus on the *pharmacologic concerns* encountered in the practice of perianesthesia nursing. These concepts are considered together because:

- anesthetic medications alter and usually depress the function of vital organ systems.
- interactions among medications produce varied patient responses indicated by allergic reactions, potentiated effects, compatibility concerns, altered neuromuscular and cardiopulmonary function, and side effects or contraindications.
- assessment, intervention and evaluation of the pharmacologic effects specifically related to anesthetic medications and techniques are *primary* and essential nursing responsibilities.

ESSENTIAL CORE CONCEPTS	AFFILIATED CORE CURRICULUM CHAPTERS
Nursing Process	
Assessment	
Planning and Implementation	Chapters 2 & 9
Evaluation	
Scope of Practice	
Standards of Care	
Pharmacologic Principles in Action	**Chapter 9**
Anatomy and Physiology	
Agonists and Antagonists	
Dose, Onset and Duration of Action, Clearance	
Neurotransmitters, Reversal and Toxicity	
Receptors, Synapses, Vascular Tone and Target Organs	
Responses: Same Medication, Different Sites	
Anesthetic Techniques	
Balanced	

- Dissociative (Neuroleptic)
- Epidural
- General
- Intravenous Regional Block
- Local Infiltration
- Spinal

Conscious Sedation
Dermatome Assessment
Efficacy, Potency and Tolerance
Enhancing and Inhibiting Pharmacologic Environments
Minimum Alveolar Concentration
Pharmacodynamics
- Clinical Consequences

Pharmacokinetics
- Absorption, Distribution and Elimination

Unique Properties and Effects

Anesthetic Medications — **Chapter 9**

Actions and Consequences for:
- Inhalation Anesthetics
  - Gaseous Inhalants
  - Volatile Liquids

Intravenous Medications
- Barbiturates, Hypnotics and Sedatives
- Dissociative and Induction Agents
- Narcotics and Antagonists
- Reversal of Effect

Local Anesthetics
- Amides and Esters
- Assessing Blockade
- Regional Techniques

Muscle Relaxants
- Assessing Neuromuscular Blockade
- Depolarizing Medications
- Nondepolarizing Medications
- Reversal Medications and Influencing Factors

Perianesthetic Medication Potpourri — Chapters 9, 10, 11 14, 15, 17, & 18

Anticholinergics
Antiemetics
Benzodiazepines
Bronchodilators
Cardioactive Drugs and Diuretics
Corticosteroids
Nonsteroidal Antiinflammatory Drugs
Oxygen
Pharmacology of Cardiac Life Support
"Tuning" Electrolyte and Acid-Base Balance

Managing Analgesia	Chapter 31
Agonistic and Antagonistic	
Management and Monitoring IV, IM, regional, PCA	
Pain Receptors	
Physiologic Stress Response	

SET I

Items 4.1-4.40

4.1. The primary neurotransmitter of the parasympathetic nervous system is:

a. acetylcholine
b. dopamine
c. epinephrine
d. norepinephrine

NOTE: Consider scenario and item 4.2 together.

A 62 year old woman is scheduled for a cystoscopy, ureteral stent placement and lithotripsy. She has mitral valve prolapse, moderate obesity and a childhood history of polio and rheumatic heart disease.

4.2. Particularly for this patient, the preanesthesia nurse recognizes the importance of prophylactic:

a. heparin anticoagulation
b. loop or osmotic diuretics
c. cardiac digitalization
d. broad-spectrum antibiotics

4.3. Eliminating the systemic effects of a volatile anesthetic medication *most* varies with:

a. alveolar ventilation
b. volume of distribution
c. renal blood flow
d. rate of hepatic clearance

4.4. To alter blood pressure, hydralazine's *primary* physiologic effect is to:

a. release renin by constricting renal vasculature
b. reduce cardiac contractile force
c. dilate arterial smooth muscle
d. increase myocardial rate

4.5. By definition, minimum alveolar concentration (MAC) is the lowest concentration of an inhalation anesthetic that:

a. allows spontaneous breathing in half of patients
b. sustains an effective half-life for Stage IV anesthesia
c. eliminates ventilation in 50% of patients at 0.5% anesthetic concentration
d. eradicates movement to pain in 50% of patients

4.6. A factor that *least* affects a patient's minimum alveolar concentration (MAC) requirement is the patient's:

a. age
b. gender
c. temperature
d. circulation

NOTE: Consider scenario and item 4.7 together.

4.7. Potential sources of electromagnetic interference that could alter the function of Mr. A's implanted DDD pacemaker include any of the following *except:*

a. succinylcholine
b. extracorporeal lithotripsy
c. mivacurium
d. mechanical ventilation

4.8. When compared with diazepam, an equipotent dose of midazolam is:

a. not comparable
b. 2-4 times greater
c. equivalent, milligram for milligram
d. one-half to two-thirds less

4.9. The "antidote" to treat anticholinesterase medication is intravenous:

a. atropine sulfate
b. edrophonium chloride
c. dexamethasone
d. azathioprine

4.10. A patient with a documented penicillin allergy should *not* receive:

a. gentamicin
b. imipenem
c. cefazolin
d. ciprofloxacin

4.11. An infant's initial response to induction of anesthesia with halothane varies from the adult's response *primarily* because the infant's:

a. tissues are highly vascular
b. vital organs slowly absorb medications
c. sensitive airway tissues easily spasm
d. metabolic rate and oxygen demand are lower

4.12. Side effects of droperidol administration result from its properties that produce:

a. parasympathetic vagal stimulation
b. alpha adrenergic blockade
c. beta adrenergic stimulation
d. sympathetic vasoconstriction

NOTE: Consider scenario and items 4.13-4.15 together.

A healthy 28 year old woman is awake, alert and oriented when admitted to Phase I PACU at 0950 after a 20 minute right carpal tunnel release. Vital signs are within 20% of other preoperative measures. Anesthesia was by intravenous regional block and conscious sedation.

4.13. At 0955, the PACU nurse notes this woman is not responsive and observes generalized tonic-clonic motor activity. The *most likely* reason for this activity is:

a. unidentified idiopathic convulsive disorder
b. extreme hyperventilation related to pain and anxiety
c. generalized central nervous system toxicity
d. hypoxemic seizure related to oversedation

4.14. An intravenous regional technique involves:

a. infiltrating the surgical site with narcotic
b. injecting local anesthetic after obliterating blood flow
c. infusing nitroprusside to suppress local blood loss
d. instilling local anesthetic into intracellular fluid

4.15. In addition to documenting this patient's level of consciousness and vital signs, the PACU nurse also documents surgery-specific observations and outcomes. After carpal tunnel release with intravenous regional block, the *most* positive patient outcomes are achieved by:

a. 100 ml fluid in a wound drain and right finger SpO_2 measures of more than 91%
b. pain level rating of "1 to 2" and gradual release of one tourniquet in Phase I PACU
c. immediate return of arm sensation and overhead suspension to limit edema
d. moderate motor control of extremity and minimal bleeding

4.16. The inhalation anesthetic that is *most likely* to induce airway spasm is:

a. desflurane
b. enflurane
c. halothane
d. isoflurane

4.17. An inhalation anesthetic is eliminated *most slowly* from:

a. renal medulla
b. cardiac tissue
c. blood-brain barrier
d. skeletal muscle

4.18. Compared with intramuscular morphine, providing analgesia with a continuous epidural morphine infusion decreases all of the following effects *except:*

a. episodic somnolence and variable duration
b. muscle activity and vomiting
c. neuroendocrine stress responses
d. incidence of pneumonia

4.19. The epidural space contains the following anatomic structures *except:*
a. blood vessels
b. adipose tissue
c. cerebrospinal fluid
d. lymph capillaries

4.20. Cocaine-induced hypertension and tachycardia occur through:
a. direct cholinergic stimulation
b. lacing cocaine doses with epinephrine
c. indirect glucocorticoid reflexes
d. blocked norepinephrine reuptake

NOTE: Consider items 4.21-4.22 together.

4.21. The PACU nurse anticipates that following administration of sublingual nifedipine, systolic blood pressure reduction will *most likely* occur within:
a. 3 minutes
b. 8 minutes
c. 15 minutes
d. 33 minutes

4.22. The *most likely* nifedipine-related cardiovascular response will be:
a. spontaneous supraventricular tachycardia
b. reflexive pulmonary hypertension
c. suppressed intraventricular conduction
d. delayed-onset cardiopulmonary edema

4.23. Safe administration of parenteral ketorolac considers all of the following factors *except:*
a. providing effective narcotic analgesia before dosing
b. reducing the dose for a 75 year old, 48 kg woman
c. limiting an intravenous loading dose to 15-30 mg
d. determining any "breathing difficulty" when using aspirin

4.24. Nalbuphine's specific opioid receptor actions include:
a. mu antagonist, kappa and sigma agonist
b. mu and sigma agonist, kappa antagonist
c. mu agonist, kappa and sigma antagonist
d. pure mu, sigma and kappa antagonist

NOTE: Consider scenario and item 4.25 together.

Mr. J sustained a tibial-fibular fracture in a motor vehicle accident 48 hours ago. He is admitted to PACU after an open reduction and internal fixation (ORIF) with tetracaine spinal anesthetic. During his first 30 minutes since admission, the PACU nurse observes increasing restlessness, disorientation and tremulousness. He is currently diaphoretic, temperature is 36° C, heart rate is 128 beats per minute, cardiac rhythm is sinus and blood pressure is 188/95.

4.25. After determining adequate respiratory quality, the nurse further considers other potential reasons for Mr. J's condition; symptoms suggest he *may have* developed:
a. tetracaine toxicity
b. cocaine overstimulation
c. alcohol withdrawal syndrome
d. deferred traumatic intraspinal bleeding

NOTE: Consider scenario and items 4.26-4.29 together.

A wildly restless, crying and confused 12 year old boy attempts to climb off the stretcher in PACU. While assuring the physical safety of staff and patient, the nurse explains possible reasons for the child's behavior to his mother, who visits in PACU.

4.26. Causes could include any of the following *except:*

a. hypoxemia
b. central cholinergic effect
c. bladder distention
d. pseudocholinesterase toxicity

4.27. After assessment, the anesthesiologist requests physostigmine 1 mg. Physiologically, this medication is used to:

a. augment the analgesic effect of narcotics at the dorsal horn
b. increase acetylcholine at the neuromuscular junction
c. reverse consciousness-depressing effects of narcotics at the hypothalamus
d. inhibit norepinephrine penetration of the blood-brain barrier

4.28. Nursing observations after administering physostigmine salicylate include monitoring:

a. temperature for hyperpyrexia
b. consciousness for atypical hyperactivity
c. cardiac rhythm for bradycardia
d. muscle function for fasciculation

4.29. Following 0.6 mg of intravenous flumazenil, the PACU nurse continues to evaluate the patient's response for evidence of flumazenil-induced:

a. muscular re-relaxation
b. emerging incisional pain
c. sinus bradycardia
d. respiratory depression

NOTE: Consider scenario and item 4.30 together.

Mr. G requires reintubation and ventilator support to reverse respiratory acidosis. He will remain intubated overnight. To facilitate intubation, Mr. G receives succinylcholine.

4.30. Succinylcholine is classified as a:

a. depolarizing muscle relaxant
b. anticholinesterase blocker
c. calcium channel inhibitor
d. nondepolarizing muscle relaxant

NOTE: Consider scenario and item 4.31 together.

Sixty minutes after bupivacaine (Marcaine) is added to an epidural infusion of morphine sulfate (Duramorph), the patient complains of vertigo and tinnitus. The nurse observes muscle tremors, hypotension and premature ventricular contractions.

4.31. These symptoms are *most likely* related to:

a. early hyperdynamic sepsis
b. local anesthetic toxicity
c. systemic allergic response
d. morphine overdose

4.32. Four year old Shannon has vomited twice since her strabismus surgery ended an hour ago. She received small amounts of halothane, fentanyl and atracurium intraoperatively. The PACU nurse administers droperidol according to established antiemetic protocol and observes her for:

a. hyperventilation
b. increased sedation
c. hypertension
d. emergence delirium

NOTE: Consider scenario and item 4.33 together.

The anesthesia provider reports Ms D received nitrous oxide, ofloxacin, alfentanil and rocuronium for her multiple dental extractions. She is wheelchair-dependent due to cerebral palsy from hypoxia at birth and had a mitral valve replacement 3 years ago.

4.33. In the immediate postanesthetic period Ms D is most *likely* to develop:

a. reflexive hyperventilation from diffusion hypoxia
b. prolonged vomiting from swallowed blood
c. malignant hypertension from autonomic dysreflexia
d. painful sensations from early narcotic metabolism

4.34. To affect postoperative nausea and vomiting (PONV), metoclopramide:

a. stimulates H_2 receptors and neutralizes gastric fluid
b. suppresses CTZ dopamine receptors and increases gastric motility
c. suppresses H_1 receptors and decreases gastric volume
d. stimulates CTZ dopamine receptors and decreases gastric emptying

4.35. Mr. S received a bolus dose of epidural morphine just prior to his arrival in PACU. The *most* critical times to assess his respiratory quality are during the first hour after injection and:

a. every hour for 18 hours
b. 2 hours after injection
c. 6-8 hours later
d. when Mr. S states itching

4.36. For a brief period following electroconvulsive therapy, a 42 year old woman is *most likely* to develop:

a. hypertension with electromechanical dissociation
b. hypotension with bundle branch block
c. hypertension and supraventricular tachycardia
d. hypotension and sinus bradycardia

NOTE: Consider scenario and item 4.37 together.

The anesthesia provider accompanies a 45 year old woman into the PACU following emergency appendectomy. The patient's medical history includes recent depression, treated with a monoamine oxidase inhibitor. She is agitated, cries "Help me," and states her pain is "8" on a verbal pain scale of 0-10

4.37. This patient's pain is best managed with any of the following medications *except:*

a. morphine sulfate
b. alfentanil
c. levo-dromoran
d. meperidine

4.38. Mr. H is 80 years old and receives IV conscious sedation in PACU to realign his dislocated artificial hip. By definition, a patient under conscious sedation may be amnesic or drowsy yet:

a. demonstrates airway patency with jaw support
b. rouses to a supraorbital stimulus
c. maintains independent, continuous airway patency
d. transfers to a stretcher with minimal aid

4.39. Medications considered appropriate for conscious sedation include:

a. thiopental and meperidine
b. diazepam and morphine sulfate
c. methohexital and ketamine
d. propofol and midazolam

4.40. Biochemically, a local anesthetic affects nerve conduction by blocking:

a. acetylcholine release at the neuromuscular junction
b. sodium entry into nerve cells to stabilize the membrane
c. calcium channels at specific osmotic junctures
d. norepinephrine effect to reverse an action potential

SET II

Items 4.41-4.82

4.41. Successful early resuscitation from cardiac arrest is best facilitated by administration of:

a. epinephrine
b. sodium bicarbonate
c. lidocaine
d. calcium gluconate

4.42. Ms X received desflurane, rocuronium and midazolam during her postpartum tubal ligation. With regard to effects of these anesthetic medications, a primary *initial* nursing priority for Ms X is *most* likely to be:

a. oxytocics to reverse uterine atony
b. prompt pain management
c. extended airway support from drowsiness
d. blood pressure support

4.43. In susceptible individuals, enflurane, desflurane and isoflurane may increase the likelihood of:

a. autonomic hyperreflexia
b. pseudocholinesterase deficiency
c. malignant hyperthermia
d. rapid muscle relaxant metabolism

4.44. Onset of a local anesthetic's effect can be changed by adjusting:

a. lipid solubility
b. alkalinity
c. osmolality
d. hydrophilia

NOTE: Consider scenario and item 4.45 together.

Seven months ago, Mr. T had a percutaneous coronary angioplasty (PTCA) after an infarction of his inferior myocardial wall. His cardiologist requests a prophylactic nitroglycerin infusion at a rate of 100 mcg/min during today's radical prostatectomy and lymphadenectomy.

4.45. This infusion's effects occur primarily by:

a. blocking cellular calcium channels
b. supporting blood pressure with contractile force
c. elevating cardiac ST segments
d. reducing myocardial demand with vascular dilation

4.46. Protocols established for advanced cardiac life support recommend that defibrillation is most effective when the time interval between doses of cardiotonic medications and defibrillation attempts is:

a. 10-15 seconds
b. 20-25 seconds
c. 35-60 seconds
d. 70-90 seconds

4.47. Adding bupivacaine to a narcotic epidural infusion will *most likely:*

a. delay ambulation
b. increase pruritus
c. relax the bladder sphincter
d. eliminate tachyphylaxis

4.48. The opioid receptors that are primarily affected by morphine are:

a. alpha
b. beta
c. sigma
d. mu

4.49. To safely administer parenteral nitroglycerin the PACU nurse:

a. limits the dose to 25 mcg/min with an infusion pump to avoid toxicity
b. interrupts the infusion hourly to reassess patient symptoms

c. uses only a glass bottle and specialized, nonplastic administration tubing
d. covers medication with a dark bag to prevent destruction of nitroglycerin molecules

4.50. The preanesthesia patient who can *most* safely receive an intubating dose of succinylcholine is a:
a. healthy 9 year old boy scheduled for a hypospadias repair
b. 25 year old woman with anterior cord syndrome and tibial fracture after a motor vehicle accident 5 days ago
c. jaundiced 48 year old man requiring laparotomy to explore his common bile duct and obtain liver biopsies
d. 72 year old woman with glaucoma and emphysema who will have a repair of her Colles' fracture

4.51. Intrathecal tetracaine's duration of action is *best* extended by:
a. delaying systemic absorption
b. buffering the solution with carbonic acid
c. specifying a quiet, sitting position to promote wide block distribution
d. diluting tetracaine in normal saline to facilitate sodium entry into the muscle cell

4.52. The PACU nurse anticipates that the peak relaxant effects of a 7 mg intubating dose of vecuronium in an average-sized adult will persist:
a. until completely removed by Hofmann elimination
b. until slight metabolic acidosis facilitates reversal
c. for approximately 30 minutes at near-normal temperatures
d. for about 90 minutes until renally excreted

NOTE: Consider scenario and item 4.53 together.

Mr. V has a history of episodic ventricular tachycardia that is not responsive to lidocaine suppression. Due to an emergency that delayed his surgeon, the preanesthesia nurse will observe Mr. V for about 30 minutes before his scheduled surgery to implant a cardiodefibrillator. He is conscious with stable vital signs.

4.53. The nurse will observe Mr. V for adverse effects related to his 1.5 mg/min bretylium infusion and anticipates the *most likely* intervention will be:
a. labetalol to suppress paroxysmal supraventricular tachycardia
b. atropine to increase intraventricular conduction
c. antiemetics to relieve unrelenting nausea associated with continuous infusion
d. fluid volume replacement to support blood pressure

4.54. Flumazenil is most effective when administered to improve:
a. postictal phase of tonic-clonic epileptic seizure
b. delayed return of muscle function after nondepolarizing neuromuscular blockade
c. hypoventilation related to benzodiazepine-induced sedation
d. strong muscle contractions associated with postanesthesia shivering

4.55. Intrathecal medications are delivered:
a. between the pia mater and arachnoid
b. over the dura mater
c. between the dura mater and arachnoid
d. under the pia mater

4.56. Medications that quickly dissolve in fatty tissue are considered:
a. hydrophilic
b. lipophobic
c. hydrophobic
d. lipophilic

NOTE: Consider scenario and item 4.57 together.

The PACU nurse observes redness and several raised, nonweeping blisters on the inner aspect of the arm of a patient who received 8 mg of intravenous morphine sulfate, in 2 mg incremental doses, during the previous 30 minutes.

4.57. These signs are *most likely* evidence of morphine's:

a. anaphylactic potential
b. systemic allergenic character
c. localized histamine release
d. ability to decrease peripheral resistance

NOTE: Consider scenario and item 4.58 together.

Mr. S is 75 years old and healthy except for back pain and increasing degeneration of his arthritic joints. He received enflurane, vecuronium, and sufentanil by continuous infusion during an anterior and posterior T-12 to L-4 spinal fusion and instrumentation. A bone graft was harvested from his iliac crest. He is currently nonresponsive and not moving. Pupils are pinpoint; respirations are spontaneous and shallow at 8 breaths per minute. Though Mr. S was awakened intraoperatively and moved his extremities, the neurosurgeon is now anxious to observe Mr. S's extremity motor and sensory function. Mr. S receives three doses of 0.01 mg naloxone and slowly rouses, has deeper respirations at a rate of 12 breaths per minute, moves his limbs, and indicates sensation.

4.58. The nurse now closely monitors Mr. S for any of the following likely occurrences *except:*

a. emerging head and hip pain
b. recurring respiratory depression
c. generalizing torso itching
d. continuing lumbar muscle tightness and shivering

NOTE: Consider scenario and items 4.59-4.60 together.

Jason was born 8 weeks prematurely and is now a healthy 6 month old who weighs 14 pounds. After today's elective repair of his umbilical hernia, the nurse measures his blood pressure at 82/50 and heart rate as 175 beats per minute. Jason flails his arms, pulls up his legs, and cries inconsolably despite his mother's calm presence. The nurse encourages Jason's mother to cradle, rock, and talk to him.

4.59. Jason's PACU nurse assures the *most* positive postoperative outcomes for Jason by arranging a hospital admission with an apnea monitor and:

a. maintaining fluid volume with lactated Ringer's solution at 40 ml/hour
b. titrating a dextrose infusion to results of serum glucose measures every 2 hours
c. administering an acetaminophen suppository to manage Jason's pain
d. rewarming Jason to 39° C with radiant heat lamps

4.60. The *most likely* explanation for Jason's current heart rate is:

a. unrelieved incisional pain
b. agitated emergence delirium
c. reflexive response to fluid volume deficit
d. falsely high, inaccurate measure

4.61. The patient with increased risk to develop malignant hyperthermia generally can safely tolerate:

a. a depolarizing muscle relaxant
b. intrathecal amide local anesthetics
c. volatile halogenated anesthetics
d. prolonged physical stress

4.62. To relax an upper airway laryngospasm, an 18 kg 6 year old child received succinylcholine 10 mg. The nurse anticipates the effects will persist for:

a. at least 1 hour
b. 12-18 minutes
c. 4-6 minutes
d. until reversed by glycopyrrolate

4.63. Factors that inhibit pseudocholinesterase effect could include any of the following *except:*

a. neostigmine used to reverse vecuronium
b. insufficient hemoglobin and serum albumin
c. hypercarbia with uncompensated acidosis
d. fluid volume deficit and oliguria

4.64. The *primary* pharmacodynamic effect of nitroprusside occurs by:

a. altering systemic vascular resistance
b. increasing renal blood flow to inhibit renin
c. reducing afterload while increasing preload
d. dilating coronary arteries to increase perfusion

NOTE: Consider items 4.65-4.67 together.

4.65. A regional anesthetic may be selected for carotid endarterectomy *primarily* to:

a. offer a lower cost treatment option
b. monitor intraoperative visual improvement
c. decrease the incidence of postoperative hypertension
d. prevent the need for an intraoperative carotid shunt

4.66. During the *initial* respiratory assessment of this patient in PACU, the nurse observes labored breathing and stridor. These symptoms *most likely* are associated with:

a. epicarotid hematoma
b. compromised autoregulation
c. cranial nerve XI trauma
d. bilateral carotid body damage

4.67. During the initial cardiac assessment of this patient, the PACU nurse observes sinus bradycardia at 43 beats per minute, without ventricular ectopy or arterioventricular conduction delays. The nurse reasons that this rhythm is *most* probably related to:

a. perianesthetic hypotensive technique
b. vasovagal response to pain
c. evolving inferior wall infarctions
d. residual effect of surgical retraction

4.68. Advanced cardiac life support (ACLS) protocols identify the *initial* priority of adult emergency care as:

a. instituting fluid replacement
b. confirming ventilations
c. assessing responsiveness
d. verifying pulselessness

NOTE: Consider scenario and items 4.69-4.71 together.

Mr. P had a heart transplant 6 months ago, requires only his immunosuppressant medications, and today needs a cholecystectomy by open laparotomy. The nurse considers any potential postoperative complications.

4.69. In the event that an alert Mr. P's heart rate measures 52 beats/ minute and his blood pressure decreases by 10%, the nurse's *most appropriate* first intervention is to provide:

a. atropine sulfate 0.4 mg intravenously
b. epinephrine infusion 3 mcg/min
c. hetastarch 300 ml
d. dopamine 12 mcg/kg/min

4.70. The cardiologist considers Mr. P's posttransplant course as uncomplicated by rejection or dysrhythmia; the nurse therefore anticipates that Mr. P's resting cardiac rhythm will be best described as:

a. sinus bradycardia at 50-60 beats per minute
b. atrial rhythm at 75 beats per minute and occasional paced complexes
c. sinus tachycardia at 100 beats per minute
d. supraventricular rhythm with occasional premature ventricular beats

4.71. The nurse is *most* likely to detect Mr. P's early hypovolemic condition by observing:

a. reflexive heart rate increases to 150 beats per minute
b. orthostatic hypotension when moved to semi-Fowler's position
c. heart rate variation when breathing
d. statements of developing precordial chest pain

4.72. The anesthesia provider administers etomidate for its:

a. hypnotic effects
b. cardiotonic strength
c. prolonged analgesic properties
d. adrenal hormone stimulation

NOTE: Consider scenario and item 4.73 together.

Ms O, age 77 years, arrived in the Emergency Department this morning complaining of severe abdominal pain and nausea. This afternoon, she is added to the surgery schedule for an exploratory laparotomy. She states that this morning she applied her usual dose of ophthalmic timolol.

4.73. Anesthetic consideration related to the effects of Ms O's ophthalmic timolol would *most* likely:

a. require cancellation of today's surgery
b. raise airway resistance and increase her potential for bronchospasm
c. cause a rapid surge in intraocular pressure
d. release stored catecholamines, markedly raising pulse and blood pressure

4.74. Thirty year old Ms C states she uses an albuterol nebulizer each day to manage her asthma. During her preanesthesia assessment, she also indictes a penicillin allergy and food allergies to bananas and avocados. The preanesthesia nurse suspects that Ms C may have increased:

a. susceptibility to develop malignant hyperthermia
b. response to histamine after receiving morphine
c. requirements for narcotic analgesics
d. sensitivity during exposure to latex

4.75. Mr. A's medical record indicates he consumes one to two cans of beer each day, including yesterday, and up to five on weekends. His chronic consumption of alcohol *most likely* will:

a. precipitate alcohol withdrawal symptoms in PACU following naloxone reversal of sufentanil
b. increase the total dose of meperidine needed to achieve effective analgesia
c. synergistically prolong motor blockade produced by bupivacaine
d. require low flows of enflurane anesthetic to maintain anesthetic depth

4.76. The *first* intervention when malignant hyperthermia is suspected is to:

a. hyperventilate with 100% oxygen
b. administer iced lactated Ringer's solution
c. medicate with dantrolene sodium 1 g
d. treat hypertension with verapamil

4.77. Progressively decreasing effect from a local anesthetic during epidural infusion defines:

a. toxicity
b. therapeutics
c. tachyphylaxis
d. tolerance

NOTE: Consider scenario and items 4.78-4.80 together.

After 90 minutes in PACU following his left femoral popliteal bypass graft and tetracaine spinal anesthetic, 62 year old Mr. P's blood pressure is consistently 75-80/40. Occasional boluses of phenylephrine (Neo-Synephrine), hetastarch, and lactated Ringer's solution briefly increase his blood pressure to 100-110/52. Tympanic temperature measured 36.3° C on admission and is 36.7° C now. Cardiac rhythm is sinus at 56 beats per minute. Mr. P is oriented but says he feels "sleepy." The nurse applies a nursing diagnosis of decreased cardiac output and continues to assess Mr. P.

4.78. The *most likely* causes related to this nursing diagnosis for Mr. P include any of the following *except:*

a. residual tetracaine motor blockade
b. perioperative myocardial infarction
c. postoperative incisional drainage
d. reversal of intraoperative hypothermia

NOTE: The scenario continues.

Within the next hour, Mr. P's blood pressure is consistently 112-120/66 after he receives 2 units of autologous packed cells. While monitoring Mr. P's EKG in Lead MCL_1 the nurse observes QRS complexes of 0.10 seconds' duration that occur at a rate of 72 beats per minute. Each is preceded by a P wave with a PR interval of 0.18 seconds. A single early QRS of 0.18 seconds' duration follows every fourth to sixth QRS.

4.79. According to advanced cardiac life support protocols, the most appropriate intervention is to:

a. eradicate ectopy immediately with lidocaine 80 mg
b. observe; intervene if wide beats occur in clusters
c. override premature beats with atropine 0.4 mg
d. suppress early beats with beta adrenergic blockade

4.80. If Mr. P were to develop a sustained rhythm of wide QRS complexes at a rate of 130 beats per minute and remain alert and conversant, the *most appropriate* immediate and simultaneous initial interventions include:

a. providing oxygen and distinguishing aberrant conduction from ventricular tachycardia
b. measuring serum potassium and infusing verapamil 5 mg over 2 minutes
c. preparing for immediate cardioversion and treating the cause of torsades de pointes
d. establishing clinical stability and injecting lidocaine 1 mg/kg

4.81. A patient who breathes isoflurane for 4 hours of a 5 hour neurosurgical procedure will *most likely:*

a. converse alertly with the PACU staff within 10 minutes after the isoflurane stops
b. develop elevated hepatic enzyme levels and jaundice
c. require frequent stimulation to breathe in PACU
d. raise his head for 5 seconds and state strong pain after isoflurane reversal

4.82. The preanesthesia nurse *avoids* administering morphine sulfate to treat a presurgical patient with:

a. acute cholelithiasis and right upper quadrant pain
b. pulmonary rales and fluid volume excess
c. renal calculi and documented morphine dependence
d. ST segment depression and substernal chest pain

Set I

Answer Key

4.1.	a
4.2.	d
4.3.	a
4.4.	c
4.5.	d
4.6.	b
4.7.	c
4.8.	d
4.9.	a
4.10.	c
4.11.	a
4.12.	b
4.13.	c
4.14.	b
4.15.	d
4.16.	a
4.17.	d
4.18.	b
4.19.	c
4.20.	d
4.21.	c
4.22.	a
4.23.	a
4.24.	a
4.25.	c
4.26.	d
4.27.	b
4.28.	c
4.29.	d
4.30.	a
4.31.	b
4.32.	b
4.33.	d
4.34.	b
4.35.	c
4.36.	c
4.37.	d
4.38.	c
4.39.	b
4.40.	b

SET I

Rationales and References

4.1. Correct Answer: **a**

Acetylcholine is the primary neurotransmitter of both preganglionic and postganglionic fibers in the parasympathetic nervous system. This chemical is stored, then released at the neuromuscular junction to facilitate transmission of neurologic impulses.

Willis, WD: The Autonomic Nervous System and Its Central Control in Physiology, *3rd ed (Berne, RM & Levy, MN, Eds). St. Louis, Mosby, pp. 253-254, 1993.*

4.2. Correct Answer: **d**

This woman should receive an antibiotic dose within 1 hour prior to surgery. Her mitral valve dysfunction is likely related to her history of rheumatic heart disease; her risk of developing bacterial endocarditis is 5-8 times greater than another patient who has no cardiac disease. Antibiotic prophylaxis is especially important when the planned surgical procedure invades the genitourinary, oral or upper respiratory systems. Patients with multiple dental caries or orthopedic hardware also may receive antibiotic pretreatment. Delivery of lithotripsy shock waves correlates with the cardiac cycle (R wave on EKG); a bradycardic, tachycardic, or irregular heart rate may be regulated by any of several cardioactive medications, not necessarily digitalis.

Burden, N: Ambulatory Surgical Nursing. *Philadelphia, Saunders, pp. 199, 207-210, & 523; Brown, M: Antibiotics and Anesthesia.* Semin Anesth *IX(3): 153-161, 1990.*

4.3. Correct Answer: **a**

Volatile (inhaled) anesthetic agents rely on respiratory quality for clearance from the brain, the target organ for effect. The solubility coefficient (minimum alveolar concentration [MAC]) of the individual anesthetic and the patient's ability to breathe influence removal. After the flow of gas (exposure) is terminated, the effects of a highly soluble drug like halothane abate rapidly. A gas anesthetic is quickly eliminated when minute ventilation (increased rate and depth to remove alveolar gas) and cardiac output (rapid circulation time to quickly lower tissue saturation) are high. Renal and liver function have minimal influence on elimination of a volatile anesthetic.

Litwack, K: Post Anesthesia Care Nursing, *2nd ed. St. Louis, Mosby, pp. 128-129, 1995; Miller, FL & Marshall, BE: The Inhaled Anesthetics in* Dripps/Eckenhoff/Vandam Introduction to Anesthesia *(Longnecker, DE and Murphy, FL, Eds). Philadelphia, Saunders, 1992, pp. 84-86; Drain, C:* The Post Anesthesia Care Unit: A Critical Care Approach to Post Anesthesia Nursing, *3rd ed. Philadelphia, Saunders, pp. 191-195, 1994.*

4.4. Correct Answer: **c**

Hydralazine is an antihypertensive that decreases peripheral resistance by acting directly on peripheral vessels to relax and dilate arterioles. As blood pressure drops, compensatory mechanisms respond to prevent dire changes in cardiac output. Heart rate, renin production, myocardial contractility, and contractile force may increase as a result.

Shannon, MT, Wilson, BA & Stang, CL: Govoni & Hayes Drugs and Nursing Implications, *8th ed. Norwalk, CT, Appleton & Lange, pp. 592-4, 1995; Morgan, GE & Mikhail, MS:* Clinical Anesthesiology. *Norwalk, CT, Appleton & Lange, pp. 169-172, 1992.*

4.5. Correct Answer: **d**

Minimum alveolar concentration (MAC) is the lowest concentration (partial pressure) of a specific inhalant anesthetic that obliterates movement in 50% of patients when a painful stimulus (like a surgical incision) is applied. MAC expresses the comparative (relative) potency of various inhalation anesthetic gases. The relationship is inverse: a low MAC indicates a very potent anesthetic.

Trevor, AJ & Miller, RD: General Anesthetics in Basic & Clinical Pharmacology, *6th ed (Katzung, BG, Ed). Norwalk, CT, Appleton & Lange, p. 387, 1995; Drain, C:* The Post Anesthesia Care Unit: A Critical Care Approach to Post Anesthesia Nursing. *Philadelphia, Saunders, p. 194, 1994.*

4.6. Correct Answer: **b**

Minimum alveolar concentration (MAC) is unaffected by anesthesia duration, a patient's sex and $PaCO_2$ levels. Age, hypothermia, central nervous system depressants and antihypertensives decrease MAC; hyperthermia, chronic alcohol use and elevated levels of monoamine oxidase (MAO) inhibitors increase MAC. Inhalation anesthetics depress cardiac function and circulation.

Trevor, AJ & Miller, RD: General Anesthetics in Basic & Clinical Pharmacology, *6th ed (Katzung, BG, Ed). Norwalk, CT, Appleton & Lange, p. 387, 1995; Miller, FL & Marshall, BE: The Inhaled Anesthetics in* Dripps/Eckenhoff/Vandam Introduction to Anesthesia, *8th ed (Longnecker, DE & Murphy, FL, Eds). Philadelphia, Saunders, pp. 85-88, 1992.*

4.7. Correct Answer: **c**

Electromechanical interference (EMI) arises from muscle activity (*conducted* EMI) or influence of an electrical or magnetic field (*radiated* EMI). *Myopotentials,* high-frequency electrical signals created by muscle activity, do not occur with mivacurium. However, seizures, muscle fasciculations during depolarization with succinylcholine, or muscle movement during mechanical ventilation *can* produce brief but strong skeletal muscle activity. In addition, either overventilation (hypocarbia) or underventilation (hypoxemia or hypercarbia) can alter the membrane potential of cardiac muscle cells—and their ability to respond to a pacing stimulus. Surgical cautery is one source of *electrical* EMI; repeated, high-frequency stimuli from an extracorporeal shock wave lithotripter (ESWL) occur near Mr. A's pacemaker housing and could damage its sensing or pacing components.

Fetzer-Fowler, S: Caring for the Ambulatory Surgical Patient Who Has a Pacemaker: Part II. J Post Anesth Nurs *8(3): 174-182, 1993; Morgan, GE & Mikhail, MS:* Clinical Anesthesiology. *Norwalk, CT, Appleton & Lange, p. 538, 1992.*

4.8. Correct Answer: **d**

Midazolam (Versed) is 2-3 times more potent than diazepam (Valium); therefore the effective dose is at least 50% less. Small doses of intravenous midazolam are administered at intervals according to effect. Midazolam is lipophilic and nearly totally bound to serum albumin. Peak effect occurs quickly, within 3-5 minutes, though *duration* is 1-4 hours; effects are further increased by narcotics and sedatives.

Nursing '94 Drug Handbook. *Des Moines, Springhouse, pp. 349-350, 1994; Drain, C:* The Post Anesthesia Care Unit: A Critical Care Approach to Post Anesthesia Nursing, *3rd ed. Philadelphia, Saunders, pp. 208-209, 1994.*

4.9. Correct Answer: **a**

Atropine sulfate (an anticholinergic) minimizes the bradycardia, salivation, gastrointestinal irritability and miosis produced when muscarinic receptors are stimulated by anticholinesterase medications. Cholinesterase-inhibiting medications include neostigmine (Prostigmin) or edrophonium (Tensilon). These medications reverse the effects of nondepolarizing muscle relaxants (NDMR) by inactivating acetylcholinesterase. As a result, concentrations of the neurotransmitter acetylcholine increase, and normal neuromuscular function resumes.

Katzung, BG: Basic and Clinical Pharmacology, *6th ed. Norwalk, CT, Appleton & Lange, pp. 102-111, 1995; Drain, C:* The Post Anesthesia Care Unit: A Critical Care Approach to Post Anesthesia Nursing, *3rd ed. Philadelphia, Saunders, pp. 208-209, 1994.*

4.10. Correct Answer: **c**

Up to 10% of patients with penicillin allergy are also sensitive to cephalosporin antibiotics. Consult with the surgeon before administering cefazolin and other antibiotics in this classification. Particularly if the patient has anaphylactic-type symptoms to penicillin, cephalosporins are usually avoided. Gentamicin and vancomycin protect against bacterial endocarditis but are associated with ototoxicity and renal failure.

Beam, TR: Anti-Infective Drugs in the Prevention and Treatment of Sepsis Syndrome. Crit Care Clin North Am *6(2): 275-291, 1994; Brown, M: Antibiotics and Anesthesia.* Semin Anesth *IX(3)L: 153-161, 1990.*

4.11. Correct Answer: **a**

Compared with the adult, a greater proportion (about twice) of an infant's body weight is comprised of "vessel-rich" vital tissues. High respiratory rate, cardiac index and rapid blood flow through vital organs like heart, kidney and liver mean rapid uptake of anesthetic medication. The result may be a quick and significant depression of cardiac function.

Litwack, K: Post Anesthesia Care Nursing, *2nd ed. St. Louis, Mosby, pp. 332-341, 1995.*

4.12. Correct Answer: **b**

As an alpha adrenergic blocker, droperidol can produce some peripheral vasodilation. The already hypovolemic, dizzy or hypotensive patient may develop even more pronounced hypotension. In addition, droperidol sedates the patient and may increase extrapyramidal activity.

Parnass, SM: Problems of Ambulatory Surgery in Post Anesthesia Care *(Vender, JS & Speiss, BD, Eds). Philadelphia, Saunders, pp.*

324-325, 1992; Skidmore-Roth, L: Mosby's 1995 Nursing Drug Reference. *St. Louis, Mosby, pp. 415-416 & 474-475, 1995.*

4.13. Correct Answer: **c**

Local anesthetic toxicity results in seizures (neurotoxicity), hypotension and bradycardia (cardiotoxicity) after initial hypertension with tachycardia. Intravenous regional block (Bier block) involves injection of large volumes of local anesthetic, usually lidocaine, into the operative extremity. Deflation of the tourniquet(s) used to obstruct blood flow and contain the local anesthetic during a Bier block can allow unmetabolized local anesthetic to suddenly enter the bloodstream. A bolus dose of local anesthetic is most likely when the tourniquet(s) is(are) deflated early (less than 30 minutes after medication injection) or too rapidly or when a tourniquet cuff has technical faults.

Burden, N: Ambulatory Surgical Nursing. *Philadelphia, Saunders, pp. 95-96, 1993; Litwack, K:* Post Anesthesia Care Nursing, *2nd ed. St. Louis, Mosby, pp. 165-166, 1995.*

4.14. Correct Answer: **b**

To establish an intravenous regional block, alias Bier block, the anesthesia provider applies a double-cuffed tourniquet to the surgical extremity. Blood is forcefully drawn from the vessels; a large bolus of local anesthetic is then injected into the venous system. The tourniquet both obstructs the extremity's blood flow and prevents movement of the anesthetic beyond the tourniquet. Anesthetic, typically lidocaine without epinephrine, then diffuses from vessels to bathe and numb tissues for approximately 90 minutes.

Brown, DL: Atlas of Regional Anesthesia. *Philadelphia, Saunders, pp. 55-61, 1992; Parnass, SM: Problems of Ambulatory Surgery in* Post Anesthesia Care *(Vender, JS & Speiss, BD, Eds). Philadelphia, Saunders, p. 318, 1992.*

4.15. Correct Answer: **d**

Ideally, a patient will have minimal bleeding and prompt return of arm function after an intravenous regional (Bier) block. However, the ongoing effect of local anesthetic medications can numb sensation and limit motor control in the extremity. Without support, protection, and cautious movement, the extremity can flail about, increasing potential for injury to the extremity or body. The PACU nurse should expect this patient to be alert but possibly have significant pain. Tourniquets create a relatively bloodless surgical field. However, if hemostasis is not assured prior to tourniquet release, significant and reportable postsurgical bleeding can occur.

Litwack-Saleh, K: Practical Points in Understanding Intravenous Regional Anesthesia. J Post Anesth Nurs *8(3): 172-173, 1993; Burden, N:* Ambulatory Surgical Nursing. *Philadelphia, Saunders, pp. 95-96, 1993.*

4.16. Correct Answer: **a**

Desflurane (Suprane) acts quickly and dissipates quickly, but is very likely to stimulate coughing and airway spasm. Inhalation anesthetics are generally known for their bronchodilating properties and low potential to irritate the airway. Halothane is a particularly appropriate choice for children and asthmatic patients. Enflurane (Ethrane) and isoflurane (Forane) have the most significant respiratory depressant effects.

Trevor, AJ & Miller, RD: General Anesthetics in Basic & Clinical Pharmacology, *6th ed (Katzung, BG, Ed). Norwalk, CT, Appleton & Lange, pp. 387-389, 1995; Drain, C:* The Post Anesthesia Care Unit: A Critical Care Approach to Post Anesthesia Nursing. *Philadelphia, Saunders, pp. 198-203, 1994.*

4.17. Correct Answer: **d**

Only about 25% of cardiac output perfuses skeletal muscle and fat, so release of any stored medication is gradual. Elimination of an inhaled anesthetic depends in part on blood flow (circulation) and also on distribution into body tissues, including brain, muscle and fat. Some inhaled anesthetic agents are quickly absorbed into fat, which has low blood flow. Body tissues that receive the greatest proportion of cardiac output (perfusion) both absorb and eliminate anesthetic gases quickly. Vital organs like the heart, brain and kidneys receive the largest blood flow, approximately 75% of cardiac output, and so quickly show both medication effects and clearance.

Litwack, K: Post Anesthesia Care Nursing, *2nd ed. St. Louis, Mosby, pp. 128-129, 1995; Drain, C:* The Post Anesthesia Care Unit: A Critical Care Approach to Post Anesthesia Nursing. *3rd ed. Philadelphia, Saunders, pp. 191-195, 1994.*

4.18. Correct Answer: **b**

Infusing a narcotic continuously into the epidural space *improves* joint and muscle movement, promotes earlier postoperative activity and provides consistent, long-term pain relief. Vomiting incidence remains high after both intramuscular or epidural morphine. Other benefits of epidural analgesia include less sedation and anxiety, decreased likelihood of pulmonary infections and deep vein thrombosis, reduced myocardial oxygen demand, and suppressed metabolic and endocrine responses to stress. Risk of respiratory depression and *progressive,* not episodic, sedation increases with epidural narcotics. Adding a local anesthetic to the narcotic solution *can* alter motor strength though, so that walking or upright positions are associated with orthostatic hypotension or muscle weakness.

Cohen, MS: Continuous Epidural Infusions of Acute Postoperative Pain Part III. Curr Rev PACN *11(12): 97-104, 1989; Gilbert, HG: Postoperative Pain Management in* Post Anesthesia Care *(Vender, JS & Speiss, BD, Eds). Philadelphia, Saunders, pp. 308-311, 1992.*

4.19. Correct Answer: **c**

The epidural space is a *potential* space between the dura mater covering the spinal canal and the epidural wall. This space is filled with nerves, lymphatic tissue and veins enmeshed in fat—but no fluid—and extends from the neck to the sacrum. Blood may appear in fluid aspirated from the epidural space after back surgery when the dura is entered.

Brown, DL: Atlas of Regional Anesthesia. *Philadelphia, Saunders, pp. 263-265 & 283-292, 1992; Drain, C:* The Post Anesthesia Care Unit: A Critical Care Approach to Post Anesthesia Nursing, *3rd ed. Philadelphia, Saunders, p. 74, 1994.*

4.20. Correct Answer: **d**

Cocaine prevents norepinephrine uptake at peripheral adrenergic nerve sites. Cocaine also directly stimulates the sympathetic nervous system, which releases catecholamines. Epinephrine (Adrenalin) surge, with severe hypertension, racing tachycardia, and cardiac failure, results.

Saleh, KL: Practical Points in Understanding Local Anesthetics. J Post Anesth Nurs *7(1): 45-47, 1991; Shannon, MT, Wilson, BA & Stang, CL:* Govoni & Hayes Drugs and Nursing Implicatoins, *8th ed. Norwalk, CT, Appleton & Lange, pp. 335–336, 1995*

4.21. Correct Answer: **c**

The nurse should begin to notice blood pressure reductions within 10-20 minutes after sublingual administration. Nifedipine is classified as a calcium channel blocker that predominantly dilates vascular smooth muscle to decrease vascular resistance and improve blood flow to coronary arteries.

Shannon, MT, Wilson, BA & Stang, CL: Govoni & Hayes Drugs and Nursing Implications, *8th ed. Norwalk, CT, Appleton & Lange, pp. 828-830, 1995; Herbert, DW:* Manual of Drugs in Anesthesia and Critical Care. *Philadelphia, Saunders, pp. 152-153, 1993.*

4.22. Correct Answer: **a**

Heart rate and cardiac output may reflexively increase in response to hypotension from nifedipine's peripheral vasodilating actions. Nifedipine's primary effect is to decrease blood pressure and improve coronary artery blood flow, relieving angina or spasm. Delays in cardiac conduction are less likely with nifedipine than with other calcium channel blockers, especially if combined with beta blockers. Nifedipine is sometimes used to treat, not cause, pulmonary hypertension and asthma.

Shannon, MT, Wilson, BA & Stang, CL: Govoni & Hayes Drugs and Nursing Implications, *8th ed. Norwalk, CT, Appleton & Lange, pp. 828-630, 1995; Skidmore-Roth, L:* Mosby's 1995 Nursing Drug Reference. *St. Louis, Mosby, pp. 771-772, 1995.*

4.23. Correct Answer: **a**

Adequate analgesia is not a prerequisite to injecting a nonsteroidal antiinflammatory drug (NSAID) like ketorolac. An NSAID does not act on opiate receptors but may *augment* the pain relief provided by a narcotic. The ketorolac dose is reduced for elderly patients, patients who weigh less than 50 kg, and patients with renal or liver insufficiency. NSAIDs also alter platelet function and so are avoided for patients with "bleeding problems" (coagulopathy), history of gastrointestinal ulcers and also renal or hepatic disease. Cross sensitivity can occur when a patient with an aspirin allergy receives NSAIDs.

Shannon, MT, Wilson, BA & Stang, CL: Govoni & Hayes Drugs and Nursing Implications, *8th ed. Norwalk, CT, Appleton & Lange, p. 666, 1995; Litwack, K & Drain, C: Pain Assessment and Management in* ASPAN's Core Curriculum for Post Anesthesia Nursing

Practice, *3rd ed (Litwack, K, Ed). Philadelphia, Saunders, pp. 658-650, 1994.*

4.24. Correct Answer: **a**

Nalbuphine (Nubain) is a strong analgesic with mixed effects at pain receptors. Agonist effects partially stimulate kappa and stimulate sigma receptors. Nalbuphine has *antagonistic* effects at *mu* pain receptors. Therefore nalbuphine antagonizes (reverses) respiratory depression created by the narcotics that stimulate mu receptors. Nalbuphine also can reverse analgesia produced by other narcotics and begin withdrawal symptoms in an addicted person. When a patient has received *no* narcotic, nalbuphine's strong analgesic effects are equal to morphine's but with less respiratory depression and less addictive potential.

Shannon, MT, Wilson, BA & Stang, CL: Govoni & Hayes Drugs and Nursing Implications, *8th ed. Norwalk, CT, Appleton & Lange, pp. 807-808, 1995; Drain, C:* The Post Anesthesia Care Unit: A Critical Care Approach to Post Anesthesia Nursing, *3rd ed. Philadelphia, Saunders, p. 220, 1994.*

4.25. Correct Answer: **c**

Severe acute alcohol withdrawal produces hallucinations, restlessness, disorientation, and tremors about 2 days after alcohol consumption stops. Concurrent sympathetic nervous system stimulation causes the tachycardia, hypertension and diaphoresis. If Mr. J abused cocaine, the nurse would more likely observe increased pulmonary congestion, hyperthermia, excessive talking and epistaxis. Confusion from local anesthetic toxicity is also associated with tremors, numbness and tinnitus. Intraspinal bleeding produces severe back pain at the site of the bleeding, as well as motor and sensory deficits. Consider fat embolism syndrome as another possible contributor to Mr. J's confusion 2 days after injury.

Drain, C: The Post Anesthesia Care Unit: A Critical Care Approach to Post Anesthesia Nursing, *3rd ed. Philadelphia, Saunders, pp. 559-560, 1994; Rogers, EJ: Postanesthesia Care of the Cocaine Abuser.* J Post Anesth Nurs *6: 102-107, 1991.*

4.26. Correct Answer: **d**

The PACU nurse should always determine that the patient breathes adequately before turning to other possible causes! Hypoxic patients first become agitated, though very high pCO_2 levels (hypercarbia) cause sedation. Sedatives, anticholinergic medications, electrolyte disrangements, pain, and a full bladder also can produce central nervous system excitement. The exact incidence of wild agitation, disorientaton, and confusion after anesthesia (emergence delirium or excitement) is unknown, but age, surgical procedure, and intraoperative medications are factors. Young children and teens or patients with psychologic depression, significant alcohol use, or preoperative anxiety seem to have a higher likelihood of significant and extended agitation.

Litwack, K: Post Anesthesia Care Unit, *2nd ed. St. Louis, Mosby, pp. 452-454, 1995; Sloan, TB: Postoperative Central Nervous System Dysfunction in* Post Anesthesia Care *(Vender, JS & Speiss, BD, Eds). Saunders, Philadelphia, p. 196, 1992.*

4.27. Correct Answer: **b**

Physostigmine, an anticholinesterase medication that penetrates the blood-brain barrier, increases the concentration of acetylcholine in the neuromuscular junction and eases impulse transmission. Small doses of physostigmine titrated to effect can counter emergence delirium. This young man's response to emergence from anesthesia may relate to pain and fear; protection, safety and emotional support may be all that are needed to "ride out" this excitement phase.

Herbert, DW: Manual of Drugs in Anesthesia and Critical Care. *Philadelphia, Saunders, pp. 58-59, 1993; Roberts, CC & Okula, SN: The Pediatric Patient in* ASPAN's Core Curriculum for Post Anesthesia Nursing Practice, *3rd ed (Litwack, K, Ed). Philadelphia, Saunders, p. 74, 1994.*

4.28. Correct Answer: **c**

Bradycardia is one cholinergic response that can occur after physostigmine administration. In effect, cholinergic responses like bradycardia, bronchospasm, nausea, salivation, or incoordination can replace anticholinergic symptoms.

Herbert, DW: Manual of Drugs in Anesthesia and Critical Care. *Philadelphia, Saunders, pp. 58-59, 1993; Drain, C:* The Post Anesthesia Care Unit: A Critical Care Approach to Post Anesthesia Nursing, *3rd ed. Philadelphia, Saunders, pp. 209-210, 1994.*

4.29. Correct Answer: **d**

Resedation, with reoccurrence of respiratory depression, is the primary potential adverse effect following flumazenil administration. The selected dose of flumazenil may return the patient to a wakeful condition but be ineffective to completely reverse residual, recurrent effects of large or long-acting doses of benzodiazepines. Flumazenil does not reverse any effects of nonbenzodiazepine medications; renarcotization is possible.

Litwack, K: Post Anesthesia Care Nursing, *2nd ed. St. Louis, Mosby, p. 141, 1995; Product information: Flumazenil (Romazicon). Nutley, NJ, Roche Laboratories, 1994.*

4.30. Correct Answer: **a**

Succinylcholine (Anectine), the only depolarizing muscle relaxant, acts like acetylcholine at the skeletal muscle cell receptor site by binding to the receptor, then depolarizes the membrane. As long as succinylcholine occupies the receptor site, repolarization is blocked and acetylcholine has no effect. Therefore the cell membrane cannot depolarize for the next muscle contraction. Paralysis, usually of short duration, results. Unlike succinylcholine, vecuronium (Norcuron) is a nondepolarizing muscle relaxant with pharmacologically reversible effects.

Litwack, K: Managing Neuromuscular Blockade. Am J Nurs *93(11): 56B, 1993; Harbut, RD: Anesthetic Agents and Adjuncts in* ASPAN's Core Curriculum for Post Anesthesia Nursing Practice, *3rd ed. (Litwack, K, Ed). Philadelphia, Saunders, p. 97, 1994.*

4.31. Correct Answer: **b**

Tinnitus, circumoral tingling, blurred vision and confusion are among the symptoms of mild local anesthetic toxicity. Though intravascular absorption seldom occurs, the large volume of medication injected for epidural use *is* a potential risk. Symptoms abate with decreasing or discontinuing the infusion rate, increasing oxygen delivery and providing emotional support. Aspirating the epidural catheter to detect cerebrospinal fluid or blood is *essential* before initiating an epidural infusion.

Brown, DL: Atlas of Regional Anesthesia. *Philadelphia, Saunders, pp. 289-91, 1992; Riegler, FX: Spinal and Epidural Anestheisa in* Dripps/Eckenhoff/Vandam Introduction to Anesthesia, *8th ed (Longnecker, DE & Murphy, FL, Eds). Philadelphia, Saunders, p. 225, 1992.*

4.32. Correct Answer: **b**

Droperidol increases effects of intraoperative narcotics, producing sedation. It is a potent antiemetic and nonanalgesic major tranquilizer that mildly blocks alpha adrenergic receptors; vasodilation with hypotension is likely. At least 50% of patients experience nausea after strabismus surgery; discomfort and delays in discharge home may result.

Brett, CM, Zwass, MS & France, NK: Eyes, Ears, Nose, Throat, and Dental Surgery in Pediatric Anesthesia, *3rd ed (Gregory, GA, Ed). New York, Churchill & Livingstone, p. 685, 1994; Shannon, MT, Wilson, BA & Stang, CL:* Govoni & Hayes Drugs and Nursing Implications, *8th ed. Norwalk, CT, Appleton & Lange, pp. 446-447. 1995.*

4.33. Correct Answer: **d**

After the small anesthetic doses needed for a brief dental extraction, Ms D should be quickly conscious and possibly in need of *analgesia*. The surgical procedure was brief, so delayed resedation or muscle weakness from residual, tissue-stored medication is unlikely. If the biochemical banlance is normal, the rocuronium (Zemuron) should clear in less than 30 minutes or with reversal medications. Alfentanil (Alfenta) is much less potent than its prototype fentanyl; small doses have an effect for only 20 to 30 minutes. Moist packing occludes the posterior throat during surgery and prevents blood from moving past the mouth; airway obstruction from unremoved throat packing or gauze to provide postoperative gum pressure poses greater risk than vomiting a stomach full of blood. Dysreflexia is unlikely with cerebral palsy. Diffusion hypoxia with *shallow* breathing is a possibility for only 5-10 minutes after nitrous oxide is discontinued and so is unlikely in the PACU. A *"balanced anesthesia technique"* capitalizes on the cumulative effects of an inhalation anesthetic like nitrous oxide, a narcotic or barbiturate, and/or a muscle relaxant.

Drain, C: The Post Anesthesia Care Unit: A Critical Care Approach to Post Anesthesia Nursing, *3rd ed. Philadelphia, Saunders, pp. 201-202, 218 & 233, 1994; Burden, N:* Ambulatory Surgical Nursing. *Philadelphia, Saunders, pp. 484-485, 1993.*

4.34. Correct Answer: **b**

Metoclopramide (Reglan) blocks dopamine receptors in the chemoreceptor trigger zone (CTZ) to decrease emesis and also increases gastrointestinal motility to decrease gastric volume. Metoclopramide does not alter histamine receptors.

Altman, DF: Drugs Used in Gastrointestinal Diseases in Basic & Clinical Pharmacology, *6th ed*

(Katzung, BG, Ed). Norwalk, CT, Appleton & Lange, pp. 953-954, 1995; Drain, C: The Post Anesthesia Care Unit: A Critical Care Approach to Post Anesthesia Nursing, *3rd ed. Philadelphia, Saunders, p. 159, 1994.*

4.35. Correct Answer: **c**

Even though Mr. S received only one intraoperative dose of morphine, the effects can persist for hours. Researchers report depressed respiratory responses to hypercarbia 6-9 hours following epidural morphine dosing. Morphine is a hydrophilic narcotic and moves cephalad through the cerebrospinal fluid toward the respiratory center in the brain stem. Migration takes approximately 3-6 hours, with respiratory depression persisting for up to 12 hours. Pruritus from epidural morphine arises from its histamine release and is unassociated with allergic respiratory distress.

Wild, L & Coyne, C: The Basics and Beyond: Epidural Analgesia. Am J Nurs *92(4): 26-36, 1992; Gilbert, HC: Postoperative Pain Management in* Post Anesthesia Care *(Vender, JS & Speiss, BD. Eds). Philadelphia, Saunders, pp. 303-306, 1992.*

4.36. Correct Answer: **c**

The seizure activity produced during electroconvulsive therapy stimulates the sympathetic nervous system and increases catecholamine release. Until these subside, the patient often is hypertensive and tachycardic. Most patients have no consequences, but the occasional patient has cardiovascular or cerebral damage from additional oxygen demand.

O'Brien, D & Burden, N: The ASC as a Special Procedures Unit in Ambulatory Surgical Nursing *(Burden, N, Ed). Philadelphia, Saunders, pp. 580-581, 1993; Castro, AD: Management of Anesthesia for Specialty Procedures in* Dripps/Eckenhoff/Vandam Introduction to Anesthesia, *8th ed (Longnecker, DE & Murphy, FL, Eds). Philadelphia, Saunders, pp. 402-403, 1992.*

4.37. Correct Answer: **d**

Hypertensive crisis, hyperthermia, seizures, and rigidity have resulted when *meperidine* is given to a patient with circulating monoamine oxidase inhibitor (MAOI). The neurologic and vascular excitation can be fatal. Reactions with other narcotics are not as severe; when morphine sulfate is used, a dose reduction is considered sufficient. MAOI levels remain in the system for 3-4 weeks even after discontinuance. In addition, accumulation of meperidine metabolites after large analgesic doses can produce seizures.

Shannon, MT, Wilson, BA & Stang, CL: Govoni & Hayes Drugs and Nursing Implications, *8th ed. Norwalk, CT, Appleton & Lange, pp. 726-728, 1995; Skoog, RE: Monoamine Oxidase Inhibitors: Pharmacology and Implications in the Perioperative Period.* J Post Anesth Nurs *4(4): 264-267, 1989; Morgan, GE & Mikhail, MS:* Clinical Anesthesiology. *Norwalk, CT, Appleton & Lange, pp. 127 & 449, 1992.*

4.38. Correct Answer: **c**

Though consciousness is drug depressed, Mr. H must retain his ability to "independently and continuously maintain a patent airway." A patient under conscious sedation also responds "appropriately" to verbal or touch stimulation. An anesthesia provider need not be present, as management and monitoring of Mr. H during his procedure is within the PACU nurse's scope of practice.

American Society of Post Anesthesia Nursing (ASPAN): Standards of Perianesthesia Nursing Practice, Resource 14. Thorofare, NJ, ASPAN, pp. 54-55, 1995; Burden, N: Ambulatory Surgical Nursing. *Philadelphia, Saunders, pp. 139-149, 1993.*

4.39. Correct Answer: **b**

Medications for conscious sedation include medications classified as narcotics and sedatives but not as anesthetics. Sedatives decrease anxiety and discomfort but stop short of obliterating airway control or consciousness. Patients can still breathe and respond appropriately to verbal stimuli. Therefore doses are titrated to response lest they oversedate and anesthetize. Thiopental, propofol, ketamine and methohexital are classified as anesthetics.

American Society of Post Anesthesia Nursing (ASPAN): Standards of Perianesthesia Nursing Practice, Resource 14. Thorofare, NJ, ASPAN, pp. 54-58, 1995; Burden, N: Ambulatory Surgical Nursing *Philadelphia, Saunders, pp. 242-247, 1993.*

4.40. Correct Answer: **b**

Rapid entry of sodium into nerve cells is blocked by local anesthetics. The cell membrane retains an ongoing resting condition and does not respond to stimuli. The normal resting condition of a cell membrane is actually an ionized charge. Potassium ion (K^+) has free "access" into the nerve cell membrane, whereas access by sodium ion (Na^+) is restricted. Normally, when a depolarizing electrical stimulus alters cell membrane permeability, sodium ions flood in, producing an action potential and muscle contraction.

Drain, C: The Post Anesthesia Care Unit: A Critical Care Approach to Post Anesthesia Nursing, *3rd ed. Philadelphia, Saunders, pp. 245-246, 1994; Fetzer-Fowler, SJ: State of the Art: Regional Anesthesia Using Anesthetic Admixtures.* J Post Anesth Nurs *7(4): 229-237, 1992.*

SET II

Answer Key

4.41. a
4.42. b
4.43. c
4.44. b
4.45. d
4.46. c
4.47. a
4.48. d
4.49. c
4.50. c
4.51. a
4.52. c
4.53. d
4.54. c
4.55. a
4.56. d
4.57. c
4.58. c
4.59. c
4.60. a
4.61. b
4.62. c
4.63. c
4.64. a
4.65. c
4.66. a
4.67. d
4.68. c
4.69. b
4.70. c
4.71. b
4.72. a
4.73. b
4.74. d
4.75. b
4.76. a
4.77. c
4.78. d
4.79. b
4.80. d
4.81. c
4.82. a

SET II

Rationales and References

4.41. Correct Answer: **a**

Stimulating alpha adrenergic receptors with epinephrine is universally accepted as a predictor of successful short-term resuscitation outcomes. By improving perfusion pressures, blood flow and oxygenation of vital organs, vasoactive drugs increase the likelihood of successful defibrillation. Sodium bicarbonate is used cautiously and sparingly during CPR to treat only documented metabolic acidosis. Lidocaine, a Class I antiarrhythmic, may increase the amount of defibrillation energy (joules) needed to reverse ventricular fibrillation.

American Heart Association: Textbook of Advanced Cardiac Life Support *(Cummins, RO, Ed). Dallas, American Heart Association, pp. 1.18 & 7.2-7.5, 1994; Herrmann, DJ & Raehl, CL: Optimizing Resuscitiation Outcomes With Pharmacologic Therapy.* Crit Care Clin North Am *5(2): 247-259, 1993.*

4.42. Correct Answer: **b**

With these short-acting, nonnarcotic medications, providing adequate analgesia will become an early nursing priority. Most likely, this patient will arrive in PACU strong, alert, hemodynamically stable, breathing well—and in pain. Desflurane, an inhalation anesthetic, rocuronium bromide (Zemuron), a nondepolarizing muscle relaxant, and midazolam (Versed), a benzodiazepine, have a brief duration of action and no analgesic properties. Any interaction between residual midazolam and narcotic analgesics given in PACU could increase the effects of both, so the PACU nurse does consider this patient's potential for new respiratory depression.

Drain, C: The Post Anesthesia Care Unit: A Critical Care Approach to Post Anesthesia Nursing, *3rd ed. Philadelphia, Saunders, pp. 198-201, 208-209, & 233, 1994; Litwack, K:* Post Anesthesia Care Nursing, *2nd ed. St. Louis, Mosby, pp. 130-132, 139-140, & 145-147, 1995.*

4.43. Correct Answer: **c**

Halothane, enflurane, isoflurane, and desflurane are volatile inhalation anesthetics that historically have induced an episode of malignant hyperthermia (MH). A rare genetic predisposition and exposure to specific stimuli may combine to produce this potentially life-threatening crisis. Often a patient has no awareness of genetic susceptibility.

Litwack, K: Post Anesthesia Care Nursing, *2nd ed. St. Louis, Mosby, pp. 470-471, 1995; Rosenberg, H: Malignant Hyperthermia in* ASPAN's Core Curriculum for Post Anesthesia Nursing Practice, *3rd ed (Litwack, K, Ed). Philadelphia, Saunders, p. 234, 1994.*

4.44. Correct Answer: **b**

Creating a more alkaline solution speeds a local anesthetic's onset of action. Bicarbonate increases the medication's pH to promote a more lipophilic environment. The cell membrane of a nerve fiber more readily admits lipid-liking solutions. As a result, sodium channels are more rapidly penetrated and blocked by lipophilic solutions. Potency and protein binding are more related to duration than onset of action.

Fetzer-Fowler, SJ: State of the Art: Regional Anesthesia Using Anesthetic Admixtures. J Post Anesth Nurs *7(4): 229-237, 1992; Covino, BG & Lambert, DM: Pharmacology of Local Anesthetics in* Dripps/Eckenhoff/Vandam Introduction to Anesthesia, *8th ed (Longnecker, DE & Murphy, FL, Eds). Philadelphia, Saunders, pp. 198-207, 1992.*

4.45. Correct Answer: **d**

Dilation of veins and large arteries is the expected response from nitroglycerin. Venous return, and therefore preload, decrease and ease myocardial work. Fluid volume shifts or stress arising from surgical manipulations and anesthetic medications can increase myocardial work and oxygen demand; as a result, a patient with a cardiac history like Mr. T's can easily develop angina.

Katzung, BG & Chatterjee, K: Vasodilators and the Treatment of Angina Pectoris in Basic and Clinical Pharmacology, *6th ed (Katzung, BG, Ed). Norwalk, CT, Appleton & Lange, pp. 172-178, 1995; Drain C:* The Post Anesthesia Care Unit: A Critical Care Approach to Post Anesthesia Nursing. *Philadelphia, Saunders, p. 102, 1994.*

4.46. Correct Answer: **c**

To best promote conversion of ventricular fibrillation, administer epinephrine and lidocaine before delivering electrical shock. Allow 30 seconds (no longer than 1 minute) of circulation time to allow the drug to have a physiologic impact and "pave the way" for the electrical defibrillation energy. Defibrillation, not the medications, will convert the rhythm.

Saver, CL: Decoding the ACLS Algorithms. Am J Nurs *94(1): 27-35, 1994; American Heart Association:* Textbook of Advanced Cardiac Life Support *(Cummins, RO, Ed). Dallas, American Heart Association, p. 1.18, 1994.*

4.47. Correct Answer: **a**

Bupivacaine, or any local anesthestic, injected into the lumbar epidural space can block motor and sensory nerves. Inability to stand and a feeling of leg heaviness may occur. Orthostatic hypotension results from the medication-induced vasodilation and impaired vascular response to decreasing venous return. All these factors will delay ambulation.

Wild, L & Coyne, C: The Basics and Beyond. Am J Nurs *92(4): 26-36, 1992; Gilbert, HG: Postoperative Pain Management in* Post Anesthesia Care *(Vender, JS & Speiss, BD, Eds). Philadelphia, Saunders, pp. 308-311, 1992.*

4.48. Correct Answer: **d**

Researchers believe opioid agonists like morphine and its derivatives act primarily on mu opioid receptors by imitating the effects of endogenous endorphins. Effects of action on mu receptors include euphoria, analgesia and respiratory depression. Kappa receptors also are stimulated, producing miosis and sedation with additional respiratory depressant and analgesic effects.

Litwack, K & Drain, CB: Pain Assessment and Management in ASPAN's Core Curriculum for

Post Anesthesia Nursing Practice, *3rd ed (Litwack, K, Ed). Philadelphia, Saunders, pp. 648-649, 1994.*

4.49. Correct Answer: **c**

Standard intravenous tubing is made of polyvinyl chloride (plastic) and absorbs nitroglycerin. Therefore nitroglycerin is prepared in a *glass* bottle and infused with a volume infusion pump through a nonabsorbing administration set.

Drain C: The Post Anesthesia Care Unit: A Critical Care Approach to Post Anesthesia Nursing. *Philadelphia, Saunders, p. 102, 1994.*

4.50. Correct Answer: **c**

Succinylcholine is widely used to facilitate intubation and is the muscle relaxant of choice for emergency intubation and to interrupt laryngospasm. However, specific patient groups should not receive this depolarizing muscle relaxant. Succinylcholine increases intracranial and intraocular pressures. Lethal hyperkalemia can result if succinylcholine is given to a patient with recent spinal cord or neuromuscular damage or catabolic conditions like burns, severe trauma or sepsis. Children and adolescents may have undiagnosed myopathies, so succinylcholine is not recommended for pediatric anesthesia *except* to manage a child's airway emergency.

Drain, C: The Post Anesthesia Care Unit: A Critical Care Approach to Post Anesthesia Nursing, *3rd ed. Philadelphia, Saunders, pp. 234-237, 1994; Harbut, RD: Anesthetic Agents and Adjuncts in* ASPAN's Core Curriculum for Post Anesthesia Nursing Practice, *3rd ed. Philadelphia, Saunders, pp. 97-101, 1994.*

4.51. Correct Answer: **a**

One determinant of a local anesthetic's duration of action is its length of contact time with a nerve fiber. Adding a vasoconstrictor like epinephrine to the solution decreases local blood flow and delays the rate of tetracaine's absorption, thereby increasing its contact time. More nerve cells can be affected by tetracaine's sodium channel blockade. A sitting position produces a more *localized,* not a widely distributed, block; adding *bicarbonate* to adjust pH and create a more alkaline solution allows rapid diffusion for earlier onset of effect.

Fetzer-Fowler, SJ: State of the Art: Regional Anesthesia Using Anesthetic Admixtures. J Post Anesth Nurs *7(4): 229-237, 1992; Riegler, FX: Spinal and Epidural Anesthetia in* Dripps/Eckenhoff/Vandam Introduction to Anesthesia, *8th ed (Longnecker, DE & Murphy, FL, Eds). Philadelphia, Saunders, pp. 218-220, 1992.*

4.52. Correct Answer: **c**

Vecuronium (Norcuron) is an intermediate-acting, nondepolarizing muscle relaxant. Adequate relaxation lasts about 30 minutes. Within 65 minutes, 95% of an injected dose of vecuronium is metabolized. Normal temperature and biochemical (acid-base and electrolytes) balance facilitate rapid metabolism. Vecuronium has no cardiovascular effects, no histamine release and little (only about 20%) biliary or renal excretion.

Litwack, K: Managing Neuromuscular Blockade. Am J Nurs *93(11): 56B, 1993; Burden, N:* Ambulatory Surgical Nursing. *Philadelphia, Saunders, p. 73, 1993.*

4.53. Correct Answer: **d**

Bretylium tosylate is very likely to produce significant hypotension. Vasopressors and fluid volume may be needed. Bretylium is a Class III antiarrhythmic used to treat lidocaine-resistant ventricular tachycardia (VT) or fibrillation (VF). Bretylium extends the repolarization phase of the cardiac cycle by increasing the length of both the action potential and the refractory period. Transient tachycardia or hypertension likely will resolve without intervention; any nausea is more related to rapid injection rather than continuous infusion of bretylium.

Herrmann, DJ: Optimizing Resuscitation Outcomes with Pharmacologic Therapy. Crit Care Clin North Am. *5(2): 257, 1993; American Heart Association:* Textbook of Advanced Cardiac Life Support *(Cummins, RO, Ed). Dallas, American Heart Association, pp. 7-9 to 7-11, 1994.*

4.54. Correct Answer: **c**

Flumazenil (Romazicon) is classified as a benzodiazepine receptor antagonist that inhibits the *respiratory depressant* effects of benzodiazepines like diazepam (Valium) or midazolam on the central nervous system. The PACU nurse should *avoid* flumazenil for the patient who regularly uses benzodiazepine medications since the risk of seizures increases. In addition, the epileptic patient or a patient with tricyclic antidepressant overdose should not receive flumazenil.

Litwack, K: Post Anesthesia Care Nursing, *2nd ed. St. Louis, Mosby, p. 141, 1995; Roche: Product information: Flumazenil (Romazicon). Nutley, NJ, Roche Laboratories, 1994.*

4.55. Correct Answer: **a**

Intrathecal medications are delivered between the pia mater and arachnoid. Injecting narcotic or local anesthetic medications into this cerebrospinal fluid–containing subarachnoid space provides spinal anesthesia. The pia mater is vascular and is most adjacent to the spinal cord. The thin arachnoid lies between the pia mater and the tougher dura mater.

Brown, DL: Atlas of Regional Anesthesia. *Philadelphia, Saunders, pp. 263-265, 1992; Stalheim-Smith, A & Fitch, GK:* Understanding Human Anatomy and Physiology. *Minneapolis/St. Paul, West Publishing, pp. 410-416, 1994.*

4.56. Correct Answer: **d**

A lipophilic, or "fat-liking" medication has a high affinity to penetrate lipid molecules. Fat-soluble medications released back into circulation can reexert physiologic effect. Lipophilic medications like fentanyl move from the circulation into the fat and then diffuse back into blood as serum concentrations metabolize and clear.

Wild, L & Coyne, C: The Basics and Beyond: Epidural Analgesia. Am J Nurs *92(4): 26-36, 1992.*

4.57. Correct Answer: **c**

Morphine causes histamine release and resultant localized redness, hives, swelling, and pruritus. Histamine's effect on H_1 receptors dilates local blood vessels and increases capillary permeability and is only a "minor contributor" to true anaphylaxis.

O'Hara, DA: Opioids in Anesthesia Practice in Dripps/Eckenhoff/Vandam Introduction to Anesthesia, *8th ed (Longnecker, DE & Murphy, FL, Eds). Philadelphia, Saunders, p. 106, 1992; Lehne, RA:* Pharmacology for Nursing Care, *Philadelphia, Saunders, pp. 676-678, 1990.*

4.58. Correct Answer: **c**

Unlike morphine, sufentanil rarely stimulates histamine release and produces little itching. Resedation and delayed, recurring hypoventilation and apnea are highly likely; naloxone's effect is shorter than the residual sufentanil's. Even though Mr. S is healthy and now appears awake, the normal physiologic changes associated with Mr. S's age *can* prolong sufentanil's action. In addition, enflurane was administered for most of Mr. S's 6 hour surgery; slow release of this medication stored in fat and muscle can further delay emergence. Enflurane is also associated with postanesthetic shivering that is unrelated to hypothermia. Naloxone can reverse analgesia while improving respiratory function; *cautiously* treat back pain or muscle spasms and hip pain (the bone graft donor site) with narcotics. Headache may indicate dural leak of cerebrospinal fluid and/or menengeal irritation.

Drain, C: The Post Anesthesia Care Unit: A Critical Care Approach to Post Anesthesia Nursing, *3rd ed. Philadelphia, Saunders, p. 218 & 544-548, 1994; Sphritz, DW: The Neurosurgical Patient in* ASPAN's Core Curriculum for Post Anesthesia Nursing Practice, *3rd ed (Litwack, K, Ed). Philadelphia, Saunders, pp. 387-392, 1994.*

4.59. Correct Answer: **c**

Acetaminophen frequently is sufficient to manage a child's postsurgical pain, though Jason could receive dilute, titrated doses of fentanyl 1-2 mcg/kg or morphine sulfate 0.05-0.1 mg/kg and astute respiratory monitoring. *Cautiously* infuse Jason's fluids to prevent fluid overload. Only 4 ml/kg/h, or 25 ml/h for Jason, is usual—he weighs only 6.3 kg. Give minute fluid boluses in about 20 ml volumes. Preventing temperature loss is critical to assure Jason's physiologic stability and metabolism of medications, but overwarming is unnecessary. Infants under stress have high glucose needs but minimal stored glucose (glycogen), so regular monitoring of serum glucose is important. However, routine infusion of glucose risks hyperglycemia, which is linked with poor resuscitation outcomes.

Cauldwell, CB: Induction, Maintenance and Emergence in Pediatric Anesthesia, *3rd ed (Gregory, GA, Ed). New York, Churchill-Livingstone, pp. 245-257, 1994; American Heart Association:* Textbook of Advanced Cardiac Life Support *(Cummins, RO, Ed). Dallas, American Heart Association, pp. 1-63 to 1-64, 1994.*

4.60. Correct Answer: **a**

Jason's rapid heart rate, near the upper limit of the infant "normal" range, likely is a response to his pain and agitation, not a reflex response to fluid deficit. Emergence delirium is more common in toddlers over 1 year and young children. Support Jason's legs with a hand or blanket after herniorrhaphy to help decrease stretching and pressure in his abdominal and inguinal tissues. Titrate small doses of analgesic medication to effect. Blood pressure is near his age-normal range and requires ongoing assessment as pain abates.

American Heart Association: Textbook of Advanced Cardiac Life Support *(Cummins, RO, Ed). Dallas, American Heart Association, pp. 1-63 to 1-64, 1994; Roberts, CC & Okula, NS: The Pediatric Patient in* ASPAN's Core Curriculum for Post Anesthesia Nursing Practice, *3rd ed (Litwack, K, Ed). Philadelphia, Saunders, pp. 63-76, 1994.*

4.61. Correct Answer: **b**

Regional anesthesia by epidural, spinal or nerve block techniques is preferred for MH-susceptible patients. Lidocaine has been considered a "weak triggering" agent of malignant hyperthermia episodes but many experts do consider it safe, particularly for regional anesthesia. Prophylactic treatment with dantrolene sodium typically precedes general anesthetic procedures. Nontriggering anesthetic medications like nitrous oxide, barbiturates, thiopental, droperidol, opioids and *non*depolarizing muscle relaxants can be safely administered to the MH-susceptible patient.

Litwack-Saleh, K: Practical Points in the Management of Malignant Hyperthermia. J Post Anesth Nurs *7: 327-329, 1992; Morgan, GE & Mikhail, MS:* Clinical Anesthesiology. *Norwalk, CT, Appleton & Lange, pp. 640-642, 1992.*

4.62. Correct Answer: **c**

Depolarizing effect of succinylcholine on the muscle lingers only briefly, only 3-8 minutes for a dose of 1-2 mg/kg. Metabolism by pseudocholinesterase begins almost immediately after injection and is extremely rapid.

Litwack, K: Managing Neuromuscular Blockade. Am J Nurs *93(11): 56B, 1993; Drain, C:* The Post Anesthesia Care Unit: A Critical Care Approach to Post Anesthesia Nursing, *3rd ed. Philadelphia, Saunders, pp. 234-237, 1994.*

4.63. Correct Answer: **c**

Acidosis related to elevated carbon dioxide *inhibits* effects of a depolarizing muscle relaxant, shortening the duration of action. Succinylcholine is hydrolyzed by a plasma enzyme, pseudocholinesterase. Anticholinesterase medications like neostigmine, reduced serum albumin, hypovolemia and dehydration, propranolol, significant anemia, and malnutrition prolong succinylcholine's action by inhibiting pseudocholinesterase.

Harbut, RD: Anesthetic Agents and Adjuncts in ASPAN's Core Curriculum for Post Anesthesia Nursing Practice, *3rd ed (Litwick, K, Ed). Philadelphia, Saunders, pp. 97-101, 1994; Morgan, GE & Mikhail, MS:* Clinical Anesthesiology. *Norwalk, CT, Appleton & Lange, pp. 138-141, 1992.*

4.64. Correct Answer: **a**

Sodium nitroprusside (Nipride) dilates both veins and arteries, thereby significantly reducing vascular resistance to cardiac ejection (afterload) and venous return (preload). Sodium nitroprusside is a "potent and efficatious" antihypertensive and has near-immediate effects.

Whalen, DA & Izzi, G: Pharmacologic Treatment of Acute Congestive Heart Failure Resulting From

Left Ventricular Systolic or Diastolic Dysfunction. Crit Care Clin North Am *5(2): 261-269, 1993; American Heart Association:* Textbook of Advanced Cardiac Life Support *(Cummins, RO, Ed). Dallas, American Heart Association, pp. 8-8 to 8-9, 1994.*

4.65. Correct Answer: **c**

A regional anesthetic technique for carotid endarterectomy apparently reduces the potential for postoperative hypertension and intraoperative myocardial infarction while decreasing the brain's metabolic demand and increasing cerebral blood flow. The need to insert a shunt into the artery to maintain cerebral blood flow during carotid occlusion is determined by balancing the risk of intraoperative embolism vs. preventing adequate cerebral blood flow.

Johnson, SM & Anderson, B: Carotid Endarterectomy: A Review. Crit Care Clin North Am *3(2): 499-505, 1991;*

4.66. Correct Answer: **a**

Rupture of the carotid artery or "blow out" of a patch graft produces rapid, airway-compressing hemorrhage into the neck. Life-threatening tracheal deviation with labored breathing, wheezing, and stridor results and may not be relieved until the wound is reopened or a tracheostomy is created. Incidence of hematoma is low, about 1-4%, and most incidences are related to hypertension and continued influence of antiplatelet medications. Carotid body damage does disturb respiratory quality, though far less acutely than hemorrhage does.

Johnson, SM & Anderson, B: Carotid Endarterectomy: A Review. Crit Care Clin North Am *3(3): 499-505, 1991; Fode, NC: Carotid Endarterectomy: Nursing Care and Controversies.* J Neurosci Nurs *22(1): 25-30, 1990.*

4.67. Correct Answer: **d**

Anatomically, the vagus nerve lies near the carotid artery and its function is easily disturbed by intraoperative retraction, edema or trauma. Bradycardia could alter cerebral blood flow and neurologic responses. Reflex hypotension with bradycardia occurs 1-5 hours postoperatively and is associated with hypovolemia or vagal stimulation after vasodilators are used to treat extreme postoperative hypertension.

Johnson, SM & Anderson, B: Carotid Endarterectomy: A Review. Crit Care Clin North Am *3(3): 499-505, 1991; Lowdon, JD & Isaacson, IJ: Postoperative Considerations After Major Vascular Surgery in* Post Anesthesia Care *(Vender, JS & Speiss, BD, Eds). Philadelphia, Saunders, pp. 120-124, 1992.*

4.68. Correct Answer: **c**

The universal algorithm for adult emergency cardiac care, one of several advanced cardiac life support (ACLS) protocols, indicates assessment of responsiveness as the very first approach to the emergency patient.

Saver, CL: Decoding the ACLS Algorithms. Am J Nurs *94(1): 27-35, 1994; American Heart Association:* Textbook of Advanced Cardiac Life Support *(Cummins, RO, Ed). Dallas, American Heart Association, p. 1-12, 1994.*

4.69. Correct Answer: **b**

Mr. P's heart will not respond to parasympathetic blockade with atropine. Should he develop clinical symptoms (hypotension or decreased sensorium) related to myocardial suppression with bradycardia, interventions include supporting heart rate and contractility with catecholamine infusion of epinephrine, cardiac pacing, or perhaps isoproterenol. A transplanted heart has no autonomic innervation because the cardiac nerve supply is severed during harvesting from the donor. Dopamine will also appropriately support his cardiac output, but the dose should be titrated at 2-10 mcg/kg, unless Mr. P develops severe hemodynamic instability.

American Heart Association: Textbook of Advanced Cardiac Life Support *(Cummins, RO, Ed). Dallas, American Heart Association, pp. 1-28 to 1-32, 1994; Weber, BL: Cardiac Surgery and Heart Transplantation in* Critical Care Nursing: A Holistic Approach, *6th ed (Hudak, CM & Gallo, BM, Eds). Philadelphia, Lippincott, pp. 374-375, 1994.*

4.70. Correct Answer: **c**

Mr. P's rhythm still should be sinus, but the PACU nurse should anticipate that his heart rate will border on tachycardia. A range of 90-110 beats per minute is usual. Lack of vagal tone (parasympathetic influence) on the denervated transplanted heart makes the heart beat more rapidly.

Weber, BL: Cardiac Surgery and Heart Transplantation in Critical Care Nursing: A Holistic Approach, *6th ed (Hudak, CM & Gallo, BM, Eds). Philadelphia, Lippincott, pp. 374-375, 1994.*

4.71. Correct Answer: **b**

Position-related orthostatic hypotension is likely; after transplantation, cardiac output changes occur gradually in response to stress or venous pooling. Changes of rate and contractile force by Mr. P's transplanted heart are not immediate. Release of catecholamines from the adrenals provide the increased cardiac output within minutes, a different response than the immediate reflex tachycardia that occurs in the innervated heart. Angina, autonomic rate changes and respiratory variation do not occur in denervated, transplanted hearts.

Weber, BL: Cardiac Surgery and Heart Transplantation in Critical Care Nursing: A Holistic Approach, *6th ed (Hudak, CM & Gallo, BM, Eds). Philadelphia, Lippincott, pp. 374-375, 1994.*

4.72. Correct Answer: **a**

Etomidate is an intravenous *hypnotic* with a brief (less than 15 minutes) duration of effect that can be safely given to neurosurgical and eye patients. Both intraocular and intracranial pressures decrease with etomidate; influence (depressant or stimulant) on the heart is minor. Etomidate is not recommended for infusion; one dose can suppress corticosteroid secretion for 8 hours and an infusion for up to 4 days. Etomidate is not an analgesic and does not alter pain perception.

Drain, C: The Post Anesthesia Care Unit: A Critical Care Approach to Post Anesthesia Nursing, *3rd ed. Philadelphia, Saunders, pp. 206-207, 1994.*

4.73. Correct Answer: **b**

Anesthetic implications related to Ms O's ophthalmic timolol arise from timolol's beta blocking effects. Topical ophthalmic medications are absorbed through ocular tissue and can produce systemic effects. Airway constriction with spasm and significant myocardial depression with bradycardia could occur. Risk increases if Ms O has a history of pulmonary edema or congestive heart failure. Timolol is a nonselective beta blocker and is often used to reduce intraocular pressure to treat glaucoma. Effects of ophthalmic doses persist for about 12 hours.

Kelsey, M: Ophthalmic Medications, Glaucoma and the Surgical Patient. J Post Anesth Nurs *7(5): 312-316, 1992; Morgan, GE & Mikhail, MS:* Clinical Anesthesiology. *Norwalk, CT, Appleton & Lange, p. 385, 1992.*

4.74. Correct Answer: **d**

A patient with multiple food and drug allergies is among patients with greater risk to develop latex allergy. Specifically, allergies to bananas, chestnuts and avocados are associated with latex hypersensitivity. The nurse should advise the anesthesia provider and surgeon of these allergies, watch Ms C for skin sensitivity and airway reactivity and prepare to remove, substitute or cover all environmental sources of latex. Direct skin contact can cause urticaria; airborne latex particles can stimulate asthma.

Benner, SD: Latex Allergy. CPANewsletter *pp. 3-4, 8 Nov, 1994; Markey, J: Latex Allergy.* J Intravenous Nurs *17(1): 35-39, 1994.*

4.75. Correct Answer: **b**

Mr. A will probably require higher narcotic levels or more frequent dosing to achieve adequate analgesia. Chronic intake of alcohol, barbiturates, opioids, or benzodiazepines increases anesthetic requirements. He has likely developed tolerance and some psychologic and physical dependence to his alcohol. His actual alcohol use may also be understated.

Morgan, GE & Mikhail, MS: Clinical Anesthesiology. *Norwalk, CT, Appleton & Lange, pp. 450-451, 1992; Drain, C:* The Post Anesthesia Care Unit: A Critical Care Approach to Post Anesthesia Nursing, *3rd ed. Philadelphia, Saunders, p. 560, 1994.*

4.76. Correct Answer: **a**

Hyperventilation assures carbon dioxide elimination, and delivering 100% oxygen promotes cellular oxygenation. The hypermetabolism of a malignant hyperthermia crisis rapidly produces acidosis. Other interventions occur simultaneously but are time consuming: ice the body with lavages and cooling blankets; infuse iced *normal saline;* prepare dantrolene, a process that requires time and many hands.

Rosenberg, H: Malignant Hyperthermia in ASPAN's Core Curriculum for Post Anesthesia Nursing Practice, *3rd ed (Litwack, K, Ed). Philadelphia, Saunders, pp. 236-237, 1994.*

4.77. Correct Answer: **c**

An *acute* decrease in response to a medication that is repeatedly injected or continuously infused is termed tachyphylaxis. The cause is unknown, though theoretically this phenomenon may relate to altered pH at the nerve cell membrane. With regard to local anesthetics, increasing the epidural dose may increase the anesthetic effect but may also significantly increase the risk of local anesthetic toxicity.

Burden, N: Ambulatory Surgical Nursing. *Philadelphia, Saunders, p. 82, 1993; Drain, C:* The Post Anesthesia Care Unit: A Critical Care Approach to Post Anesthesia Nursing, *3rd ed. Philadelphia, Saunders, p. 181, 1994.*

4.78. Correct Answer: **d**

Hypotension often *is* associated with thermal rewarming, though Mr. P's tympanic temperature, a reflection of his core body temperature, has been near normal since admission to PACU. Even his temperature rise over the 90 minute PACU stay was small and probably would not account for marked rewarming vasodilation. Residual tetracaine effect is more likely than rewarming to produce ongoing vasodilation, hypotension and heat *loss* for Mr. P. Undetected and continuing volume loss (bleeding or perhaps fluid translocation) must be considered when a patient has persistent, unresolving hypotension. The PACU nurse should look closely for bleeding into Mr. P's tissues, beneath him for hidden pools of drainage, for oozing from suture sites and at the rate and volume of drainage collecting in any wound drain. A new myocardial infarction with "pump failure" may also account for persistent hypotension. Though postoperative hypotension remains a common, almost daily occurrence in PACU, Mr. P's situation calls for diligent scrutiny for the cause. After 90 minutes, a continued (automatic) response with vasopressors and hydration is not sufficient.

Litwack, K: Post Anesthesia Care Nursing, *2nd ed. St. Louis, Mosby, pp. 462-470, 1995.*

4.79. Correct Answer: **b**

Single, isolated premature ventricular contractions (PCVs), like Mr. P's wide, early QRS complexes, usually are observed and not immediately treated with medication. PVCs, or "warning arrhythmias," may signal electrolyte imbalance, hypoxemia, or myocardial muscle damage. The PACU nurse should administer oxygen and treat the cause of the PVC rather than suppress the arrhythmia. Even during an evolving myocardial infarction, lidocaine is only used if PVCs are associated with angina or recurring hypotension. Overriding "escape" PVCs by increasing heart rate with atropine is appropriate with symptomatic bradycardia—often a heart rate of 40-50 beats per minute and hypotension; lidocaine is *never* used to suppress PVCs related to bradycardia with ventricular escape beats.

American Heart Association: Textbook of Advanced Cardiac Life Support *(Cummins, RO, Ed). Dallas, American Heart Association, pp. 1-29 to 1-31, 3-7 to 3-9, & 9-3 to 9-4, 1994.*

4.80. Correct Answer: **d**

The advanced cardiac life support tachycardia algorithm recommends providing oxygen, determining hemodynamic stability and administering lidocaine 1-1.5 mg/kg as the first-choice medication for the *stable* patient with ventricular tachycardia. Lidocaine is also appropriate when the origin (ventricular vs. supraventricular) of a wide QRS tachycardia is not clearly established. A series of wide QRS complexes that occur regularly between 100-220 times per minute describes ventricular tachycardia. The PACU nurse must *never give verapamil* to a patient with ventricular tachycardia; use verapamil only when absolutely certain the rhythm is *supra*ventricular. Immediate cardioversion is recommended only for the hemodynamically *un*stable patient or when ventricular tachycardia exceeds 150 beats per minute.

American Heart Association: Textbook of Advanced Cardiac Life Support *(Cummins, RO, Ed). Dallas, American Heart Association, pp. 1-37 to 1-38, 3-6 to 3-7 & 3-19 to 3-20, 1994.*

4.81. Correct Answer: **c**

Administering isoflurane (Forane) for longer than 60 minutes is likely to delay emergence. Normally, patients waken quickly (within one half hour) after the flow of isoflurane gas stops. For lengthy surgical procedures, however, ongoing exposure to isoflurane is needed to maintain brain saturation and anesthesia; isoflurane then "deposits" into less vascular tissues like muscle, fat, or skin, potentially saturating those tissues as well. The inhaled anesthetic must redistribute from tissues back into the blood to circulate to the lungs for elimination. Isoflurane's ready solubility and low blood-gas partition coefficient mean the patient receives a large dose of the inhalation anesthetic to maintain saturation and clinical effect. Halothane, not isoflurane, has been (controversially) associated with clinical evidence of hepatitis.

Drain, C: The Post Anesthesia Care Unit: A Critical Care Approach to Post Anesthesia Nursing, *3rd ed. Philadelphia, Saunders, pp. 192-194 & 200, 1994.*

4.82. Correct Answer: **a**

Morphine sulfate can increase spasm of the sphincter of Oddi, which can further increase the pain of a preoperative patient with biliary obstruction or gall bladder disease. The intense symptoms of this spasm can resemble cardiac pain. Morphine is specifically selected for both its analgesic and hemodynamic effects for patients with evolving myocardial infarction and acute pulmonary edema.

American Heart Association: Textbook of Advanced Cardiac Life Support *(Cummins, RO, Ed). Dallas, American Heart Association, pp. 1-50 to 1-51, 1994; O'Brien, DD: The Gastrointestinal Surgical Patient in* ASPAN's Core Curriculum for Post Anesthesia Nursing Practice, *3rd ed (Litwack, K, Ed). Philadelphia, Saunders, p. 451, 1994.*

Section 5

The Spectrum of Perianesthesia Clinical Practice

Scenarios and items in this section represent situations that illustrate perianesthesia nursing practice. This specialty is defined by a set of knowledge and skills related to *anesthetic medications, techniques* and *surgical manipulations* that significantly alter a patient's organ systems. These concepts are considered together because the clinical nurse:

- focuses on anesthesia-induced alterations of airway, circulation, consciousness and neurologic function that require astute nursing consideration, whether for 5 minutes or 5 hours
- hones this unique body of knowledge for an infinite number of highly individual patient situations
- synthesizes and applies concepts from multiple clinical disciplines to a diverse clinical spectrum, perhaps an infant, a critically ill trauma patient, a frail elderly woman after eye surgery and a depressed patient after electroshock therapy—all in one day
- distinguishes priorities from a potpourri of varied and often simultaneous concerns

Essential Core Concepts	Affiliated Core Curriculum Chapters
Nursing Process	
Assess	
Plan and Implement	Chapters 2 & 14
Evaluate	
Perianesthesia Spectrum	
Situational Applications	
Anesthetics	
Minimum Alveolar Concentration, Potency	
Pharmacodynamics	
Pharmacokinetics	
Receptors and Blocks	
Regional, Local General or Balanced	
Standards	
Perianesthesia Units and Beyond	
Preanesthesia to Discharge Education	
Priorities: Imminent Need, or Remote Potential	

Surgical Manipulations
- Cautery and Blood Loss
- Position, Injury and Pain

Clinical Continuums

Airway: From Patency to Obstruction
Awareness: From Delays to Delirium
Cardiac: From Heartbeat to Heart Failure
Consciousness: From Sedation to Self-Awareness
Hemodynamics: From Hemorrhage to Hemostasis
- From Hypotension to Hypertension
- From Vessel Patency to Stagnation

Immunity: From Allergy to Sepsis
Nausea: From Retching to Relief
Neurologic: From Deficit to Function
Oxygenation: From Hypoxia to Toxicity
Pain: From Angst to Contentment
Pulmonary: From Ventilation to Apnea
- From Croup to Aspiration

Temperature: From Shivers to Sweats

SET I

Items 5.1-5.30

5.1. Of the following four postanesthesia patients in PACU, the patient with the *greatest* risk of pulmonary aspiration is:

a. receiving parenteral nutrition and swallows before extubation
b. elderly, weighs 40 kg, and rests in semi-Folwer's position
c. a smoker with a harsh, dry cough and who received metoclopramide
d. healthy, drowsy, and 6 months pregnant

NOTE: Consider scenario and items 5.2-5.4 together.

It's 1 AM in PACU and a combative and frightened young woman states severe back pain and right leg numbness. Two hours ago her fourth back surgery, a T-3 to L-1 spinal fusion with insertion of rods and bolts, ended. The neurosurgeon elects to repeat computed tomography (CT) scanning and magnetic resonance imaging (MRI). The PACU nurse administered midazolam 1 mg intravenously after collaboration with the anesthesiologist and intends to accompany the patient to the radiology department.

5.2. The *most immediate* nursing priority for this patient is to:

a. provide amnesia for a claustrophobic event
b. continue chemical restraint to prevent injury
c. assess respiratory quality for altered function
d. monitor neurologic status to detect deterioration

5.3. This midazolam dose will *most* affect this patient's recall of:

a. claustrophobic feelings during the MRI
b. recognition of her husband for 4 hours after MRI
c. combative emergence behaviors in PACU
d. intraoperative wake-up during today's surgery

5.4. To deliver the safest care to this patient during this procedure, the nurse and physician consult and plan that:

a. midazolam will be repeated at 5 minute intervals
b. the anesthesiologist will reintubate this woman
c. respiratory monitoring will continue during MRI
d. midazolam reversal will occur after MRI completion

NOTE: Consider scenario and item 5.5 together.

During the admission report of a drowsy, actively shivering patient, the anesthesia provider states that intraoperative electrocautery was used. The PACU nurse determines an apical pulse and assesses this patient's DDI pacemaker function on EKG.

5.5. The nurse now expects to observe the following pacemaker responses *except:*

a. magnet-protected DDI programming
b. fixed rate function
c. pacing in the VOO mode
d. absent stimulation

NOTE: Consider scenario and item 5.6 together.

Thirty minutes after arrival in PACU following general anesthesia, Ms. D remains nonresponsive to voice or touch stimuli, has pinpoint, equal pupils and consistent vital signs. BP = 104/56, heart rate = 96 and regular, respiratory rate = 12 breaths per minute.

5.6. Determining reasons for Ms. D's delayed arousal, the PACU nurse considers adequate ventilation and any of the following factors *except:*

a. insulin-dependent diabetes mellitus
b. coagulopathy or creatinine elevation
c. intraoperative radiant heat transfer
d. gastric distention or low magnesium

NOTE: Consider scenario and item 5.7 together.

Mr. P received bupivacaine spinal anesthesia for a right cystectomy to resect a bladder tumor. Ten minutes after admission to PACU he complains of nausea and vomits 90 ml of bile-colored fluid.

5.7. While assessing this situation, the PACU nurse considers Mr. P's nausea is *most likely* associated with:

a. droperidol deficiency
b. intraoperative position
c. bupivacaine toxicity
d. vascular tone inadequacy

NOTE: Consider scenario and item 5.8 together.

Mr. C's medical history includes depression and smoking. For bilateral bunionectomy and arthrodesis, he received a general anesthetic with inhaled gas and narcotic medications. Upon admission to PACU, he is extubated, breathes spontaneously, makes audible crowing sounds, is disoriented and moves about on the stretcher. With difficulty, one SpO_2 measure was obtained, indicating a saturation of 93% with 40% oxygen delivered by face tent.

5.8. Mr. C's agitation makes lung auscultation difficult. The *most appropriate initial* nursing and medical interventions are to:

a. suction nasotrachea vigorously
b. sedate with morphine sulfate 4 mg
c. oxygenate with positive pressure ventilation
d. insert nasopharyngeal airway

5.9. The nurse suspects laryngospasm in a minimally responsive patient when assessment reveals:

a. lower lobe consolidation on x-ray
b. bilaterally absent breath sounds
c. restlessness; a sedated patient cannot spasm
d. no resistance during bag-valve-mask ventilation

NOTE: Consider scenario and item 5.10 together.

The site coordinator of a collaborative medical-nursing research project invites a PACU staff nurse to collect data. The study proposes to compare analgesic effects and patient responses to a narcotic and a nonsteroidal medication. The PACU nurse will document each patient's relevant physiologic data and response to a visual analog scale (VAS), a four item questionnaire using images of pain-indicating facial expressions.

5.10. Before participating, the nurse questions the researcher to assure:

a. approval of the facility's internal review panel
b. completion of a comprehensive literature review
c. recent adaptation of the data collection tool for a PACU setting
d. equal distribution of subjects between study groups

NOTE: Consider scenario and items 5.11 together.

During initial PACU admission assessment, the nurse observes 6 premature ventricular contractions per minute on a barely arousable elderly woman's EKG. During her 3 hour surgery, she initially received thiopental and oxygen with nitrous oxide, then atracurium, fentanyl, halothane, and droperidol. Blood pressure is 60/40, measured by a noninvasive automatic method. The anesthesiologist orders a 200 ml fluid challenge and considers pharmacologic intervention.

5.11. With regard to her inhalation anesthetic, this patient should now receive reduced doses of:

a. dobutamine
b. lidocaine
c. epinephrine
d. isoproterenol

NOTE: Consider scenario and items 5.12-5.13 together.

Following endoscopy with midazolam sedation to evaluate the status of gastrointestinal bleeding, an 80 year old woman becomes gradually more sedated and finally apneic. The patient's usual medications, prednisone, warfarin, and triazolam, continue during hospitalization. The nurse and anesthesiologist provide immediate respiratory support and administer flumazenil 0.4 mg intravenously.

5.12. The nurse monitors this woman's level of consciousness and respiratory quality and observes for:

a. petechiae
b. hypoglycemia
c. seizures
d. hypertension

5.13. The nurse anticipates this woman could develop any of the following additional symptoms *except:*

a. diaphoresis
b. endoscopic recall
c. hiccoughs
d. light-headedness

5.14. Collaborative nurse-physician considerations following ketamine anesthesia should include:

a. limiting verbal, tactile and visual stimulation
b. racemic epinephrine for anticipated bronchospasm
c. flumazenil to reverse sedative effects
d. encouraging activity to promote transfer from PACU

5.15. The most common symptom indicating latex reaction is:

a. tachyphylaxis
b. urticaria
c. bronchospasm
d. hypotension

5.16. One *early* sign of impending respiratory impairment in a patient receiving morphine sulfate by patient-controlled analgesia (PCA) is:

a. shallow respirations
b. lethargy
c. pruritus
d. bradycardia

5.17. After rhytidectomy and blepharoplasty, effective management of postoperative nausea and vomiting is essential to prevent:

a. intractable pain
b. subdermal infection
c. disrupted sutures
d. metabolic acidosis

5.18. In the immediate postanesthetic period, nausea appears to be *least* associated with:

a. laparoscopic tubal sterilization
b. propofol induction
c. nitrous oxide inhalation
d. fluid volume deficit

5.19. During the immediate postoperative period, effective pain management for the patient who uses heroin includes:

a. only nonsteroidal antiinflammatory drugs (NSAIDs)
b. providing opioid narcotics in large doses
c. substituting equivalent volumes of methadone
d. agonist/antagonist narcotic reversal

5.20. The PACU nurse effectively reduces personal legal risk by all of the following *except:*

a. encouraging early mobility, self-care and discharge after a bupivacaine-fentanyl epidural
b. congenial interactions with waiting family members about surgical delays

c. detailed and objective documentation of actions and responses during a hypotensive occurrence
d. strictly insisting upon physician consultation before releasing a vomiting Phase II patient

5.21. Natural substances with morphine-like properties that moderate pain messages are:
a. enkephalins
b. morphinomimetics
c. endomorphamines
d. prostaglandins

NOTE: Consider scenario and item 5.22 together.

Ms. Z received a 15 minute anesthetic with nitrous oxide, oxygen, and thiopental in PACU to reseat her left total hip joint that dislocated during a fall on the ice.

5.22. With regard to her nitrous oxide inhalation, the PACU nurse assures that Ms. Z receives oxygen and:
a. active rewarming to suppress inevitable shivering
b. frequent stimulation with reminders to sigh deeply
c. close scrutiny for likely ventricular ectopy
d. a quiet environment with minimal disturbance

5.23. Physiologic consequences of acute pain include:
a. adrenergic stimulation
b. catecholamine suppression
c. peripheral vasodilation
d. cholinergic crisis

NOTE: Consider items 5.24-5.25 together.

5.24. A breathing pattern the PACU nurse would most likely observe during malignant hyperpyrexia is:
a. Kussmaul's
b. Cheyne-Stokes
c. Adams-Stokes
d. Biot's

5.25. This respiratory pattern is most likely due to:
a. fever-induced effect on the thalamus
b. proactive hyperventilation to decrease anxiety
c. anticipatory hypoventilation related to alkalosis
d. compensatory attempt to reverse lactic acidosis

NOTE: Consider scenario and items 5.26-5.27 together.

Mr. S received 200 mcg fentanyl intraoperatively and is now aware and follows commands. Respiratory rate is 14 breaths per minute; SpO_2 is 96%. He complains of nausea. The PACU nurse administers droperidol 0.5 mg intravenously.

5.26. In addition to reevaluating Mr. S's nausea after this intervention, the PACU nurse's plan of care includes observation for progressive:
a. hypertension
b. muscle relaxation
c. dissociative psychosis
d. hypoventilation

5.27. When administered to patients with parkinsonian tremors, droperidol:
a. increases histamine release
b. counteracts antiemetic effects
c. augments tremors
d. causes hypertension

NOTE: Consider scenario and items 5.28-5.30 together.

The anesthesiologist orders a continuous epidural infusion of fentanyl for a 37 year old woman following an abdominoplasty. The patient complains of pain upon arrival in PACU and the anesthesiologist administers a bolus dose of 2 ml epidural fentanyl.

5.28. The nurse expects the patient will experience some *initial* pain relief within:
a. 5-15 minutes
b. 25-35 minutes
c. 45-55 minutes
d. 65-90 minutes

5.29. While connecting the infusion, the PACU nurse considers fentanyl's characteristics as a synthetic opioid, which:

a. reverses with intramuscular phentolamine (Regitine)
b. is less potent than epidural morphine
c. redistributes rapidly for analgesia at distant dermatomes
d. is lipid soluble with localized effects

NOTE: The scenario continues.

Thirty minutes after the bolus injection and beginning of the epidural fentanyl infusion, the nurse reassesses the patient. He is drowsy and his respiratory rate is 8 breaths per minute. The nurse decreases the fentanyl infusion rate and assures an appropriate reversal medication is at the bedside.

5.30. If necessary, the effects of fentanyl are best reversed with:

a. flumazenil
b. butorphanol
c. naloxone
d. neostigmine

SET II

Items 5.31-5.60

5.31. Outcomes related to intraoperative hypothermia include shivering, increased oxygen consumption and:
a. neurogenic seizure
b. ventricular dysrhythmias
c. central vasodilation
d. respiratory alkalosis

5.32. An independent intervention by the PACU nurse to alter a patient's reflexive pain response is:
a. extending the epidural morphine dose range
b. ordering transcutaneous electrical nerve stimulator (TENS) limits
c. teaching relaxation and imagery techniques preoperatively
d. establishing patient-controlled analgesia (PCA) parameters

5.33. The surgical patient with *least* risk for latex reactivity is a:
a. 60 year old chemically dependent man who had three arm fasciotomies last week
b. 14 year old diabetic girl with sacral meningomyelocele
c. 25 year old woman during vaginal delivery of a healthy boy
d. 42 year old male Operating Room nurse who requires an emergency appendectomy

NOTE: Consider scenario and item 5.34 together.

Ms. A, an elderly nursing home resident with dementia, received midazolam in the Emergency Department. In the preanesthesia area during preparation for exploratory laparotomy for suspected acute small bowel obstruction, she rouses only to strong voice and touch stimulation. The nurse then notes that no surgical consent was signed and no family members are present.

5.34. In this circumstance, proceeding with the planned surgical procedure is legally considered:
a. assault
b. fealty
c. prudent
d. battery

NOTE: Consider scenario and items 5.35-5.36 together.

The Emergency Department nurse accompanies an 18 year old patient to the preanesthesia area before repair of stabbing injuries. The nurse reports this young woman "took an unknown street drug." Currently, she is chatty and moving about expressively. Temperature is 38° C, blood pressure 186/98, heart rate 125 beats per minute in sinus tachycardia. Pupils are equal and dilated.

5.35. The PACU nurse suspects this patient has recently used:
a. morphine
b. heroin
c. cocaine
d. methadone

NOTE: The scenario continues.

Upon arrival in PACU 2 hours later, this patient is minimally responsive with shallow, regular respirations, constricted pupils and an oral airway. The anesthesia provider reports stable intraoperative vital signs, a brief episode of epistaxis, and 2 ml fentanyl dose. The surgeon suspects the patient also uses opiates.

5.36 During the immediate postanesthesia period, the nurse plans close blood pressure and heart rate observation plus:

a. limited sensory stimulation and monitoring for PVCs
b. low-dose methadone analgesia and assessment for lung congestion
c. frequent "stir-up" activity and nalbuphine
d. seizure precautions and naloxone reversal

NOTE: Consider scenario and items 5.37-5.38 together.

A 74 year old man with hypertension arrives in PACU Phase I alert and pain free after a propofol and midazolam anesthetic for cystoscopy and laser ablation of recurrent bladder tumors. During surgery, bradycardia followed by hypotension occurred; atropine 0.4 mg increased the heart rate to 140 beats/minute. Neosynephrine 0.3 mg significantly improved blood pressure. A 12-lead EKG shows supraventricular tachycardia at 120 beats per minute and PR 0.08, QRS 0.18 and ST depression in precordial leads.

5.37. The greatest current collaborative nursing-physician priority for this patient is:

a. bleeding prophylaxis
b. heart rate reduction
c. renal and cerebral perfusion
d. resedation prevention

5.38. The consulting cardiologist wishes to administer metoprolol 5 mg intravenously over 1 minute. Prior to injecting the medication, the PACU nurse assesses that the patient has:

a. adequate fluid volume
b. absence of asthma
c. a urinary catheter
d. no seizure history

5.39. The legally accepted way to amend a documentation error on the PACU record is to:

a. mask misentries and clearly write corrections above
b. mark errors with one line and initial new entry
c. recopy entire page and incorporate correct data
d. copy an incident report to insert data omissions

5.40. When providing patient education, the preanesthesia nurse is aware that the Patient Self-Determination Act of 1991 requires the hospital to:

a. continue resuscitative efforts despite medical futility
b. expect a patient to appoint a surrogate in a living will
c. only intubate a perioperative patient who requests "no-CPR"
d. provide written information about the right to an advance directive

5.41. A 48 year old woman receives methohexital, succinylcholine and atropine during her electroconvulsive therapy (ECT) on the mental health unit. A PACU nurse cares for her in PACU until this woman returns to her room. Joint Commission on Accreditation of Heath Care Organizations (JCAHO) criteria require that the nurse's discharge documentation include:

a. oxygen saturation, ECT energy delivered, and resolution of agitation
b. physiologic stability, fluid volume administered, and compliance with PACU discharge criteria
c. psychiatrist evaluation, clear memory, and admission and discharge vital signs
d. complication treatments only, medications given, and a statement of respiratory quality

NOTE: Consider scenario and items 5.42-5.44 together.

Ms. C received a single dose of epidural fentanyl 100 mcg at 10 AM during inhalant, narcotic and muscle relaxant anesthesia for abdominoperineal resection. She arrives in PACU at noon, aware, breathing adequately, and comfortable. The pharmacist is preparing her epidural fentanyl infusion, which will be titrated for postoperative pain management. At 12:20 PM, blood pressure and heart rate are unchanged from PACU admission measures, though Ms. C's respiratory rate is 8 breaths per minute and she is difficult to arouse.

5.42. After consultation with the anesthesiologist, the PACU nurse administers naloxone 0.1 mg and Ms. C is quickly more responsive. Over the next hour, the PACU nurse observes Ms. C for postreversal evidence of:

a. hyperventilation and tachycardia
b. emergence delirium and nausea
c. hypoventilation and lethargy
d. hyperthermia and hypotension

5.43. One potential outcome related to naloxone's effect is:

a. torso erythema with pruritus
b. profound hypotension
c. acute pulmonary thrombosis
d. inadequate analgesia

NOTE: The scenario continues.

Ms. C's epidural fentanyl infusion was started 1 hour ago and she reports significant pain relief, rating pain a 3 on a Likert-like pain scale of 0-10. After phoning a PACU discharge report, the nurse prepares Ms. C for transport and observes that she is more drowsy but rouses to touch, then drifts back to sleep. Ms. C's neurologic assessment is otherwise unchanged. Respirations are shallow at a rate of 9 breaths per minute, with no wheezes or crackles. SpO_2 is 95% with supplemental oxygen provided at 3 liters per minute by nasal cannula.

5.44. The *most appropriate* nursing action at this time is to delay transfer and:

a. ready the standby ventilator
b. administer naloxone 0.8 mg per PACU protocol
c. decrease the epidural infusion rate by 50%
d. assess Ms. C for total spinal anesthesia

5.45. Compared with 0.1 mg fentanyl, an equipotent analgesic dose is:

a. meperidine 125 mg
b. morphine 10 mg
c. butorphanol 10 mg
d. methadone 20 mg

5.46. The patient most ready for extubation meets criteria including:

a. vital capacity <15 ml/kg, inspiratory force <–20 cm H_2O, ability to maintain head lift for 1 minute
b. vital capacity >15 ml/kg, inspiratory force >–20 cm H_2O, respiratory rate of 28 breaths per minute
c. vital capacity >15 ml/kg, inspiratory force >–20 cm H_2O, ability to maintain head lift for 5 seconds
d. vital capacity <15 ml/kg, inspiratory force >–20 cm H_2O, heart rate 125 beats per minute

NOTE: Consider scenario and item 5.47 together.

Ms. K's cardiac monitor shows sinus bradycardia with a rate of 41 beats/minute. She rouses quickly and states she "feels OK" except for "slight" abdominal pain after her laser-assisted vaginal hysterectomy. Her blood pressure is 102/54 and SpO_2 is 98% while breathing oxygen at 40% by face tent. Preanesthetic blood pressure was 112/58.

5.47. The *most appropriate* intervention by the PACU nurse is to consult the anesthesiologist and anticipate:

a. continued PACU stimulation and observation
b. neostigmine to counteract residual muscle relaxant
c. warmed fluids to inhibit pseudocholinesterase
d. fluid volume expansion and intravenous atropine 4 mg

NOTE: Consider scenario and items 5.48-5.51 together.

Upon admission to PACU, a 45 year old male patient emerging from general anesthesia shakes violently, triggering the alarm systems of the monitoring equipment. The patient states that he is feeling cold, and tympanic temperature measurement is 35.5° C.

5.48. When planning patient care for this patient, the nurse considers that postanesthesia shaking:

a. universally indicates hypothermia
b. normally occurs in geriatric men
c. typically develops for unknown reasons
d. usually depletes neuromuscular acetylcholine stores

5.49. Minimizing adverse outcomes related to this patient's postanesthesia shivering *most requires* nursing interventions that:

a. continue oxygenation and respiratory quality
b. minimize shaking-related muscle aches
c. resedate to achieve light, Stage II anesthesia
d. relax and suppress physiologic stress

5.50. The preoperative nurse informed the postanesthesia staff that a patient scheduled for myomectomy also has a medical history of asthma and hepatitis C. The PACU plans to care for this patient by:

a. disposing of fecal-contaminated linen in two bags
b. wearing an air-purifying respirator
c. breaking contaminated needles from the hub
d. donning a face shield and latex gloves

5.51. Pruritus associated with epidural morphine infusion is best relieved by:

a. metoclopramide
b. diphenhydramine
c. hydroxyzine
d. naloxone

NOTE: Consider scenario and items 5.52-5.54 together.

After left shoulder reconstruction, the patient states severe pain that is unrelieved by large narcotic doses. The anesthesiologist elects to provide a brachial plexus block by interscalene approach. During the procedure, the patient mentions momentary tingling in her left arm.

5.52. The PACU nurse promptly:

a. informs the physician who aborts the block
b. assures the patient that brief-paresthesia is normal
c. prepares supplies to support ventilation
d. repositions the patient's head and neck

5.53. The PACU nurse expects Horner's syndrome may occur in this patient, evidenced by:

a. increased skin temperature of left arm, constriction of left pupil and ptosis of left eyelid
b. left arm erythema, dilation of right pupil and ptosis of right eyelid
c. pallor of left arm skin, constriction of left pupil and ptosis of left eyelid
d. decreased skin temperature of left arm, dilation of right pupil and left facial droop with ptosis

5.54. In addition to ongoing neurovascular assessment, the PACU nurse:

a. provides anatomic arm alignment unimpeded by the stretcher siderail
b. withholds any narcotic analgesia to prevent potentiated effects
c. encourages active arm lifts and motion to reduce adhesions
d. delays patient transfer from PACU until finger numbness abates

5.55. A latex-limiting perianesthesia environment may include any of the following *except:*

a. Steri-Strip dressings
b. vinyl tourniquets

c. piggybacked intravenous solutions
d. regular cimetidine infusions

NOTE: Consider scenario and item 5.56 together.

The anesthesiologist elected to administer incremental doses of nalbuphine 2 mg, up to a 10 mg total dose, to a woman with documented allergy to meperidine and morphine. The patient received intraoperative propofol and succinylcholine.

5.56. Anticipated nalbuphine-related effects include:
a. augmented pain
b. morphinelike analgesia
c. ventricular irritability
d. hallucinations

NOTE: Consider scenario and item 5.57 together.

The anesthesiologist accompanies a 45 year old woman into the PACU following emergency appendectomy. The patient's medical history includes recent depression, treated with a monoamine oxidase inhibitor.

5.57. This patient's pain management may include any of the following medications *except:*
a. hydromorphone
b. droperidol
c. ketorolac
d. meperidine

5.58. Methods specific to preventing transmission of active tuberculosis require patient isolation and:
a. positive pressure room air exchange
b. high-filtration nose and mouth protection
c. double gloving technique when sampling blood
d. universal precautions according to PACU protocol

5.59. Clinical research consistently indicates postanesthesia shivering decreases after:
a. intravenous morphine sulfate 2 mg
b. 10 minutes by spontaneous resolution
c. intravenous meperidine 12.5 mg
d. warmed blankets to the head every 5 minutes

5.60. For a brief period following electroconvulsive therapy, the patient is most likely to develop:
a. hypertension with electromechanical dissociation
b. hypotension with bundle branch block
c. hypertension and supraventricular tachycardia
d. hypotension and sinus bradycardia

SET III

Items 5.61-5.75

NOTE: Consider scenario and items 5.61-5.62 together.

A 43 year old woman arrives in PACU after a 2 hour surgery for left total knee replacement. She received a spinal anesthesia $\frac{1}{2}$ hour preoperatively with 0.5% tetracaine (Pontocaine) with epinephrine 1:100,000; she received 4 mg of intravenous midazolam during surgery. Assessment indicates an alert, oriented and chatty woman who is unable to move her legs; her sensation ceases at the T-6 dermatome.

5.61. The patient expresses concern that she's still unable to move her legs. When planning a response, the PACU nurse anticipates residual effects of this spinal anesthetic:

a. will likely persist at least 3 more hours
b. may resolve within about 45-60 minutes
c. should have resolved by now
d. will surely resolve in 30 minutes

5.62. Thirty minutes later, this patient mentions a frontal headache, nausea and left hip pain. The nurse's most effective interventions include analgesia and:

a. seizure precautions
b. flat, supine position
c. emetic therapy
d. high-Fowler's position

5.63. Intraoperative extension of the supine patient's arm to 110 degrees:

a. is the position of choice
b. facilitates intravenous catheter patency
c. compresses the radial nerve
d. may injure the bracheal plexus nerve

5.64. Clinical evidence of aspiration include all of the following *except:*

a. tachycardia
b. bronchial wheeze
c. pCO_2 = 35 mm Hg
d. acute Mobitz II block

NOTE: Consider scenario and items 5.65-5.67 together.

A 56 year old man is admitted to PACU following repair of a dissecting suprarenal abdominal aneurysm. The nurse observes that he is nonresponsive, pulseless, and hand ventilated with a bag-valve-mask apparatus. A pulmonary artery and radial artery catheter are in place. EKG pattern in Lead II shows the rhythm below.

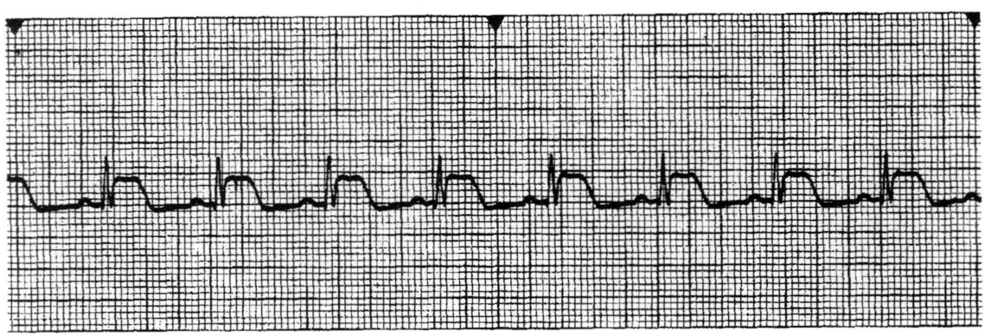

Figure 5.1. From Wiederhold, R. (1989). *Electrocardiography: The Monitoring Lead,* p. 243. Philadelphia: W.B. Saunders.

5.65. The PACU nurse interprets this pattern as:

a. sinus rhythm with evolving infarction
b. first degree atrioventricular block
c. pulseless electrical activity
d. atrial flutter with 2:1 conduction

5.66. The most appropriate nursing intervention is to:

a. initiate one-person cardiopulmonary resuscitation
b. cardiovert with 200 joules
c. begin a nitroglycerin infusion
d. deliver 100% oxygen and infuse isoproterenol

5.67. Clinical situations most associated with pulseless electrical activity include all of the following *except:*

a. evolving myocardial infarction
b. acute pulmonary embolism
c. profound hypovolemic shock
d. unrelenting laryngeal obstruction

5.68. A male patient whose blockade after spinal anesthesia is assessed at the T-4 dermatome has increased risk to develop:

a. postdural puncture headache
b. vagal-mediated reflex tachycardia
c. postspinal hypertension
d. respiratory insufficiency

5.69. Vigorous handwashing, once an elemental and essential principle of infection control, is:

a. unnecessary when applying universal precautions
b. mandatory before and after any patient contact
c. an obsolete practice when skin on hands is intact
d. most effective when sustained for at least 1 minute

5.70. Studies most consistently correlate development of postanesthesia shivering with:

a. peripheral vasoconstriction
b. inhalation anesthetics
c. intraoperative oxygen debt
d. increased parasympathetic activity

5.71. Definitive medical intervention for a postdural puncture headache is:

a. intravenous narcotic resedation
b. autologous epidural blood patch
c. spinal reanesthesia with hyperbaric solution
d. intravascular expansion with colloid infusion

5.72. The most ominous predictor of imminent cardiac arrest in a healthy postoperative 6 year old child is:

a. ventricular couplets
b. aberrant conduction
c. sinus bradycardia
d. supraventricular tachycardia

NOTE: Consider scenario and item 5.73 together.

A 5 year old insulin-dependent diabetic child is scheduled at 8 AM for a tonsillectomy. The child and parents have participated in the preoperative education program. Records indicate a history of blood glucose stability. A blood glucose drawn at 7:30 AM was 120 mg/dl.

5.73. Recommended preoperative preparation *best* includes infusion of:

a. 5% dextrose in water at 50 ml/hour
b. lactated Ringer's solution at a "keep open" rate
c. 200 ml bolus of 10% dextrose in 0.225% saline
d. 0.9% saline at 100 ml/hour

NOTE: Consider scenario and item 5.74 together.

The physician determines that a 42 year old businessman can be discharged home after his cardioversion with midazolam and propofol anesthesia rather than enter the hospital overnight as originally planned. The patient is ecstatic and insists he can take a cab as he has no ride home.

5.74. To ensure the patient's safety, the PACU nurse:

a. observes the cardiac rhythm one additional hour, then contacts the cab company.
b. tests the patient's psychomotor ability and documents impairment, then schedules overnight telemetry observation
c. calmly explains the facility policy, then contacts facility resources to arrange an adult escort
d. assures the patient can ambulate and void, then discharges him with his 14 year old son

5.75. The postoperative diabetic patient's potential for glucose-insulin imbalance increases *most* with:

a. hypothermia and prostatectomy
b. hypertension and hypoxemia
c. infection and physiologic stress
d. depression and hypophysectomy

Set I

Answer Key

5.1.	d
5.2.	c
5.3.	a
5.4.	c
5.5.	a
5.6.	d
5.7.	d
5.8.	c
5.9.	b
5.10.	a
5.11.	c
5.12.	c
5.13.	b
5.14.	a
5.15.	b
5.16.	b
5.17.	c
5.18.	b
5.19.	b
5.20.	a
5.21.	a
5.22.	b
5.23.	a
5.24.	a
5.25.	d
5.26.	d
5.27.	c
5.28.	a
5.29.	d
5.30.	c

SET I

Rationales and References

5.1. Correct Answer: **d**

Though any patient has potential to vomit and aspirate gastric contents after general anesthesia, anatomic and physiologic changes during pregnancy add to this risk. Drug-inhibited protective reflexes, tracheal or stomach tubes, trauma, gastric reflux, full stomach, some surgical procedures and Trendelenburg's position also increase aspiration risk. A head-elevated position, histamine receptor (H_2) blockade and consciousness with intact airway-protective reflexes reduce aspiration risk. Pregnancy decreases gastric motility and, like obesity, increases intraabdominal pressure.

Litwack, K: Post Anesthesia Care Nursing, *2nd ed. St. Louis, Mosby, pp. 404-405, 1995; Pelligrini, C: Postoperative Complications in* Current Surgical Diagnoses and Treatment *(Way, LW, Ed). Norwalk, CT, Appleton & Lange, p. 28, 1992.*

5.2. Correct Answer: **c**

Monitoring the sedated patient's airway for obstruction, hypoxia and apnea must become the nurse's primary focus even though midazolam was administered to decrease restlessness and anxiety so the procedures could be completed. Midazolam's potent action produces quick sedation and can rapidly alter respiratory function. Hypotension with tachycardia is also possible. In addition, the nurse can expect that midazolam will potentiate the depressant effects of residual intraoperative medications.

Litwack, K: Post Anesthesia Care Nursing, *2nd ed. St. Louis, Mosby, pp. 139-140, 1995; Kennedy, SK: Nonopioid Intravenous Anesthetics and Murphy, FL: Conduct of General Anesthesia in* Dripps/Eckenhoff/Vandam Introduction to Anesthesia, *8th ed (Longnecker, DE & Murphy, FL, Eds). Philadelphia, Saunders, pp. 98-99 & 157-158, 1992.*

5.3. Correct Answer: **a**

Amnesia produced by midazolam is dose related. Only memory of events that occur within minutes *after* dosing is affected (anterograde amnesia). Midazolam affects the receptors in the limbic system and so alters awareness.

Drain, C: The Post Anesthesia Care Unit: A Critical Care Approach to Post Anesthesia Nursing Practice, *3rd ed. Philadelphia, Saunders, pp. 208-209, 1994; Edwards, MW: Premedication in* Dripps/Eckenhoff/Vandam Introduction to Anesthesia, *8th ed (Longnecker, DE & Murphy, FL, Eds). Philadelphia, Saunders, p. 33, 1992.*

5.4. Correct answer: **c**

Nursing assessment of adequate ventilation continues during transport and this woman's CT scan and MRI. She remains a postanesthesia patient and receives care that aligns with PACU standards, even in a non-PACU setting and at any hour or any day of the week. Prior to leaving PACU, the nurse must assure, not assume, that oxygen delivery can continue and that monitoring, intubating and resuscitation supplies are immediately available. The nurse can expect midazolam's peak effects, and the greatest respiratory risk and amnesia effects, will occur between 5 and 30 minutes after a single dose. Repeated doses of midazolam, reintubation, or reversal may, or may not, be necessary.

Shannon, MT, Wilson, BA & Stang, CL: Govoni & Hayes Drugs and Nursing Implications, *8th ed. Norwalk, CT, Appleton & Lange, pp. 780-781, 1995; American Society of Anesthesiologists: Standards for Postanesthesia Care in* ASPAN's Standards of Perianesthesia Nursing Practice, *Resource 11. Thorofare, NJ, ASPAN, pp. 49-50, 1995.*

5.5. Correct Answer: **a**

After exposure to cautery or rapid muscle fasiculations, a specific pacemaker's response is unpredictable and *the nurse cannot assume its original programming and function were preserved.* Placing a magnet over a pacemaker will interrupt the pacemaker's sensing ability but *does not eliminate the risk of interference response.* Random "reprogramming" by noncardiac electrical activity can mimic a variety of pacemaker commands. This pacemaker may now regularly pace ventricles in a fixed rate VOO mode, either as a response to EMI or after intentional reprogramming to reduce risk of unexpected asystole. Accelerated rate and failure to sense, stimulate and capture are among possible pacemaker responses to EMI; all have hemodynamic consequences for the patient.

Fetzer-Fowler, S: Caring for the Ambulatory Surgical Patient Who Has a Pacemaker: Part I & II. J Post Anesth Nurs *8(2-3): 116-124 & 174-180, 1993.*

5.6. Correct Answer: **d**

Always consider inadequate ventilation *first* when evaluating possible reasons for delayed arousal after general anesthesia. A sedated patient becomes hypoxic and also retains carbon dioxide (hypercarbia). This delays elimination of any inhalation anesthetics or narcotics and extends hypnotic and narcotic effects. Prolonged drug effects may require reversal. Then consider specific surgery-related *metabolic or electrolyte disturbances or neurologic injury.* Dilutional hyponatremia, calcium deficit, diabetic hypoglycemia, or undetected intracranial bleeding can delay awakening. Liver or renal disease and heat transfer (hypothermia) delay drug excretion and can prolong sedation or muscle weakness.

Litwack, K: Post Anesthesia Care Nursing, *2nd ed. St. Louis, Mosby, pp. 45-48, 1995; Belatti, RG: Common Post Anesthetic Problems in* Post Anesthesia Care *(Vender, JS & Speiss, BD, Eds). Philadelphia, Saunders, pp. 9-11, 1992.*

5.7. Correct Answer: **d**

Occurrence of nausea and vomiting in patients with spinal blocks suggests new, unrecognized hypotension related to vascular dilation. Cerebral hypoperfusion accompanies the hypotension. Vomiting center hypoxia and/or heightened vagal tone in the gastrointestinal tract results in nausea. One study revealed a 21% incidence of emesis among spinal anesthesia patients, particularly when blood pressure falls to less than 80 mm Hg systolically; delivery of 100% oxygen decreased emesis. Fluid volume, vasopressors, and a foot-elevated position increase blood pressure and may reduce the sensations of nausea.

Belatti, RG: Common Post Anesthetic Problems in Post Anesthesia Care *(Vender, JS & Speiss, BD, Eds). Philadelphia, Saunders, pp. 13-18, 1992; Riegler, FX: Spinal and Epidural Anesthesia in* Dripps/Eckenhoff/Vandam Introduction to Anesthesia, *8th ed (Longnecker, DE & Murphy, FL, Eds). Philadelphia, Saunders, pp. 221-222, 1992.*

5.8. Correct Answer: **c**

Preventing hypoxemia and hypercarbia are immediate nursing and medical goals. Moving oxygen past the obstruction assures alveolar ventilation. Laryngeal stimulation has triggered this response of spasm and partial obstruction. Suction, airway placement, or reintubation will only increase irritation and should not be performed routinely or indiscriminately. Avoid narcotics and sedatives that suppress respiratory effort until oxygenation is assured. Succinylcholine may be needed to relax the musculature and release the spasm for adequate ventilation; close monitoring of muscle strength is then essential.

Litwack, K: Post Anesthesia Care Nursing, *2nd ed. St. Louis, Mosby, pp. 398-399, 1995; Peruzzi, WT & Vender, JS: Respiratory Care: Oxygenation, Bronchial Hygiene, and Mechanical Ventilation in* Post Anesthesia Care *(Vender, JS & Speiss, BD, Eds). Philadelphia, Saunders, pp. 113-115, 1992.*

5.9. Correct Answer: **b**

Absent breath sounds, quickly evolving hypoxemia or inability to ventilate with a bag-valve-mask device point to laryngospasm and complete airway obstruction. Nursing observation is crucial; a sedated or still anesthetized patient may not show the restlessness and air hunger of a more aware patient. Extubation during light anesthesia can sufficiently irritate the airway and prompt the reflex of airway spasm.

Litwack, K: Post Anesthesia Care Nursing, *2nd ed. St. Louis, Mosby, pp. 398-399, 1995; Fetzer-Fowler, SJ & Mullen, CA: Laryngospasm-Induced Pulmonary Edema: Case Report.* J Post Anesth Nurs *5(4): 222-227, 1990.*

5.10. Correct Answer: **a**

Ethical concerns should be this nurse's primary interest before participating as a data collector for this study. Human research subjects must provide informed consent and be protected from harm during experimentation, and their identities, responses, and results must remain confidential. Therefore research proposals must be scrutinized and approved by the facility's internal review board, sometimes also called a human subjects committee, or a research or ethics panel. Literature review, study methods, the tool's validity and reliability and sampling techniques may interest the nurse participant but not preclude participation.

Summers, S: Nursing Research in ASPAN's Core Curriculum for Post Anesthesia Nursing Practice, *3rd ed (Litwack, K, Ed). Philadelphia, Saunders, pp. 15-22, 1994.*

5.11. Correct Answer: **c**

Halothane, to a much greater extent than other inhalant anesthetics, sensitizes the heart to catecholamines. Administering epinephrine, a catecholamine with strong alpha and beta adrenergic effects, to a patient who still has significant residual concentrations of halothane can produce serious catecholamine-related rhythm disturbances. Until residual halothane clears (30 minutes or more after delivery ceases), diluting any epinephrine to a concentration of between 1:100,000 and 1:200,000 is recommended.

Drain, C: The Post Anesthesia Care Unit: A Critical Care Approach to Post Anesthesia Nursing, *3rd ed. Philadelphia, Saunders, pp. 198-203, 1994; Morgan, GE & Mikhail, MS:* Clinical Anesthesiology. *Norwalk, CT, Appleton & Lange, pp. 107-109, 1992.*

5.12. Correct Answer: **c**

Seizures can occur after flumazenil administration, particularly when a patient regularly uses benzodiazepine-based medications such as triazolam (Halcion) or diazepam or large doses of nonbenzodiazepine tricyclic antidepressant medications. Flumazenil's benzodiazepine receptor antagonist action disrupts the action of benzodiazepines on gamma aminobutyric acid (GABA) receptors.

Nursing '94 Drug Handbook. *Des Moines, Springhouse, pp. 1090-1091, 1994; Burden, N:* Ambulatory Surgical Nursing. *Philadephia, Saunders, pp. 68-69, 1993.*

5.13. Correct Answer: **b**

Flumazenil only reverses the physiologic sedative and respiratory actions of benzodiazepine. Amnesia for procedural effects is unaffected. Dizziness, sweating, vision disturbance, hiccoughs, nausea, and labile emotions commonly occur.

Shannon, MT, Wilson, BA & Stang, CL: Govoni & Hayes Drugs and Nursing Implications, *8th ed. Norwalk, CT, Appleton & Lange, pp. 528-529, 1995; Burden, N:* Ambulatory Surgical Nursing. *Philadephia, Saunders, pp. 68-69, 1993.*

5.14. Correct Answer: **a**

Minimizing verbal, tactile and visual stimuli helps minimize neurologic effects after ketamine administration. Ketamine hydrochloride is a dissociative anesthetic that may make a patient feel unattached to the environment. Dreams, delirium or hallucinations may occur and contribute to restless agitation, or emergence delirium, in PACU.

Omoigui, S: The Anesthesia Drug Handbook. *St. Louis, Mosby, pp. 98-99, 1992; Drain, C:* The Post Anesthesia Care Unit: A Critical Care Approach to Post Anesthesia Nursing, *3rd ed. Philadelphia, Saunders, pp. 212-213, 1994.*

5.15. Correct Answer: **b**

Urticaria with itching, erythema, edema and/or pustules most frequently indicates a localized chemical allergic response when skin contacts latex. This contact dermatitis is considered a Type VI reaction. Such a hypersensitivity response may develop within 6-48 hours after latex contact. Most local allergies clear spontaneously or with medications such as antihistamines or hydrocortisone.

Gold, J: Ask About Latex. RN *94(6): 32-35, 1994; Markey, J:*

Latex Allergy. J Intravenous Nurs *17(1): 35-39, 1994.*

5.16. Correct Answer: **b**

Increasing sedation is an early indicator of looming respiratory compromise; rate often decreases before depth. Pain maintains conscious awareness and so can help stimulate respiration. As pain is relieved and the patient relaxes, drowsiness can decrease the patient's response to hypoxia. Therefore oxygen delivery, close respiratory observation, reminders to breathe and move ("stir up"), and pulse oximetry measures are essential nursing responsibilities. This is particularly true when a patient is just beginning to receive a narcotic and the individual response to narcotics is unknown.

Willens, JS: Giving Fentanyl for Pain Outside the OR. Am J Nurs *94(2): 24-28, 1994; Gilbert, H: Postoperative Pain Management in* Post Anesthesia Care *(Vender, JS & Speiss, BD, Eds). Philadelphia, Saunders, 296-303, 1992.*

5.17. Correct Answer: **c**

Bleeding and tension on fine facial sutures are undesired outcomes of postoperative retching and vomiting. Agitation, hypertension, urinary retention and coughing also strain incisions. Bleeding, with or without hematoma, is the most common complication after facial reconstructive (plastic surgery) procedures. Significant pain and infection are rareoutcomes. Protracted vomiting is more likely to produce metabolic alkalosis than acidosis.

Burden, N: Ambulatory Surgical Nursing. *Philadelphia, Saunders, pp. 491-493, 1993; Fritsch, DE: The Plastic Surgery and Burn Patient in* ASPAN's Core Curriculum for Post Anesthesia Nursing Practice, *3rd ed (Litwack, K, Ed). Philadelphia, Saunders, pp. 603-611, 1994.*

5.18. Correct Answer: **b**

Incidence of nausea and vomiting is low among patients who receive propofol. Abdominal laparoscopic procedures seem to increase the incidence of nausea. Rapid correction of hypovolemia and a gradual, nonabrupt rise to upright position appear to reduce nausea. Nitrous oxide is associated, albeit controversially, with postoperative nausea and vomiting.

Burden, N: Ambulatory Surgical Nursing. *Philadelphia, Saunders, pp. 66-67 & 301-302, 1993; Belatti, RG: Common Post Anesthetic Problems in* Post Anesthesia Care *(Vender, JS & Speiss, BD, Eds). Philadelphia, Saunders, pp. 13-18, 1992.*

5.19. Correct Answer: **b**

Tolerance to an addictive substance often means an (ab)user requires more narcotic to manage pain than a nonaddicted patient needs. Cross tolerance among opioids is likely. Heroin, an analgesic derived from morphine (and twice as potent), breaks down in the body to morphine. Antagonist effects of narcotic reversal medications can precipitate acute withdrawal from heroin, or any addictive or chronically used narcotic, with serious consequences. Methadone or NSAID substitution await addiction treatment for physiolgic and psychologic dependence—which does not begin in PACU. Irritability of the central nervous system, tremors, panic, sweating and muscle pain herald withdrawal.

O'Hara, DA: Opioids in Anesthesia Practice in Dripps/Eckenhoff/Vandam Introduction to Anesthesia, *8th ed (Longnecker, DE & Murphy, FL, Eds). Philadelphia, Saunders, pp. 106-107, 1992; Drain, C:* The Post Anesthesia Care Unit: A Critical Care Approach to Post Anesthesia Nursing, *3rd ed. Philadelphia, Saunders, pp. 557-559, 1994.*

5.20. Correct Answer: **a**

Early return of complete motor, sensory and sympathetic function is unlikely after a bupivacaine-fentanyl combination for epidural injection. Expect prolonged effect. Though individual responses vary, encouraging self-care and early discharge is probably unsafe, poor judgment, and a legal risk. Some legalists regard a clearly written, objective, accurate record as the health care worker's strongest legal defense. Document patient occurrences, health care team observations, responses, interventions, and patient outcomes. Knowledge of patient rights, cordial communications, advocacy and practicing within facility procedural guidelines also minimize legal risk.

Calloway, SD: Legal Issues in Post Anesthesia Care Nursing in ASPAN's Core Curriculum for Post Anesthesia Nursing Practice, *3rd ed (Litwack, K, Ed). Philadelphia, Saunders, pp. 26-29, 1994; Niehaus, D: The Surgical Patient in the Ambulatory Short-Stay Setting in Post Anesthesia Care Nursing in* ASPAN's Core Curriculum for Post Anesthesia Nursing Practice, *3rd ed (Litwack, K, Ed). Philadelphia, Saunders, pp. 633-639, 1994.*

5.21. Correct Answer: **a**

When released from nociceptors in response to a nerve impulse, naturally occurring endorphins, including enkephalins, beta endorphins and dymorphins, inhibit nerve cell response. These endorphins seem to interrupt further transmission of a painful impulse along nerve pathways tothe brain. Serotonin acts similarly to interrupt transmission of painful signals.

Puntillo, KA: Pain in AACN's Clinical Reference for Critical-Care Nursing, *3rd ed (Kinney, MR, Packa, DR & Dunbar, SB, Eds). St. Louis, Mosby, pp. 329-333, 1993; Wild, L: Pain Management.* Nurs Clin North Am *2(4): 537-538, 1990.*

5.22. Correct Answer: **b**

After receiving nitrous oxide, a patient requires oxygen support and frequent stimulation to breathe deeply for at least 5-10 minutes after discontinuing a nitrous oxide/oxygen mix. More than other inhaled anesthetics, nitrous oxide administration is associated with diffusion hypoxia. Alveoli are quickly flooded when nitrous oxide rapidly moves (diffuses) from blood into the lungs for elimination. By diluting carbon dioxide also awaiting elimination, pCO_2 decreases, briefly suppressing the ventilatory drive. Nitrous oxide is relatively nonirritating and not associated with shivering or cardiac effects.

Burden, N: Ambulatory Surgical Nursing. *Philadelphia, Saunders, pp. 70-71, 1993; Drain, C:* The Post Anesthesia Care Unit: A Critical Care Approach to Post Anesthesia Nursing, *3rd ed. Philadelphia, Saunders, pp. 201-202, 1994.*

5.23. Correct Answer: **a**

Pain alters physiologic responses and increases physiologic stress. Reflex autonomic nervous system consequences of pain include adrenergic stimulation. Blood pressure, heart rate, cardiac output, oxygen consumption, and peripheral resistance increase; metabolic changes include acidosis and release of catecholamines.

Heffline, MS: Exploring Nursing Interventions for Acute Pain in the Postanesthesia Care Unit. J Post Anesth Nurs *5(5): 321-328, 1990; Litwack, K & Drain, CB: Pain Assessment and Management in* ASPAN's Core Curriculum for Post Anesthesia Nursing Practice, *3rd ed (Litwack, K, Ed). Philadelphia, Saunders, p. 646, 1994.*

5.24. Correct Answer: **a**

Malignant hyperthermia produces profound metabolic acidosis. The body compensates with consistently rapid and deep respirations (Kussmaul's) to exhale carbon dioxide. Through carbonic acid (H_2CO_3), the body's bicarbonate buffer system seeks to equilibrate hydrogen ion (H^+) and bicarbonate ion (HCO_3^-) concentrations and CO_2 to reverse acidosis.

Litwack, K: Post Anesthesia Care Nursing, *2nd ed. St. Louis, Mosby, pp. 470-475, 1995; Baumgardner, JE: Interpretation of Arterial Blood Gas annd Acid-Base Data in* Dripps/Eckenhoff/Vandam Introduction to Anesthesia, *8th ed (Longnecker, DE & Murphy, FL, Eds). Philadelphia, Saunders, pp. 11-15, 1992.*

5.25. Correct Answer: **d**

Increased respiratory rate (tachypnea) and depth is one way the body attempts to decrease its rapidly developing acidic condition during an episode of malignant hyperthermia (MH). Metabolic acidosis occurs when extracellular pH decreases after bicarbonate (HCO_3^-) loss or increase in hydrogen ion concentration (H^+). The acidic environment stimulates chemoreceptors in the medulla, which prompts increased respiratory rate and depth. Compensatory hyperventilation alone cannot restore normal pH. Often, the patient is already intubated, particularly during an intraoperative MH crisis, and receives 100% oxygen and manual hyperventilation with a bag-valve-mask device.

Litwack, K: Post Anesthesia Care Nursing, *2nd ed. St. Louis, Mosby, pp. 470-474, 1995; Rothenberg, DM: Postoperative Acid-Base Disorders: Recognition and Management in* Post Anesthesia Care *(Vender, JS & Speiss, BD, Eds). Philadelphia, Saunders, pp. 102-106, 1992.*

5.26. Correct Answer: **d**

When combined with fentanyl, droperidol prolongs narcotic effect and increases the potential for resedation and hypoventilation. Droperidol is classified as a neuroleptic, antipsychotic medication and tranquilizer. When administeredin small doses of 0.125-0.25 mg to suppress emesis, droperidol's alpha adrenergic effects inhibit dopamine receptor action in the chemoreceptor trigger zone (CTZ) and may produce hypotension.

Drain, C: The Post Anesthesia Care Unit: A Critical Care Approach to Post Anesthesia Nursing, *3rd ed. Philadelphia, Saunders, pp. 210-212, 1994; Herbert, DW:* Manual of Drugs in Anesthesia and Critical Care. *Philadelphia, Saunders, pp. 13-14, 1993.*

5.27. Correct Answer: **c**

Droperidol is *not* administered to patients with Parkinson's disease because droperidol further disrupts the already diseased extrapyramidal system. Tremulous movements and facial, tongue and laryngeal rigidity and spasm can increase. These may be sufficiently severe to require ventilatory support. Hypotension and sedation are also likely effects.

Herbert, DW: Manual of Drugs in Anesthesia and Critical Care. *Philadelphia, Saunders, pp. 13-14, 1993; Smith, DS & Fisher, SM: Neuroanesthesia and Neurologic Diseases in* Dripps/Eckenhoff/Vandam Introduction to Anesthesia, *8th ed (Longnecker, DE & Murphy, FL, Eds). Philadelphia, Saunders, pp. 394-395, 1992.*

5.28. Correct Answer: **a**

As a lipid-soluble medication, fentanyl's effect occurs promptly, and duration of effect is long. After a 50-100 mcg (1-2 ml) dose of epidural fentanyl, the patient may notice a slight effect within 15 minutes after injection; effects may last several hours. Achieving adequate relief of pain may require up to 1-2 hours with epidural medications; meanwhile an intravenous narcotic may supplement analgesia.

Sevarino, F & Preble, L: A Manual for Acute Postoperative Pain Management. *New York, Raven Press, p. 210, 1992; VadeBoncouer, TR: Management of Postoperative Pain in* Dripps/Eckenhoff/Vandam Introduction to Anesthesia, *8th ed (Longnecker, DE & Murphy, FL, Eds). Philadelphia, Saunders, pp. 448-450, 1992.*

5.29. Correct Answer: **d**

Fentanyl affects only a limited number of spinal segments. Fentanyl, like sufentanil and meperidine, is lipid soluble. It quickly and easily diffuses into spinal cord blood vessels and does not linger for long in cerebrospinal fluid (CSF) nor migrate through the CSF to affect more distant spinal nerves. Lipid solubility or insolubility is the most significant factor affecting onset and duration of analgesic action.

Sevarino, F & Preble, L: A Manual for Acute Postoperative Pain Management. *New York, Raven Press, p. 210, 1992; VadeBoncouer, TR: Management of Postoperative Pain in* Dripps/Eckenhoff/Vandam Introduction to Anesthesia, *8th ed (Longnecker, DE & Murphy, FL, Eds). Philadelphia, Saunders, pp. 448-450, 1992.*

5.30. Correct Answer: **c**

Naloxone is a pure narcotic antagonist and is used to reverse the sedative and respiratory depressant effects of narcotics. Small intravenous doses of 0.05-0.1 mg each are titrated to effect adequate respiration and awareness while retaining some analgesia. Flumazenil reverses benzodiazepines, and neostigmine reverses muscle relaxant effects.

Sevarino, F & Preble, L: A Manual for Acute Postoperative Pain Management. *New York, Raven Press, p. 210, 1992; McHenry, LM & Salerno, E:* Mosby's Pharmacology in Nursing, *18th ed. St. Louis, Mosby Year Book, pp. 214-222, 229-230 & 147-148, 1992.*

SET II

Answer Key

5.31. b
5.32. c
5.33. c
5.34. d
5.35. c
5.36. a
5.37. b
5.38. a
5.39. b
5.40. d
5.41. b
5.42. c
5.43. d
5.44. c
5.45. b
5.46. c
5.47. a
5.48. c
5.49. a
5.50. d
5.51. d
5.52. b
5.53. a
5.54. a
5.55. c
5.56. b
5.57. d
5.58. b
5.59. c
5.60. c

Set II

Rationales and References

5.31. Correct Answer: **b**

Shivering related to hypothermia may increase oxygen consumption as much as 500%. This "cold stress" increases cardiac work and can result in hypoxia and metabolic acidosis, which are precursors to dysrhythmias.

Winter, MG: Effects of Irrigation Fluid Warming on Hypothermia During Urologic Nursing. Urol Nurs *14: 6-8, 1994; Drain, C:* The Post Anesthesia Care Unit: A Critical Care Approach to Post Anesthesia Nursing, *3rd ed. Philadelphia, Saunders, pp. 563-564, 1994.*

5.32. Correct Answer: **c**

Teaching imagery and relaxation are independent nursing activities. Nursing responsibilities can be classified as dependent, interdependent or independent actions. Independent nursing functions are nurse-identified, nurse-treated and nurse-evaluated and include patient education, imagery, or therapeutic touch. Interdependent nursing roles are collaborative nurse-physician functions like titrating a physician-ordered nitroprusside infusion to effect. Carrying out a specific physician order, like setting or extending medication doses, is a dependent nursing role.

Heffline, MS: Exploring Nursing Interventions for Acute Pain in the Postanesthesia Care Unit. J Post Anesth Nurs *5(5): 321-328, 1990; Litwack, K & Drain, CB: Pain Assessment and Management in* ASPAN's Core Curriculum for Post Anesthesia Nursing Practice, *3rd ed (Litwack, K, Ed). Philadelphia, Saunders, pp. 654-655, 1994.*

5.33. Correct Answer: **c**

Increased sensitivity to latex seems to occur in individuals repeatedly exposed to latex-containing products like surgical gloves or catheters. Ongoing and prolonged latex contact occurs in individuals with occupational exposure like health care workers (up to 5.6% of OR nurses, 7.5% of surgeons) and in patients who need multiple surgeries. Patients with spina bifida comprise another high-risk group; reportedly between 18-40% develop latex reactions. In addition, allergy to bananas, avocados and chestnuts also is associated with higher incidence of latex reactivity.

Benner, SD: Latex Allergy. CPANewsletter, *pp. 3-4, 8 Nov, 1994; Markey, J: Latex Allergy.* J Intravenous Nurs *17(1): 35-39, 1994.*

5.34. Correct Answer: **d**

Battery is willful and intentional touch or invasion of another person without their consent. Both the midazolam and dementia render Ms. A incompetent to legally provide informed consent for her surgical procedure.

Calloway, SD: Legal Issues in Post Anesthesia Care Nursing in ASPAN's Core Curriculum for Post Anesthesia Nursing Practice, *3rd ed (Litwack, K, Ed). Philadelphia, Saunders, pp. 26-29, 1994.*

5.35. Correct Answer: **c**

Excessive talking, high energy, pupillary dilation, tachycardia, hyperthermia and hypertension are among indicators of cocaine high. Cocaine stimulates the central nervous system and alters mood. Adrenergic responses and pulmonary and cardiovascular vasoconstriction can produce hypoxia, lethal arrhythmias, severe hypertension, seizures or intracerebral bleeding or infarction.

Rogers, E: Postanesthesia Care of the Cocaine Abuser. J Post Anesth Nurs *6(2): 102-107, 1991; Saleh, KL: Practical Points in Understanding Local Anesthetics.* J Post Anesth Nurs *7(1): 45-47, 1992.*

5.36. Correct Answer: **a**

Provide oxygen, a safe, calm and quiet environment while monitoring signs of pulmonary congestion and cardiac ischemia and stress, including ventricular ectopy (PVCs) and cardiac arrest. The amount of this patient's cocaine and narcotic use is unclear; determining duration of effect is difficult but will likely continue into the postoperative period. Cocaine use is associated with seizures from central nervous system stimulation, pulmonary edema from constriction of pulmonary vessels, easy epistaxis from ischemia of nasal mucosa, and withdrawal lethargy when dopamine and norepinephrine reserves are depleted. Administration of naloxone or nalbuphine may prompt acute opiate withdrawal and is not advised; this patient appears to breathe adequately without intervention. Unrehabilitated narcotic-addicted patients often require very large amounts of narcotic; methadone substitution is not an immediate postoperative priority.

Litwack, K: Post Anesthesia Care Nursing, *2nd ed. St. Louis, Mosby, pp. 100 & 160, 1995; Rogers, E: Postanesthesia Care of the Cocaine Abuser.* J Post Anesth Nurs *6(2): 102-107, 1991.*

5.37. Correct Answer: **b**

Intraoperative events (bradycardia and hypotension) and the rapid tachycardia promote cardiac hypoxia; EKG documents cardiac muscle ischmeia (ST depression). Now, heart rate reduction after neosynephrine and atropine is important to decrease myocardial work, oxygen demand and additional injury. The patient has no angina, is alert and appears unsedated; adequate coronary and cerebral perfusion can be presumed for now. Surgical laser treatment minimizes bleeding. Though not the most immediate priorities for this patient, it is important to regularly reassess bleeding, coronary perfusion and resedation while his heart rate decreases in PACU.

McGaffigan, PA & Christoph, SB: Assessment and Monitoring of the Post Anesthesia Patient in The Post Anesthesia Care Unit: A Critical Care Approach to Post Anesthesia Nursing, *3rd ed (Drain, C, Ed). Philadelphia, Saunders, p. 275, 1994; Purcell, JA: Cardiac Electrical Activity in* AACN's Clinical Reference for Critical-Care Nursing, *3rd ed (Kinney, MR, Packa, DR & Dunbar, SB, Eds). St. Louis, Mosby, pp. 236-237, 1993.*

5.38. Correct Answer: **a**

Hypotension is a likely consequence after a beta-blocking medication like metoprolol (Lopressor). Assuring adequate fluid volume supports hemodynamic stability during intentional heart rate reduction; metoprolol will block the normal tachycardic response that compensates for falling blood pressure. At low doses, metoprolol is a selective beta-1 adrenergic blocker and inhibits inotropic (contractile) and chronotropic (rate increasing) responses. As metoprolol has no beta-2 effects, asthma-stimulating bronchoconstriction is unlikely.

American Heart Association: Textbook of Advanced Cardiac Life Support *(Cummins, RO, Ed). Dallas, American Heart Association, pp. 8.11-8.12, 1994; Shannon, MT, Wilson, BA & Stang, CL:* Govoni & Hayes Drugs and Nursing Implications, *8th ed. Norwalk, CT, Appleton & Lange, pp. 770-771, 1995.*

5.39. Correct Answer: **b**

During legal scrutiny of the patient's record, erasures, obliterations, squeezed in entries, misspellings and entering that an occurrence (incident) report was completed might raise questions about documentation accuracy. The patient's record reflects the health care interventions received and is a legal document. Detail, clarity and quality of entrieswritten into this document provide information, or lack of, about significant patient care events and can affect outcomes of lawsuits.

Calloway, SD: Legal Issues in Post Anesthesia Care Nursing in ASPAN's Core Curriculum for Post Anesthesia Nursing Practice, *3rd ed (Litwack, K, Ed). Philadelphia, Saunders, pp. 26-29, 1994.*

5.40. Correct Answer: **d**

The Patient Self-determination Act of 1991 details the legal expectation that a patient understand his or her personal right to determine treatment limits. Hospitals must establish written policies and procedures to inform patients about options, including the right to refuse or accept any medical or surgical intervention, resuscitation choices, advance directives or living wills. Freestanding ambulatory surgery units are currently exempt from this requirement, but often voluntarily provide relevant written material that is available upon patient request.

American Heart Association: Ethical Considerations in Resuscitation. JAMA *268(16): 2282-2287, 1992; Burden, N:* Ambulatory Surgical Nursing. *Philadelphia, Saunders, p. 203, 1993; Irvin, SM: Can Advance Directives Assure That Patients' Decisions Will Be Considered?* J Post Anesth Nurs *10(2): 79-83, 1995.*

5.41. Correct Answer: **b**

JCAHO expects the patient who receives ECT to meet the same discharge criteria as any postoperative patient who leaves PACU. Any patient who receives sedative or anesthetic medications for a procedure *must* receive the same level of care, whether provided in surgery, PACU, radiology or a mental health unit. Minimum documentation includes vital signs and pulse oximetry measures, level of consciousness, crystalloid and colloid solutions and any medications given, postprocedure events or complications, the interventions and response and compliance with PACU discharge criteria or physician assessment.

Joint Commission on Accreditation of Health Care Organizations: Accreditation Manual for

Hospitals. *Oakbrook Terrace, Ill., JCAHO, pp. 1-12, 1994.*

5.42. Correct Answer: **c**

Renarcotization with lethargy and respiratory depression can reoccur after a dose of naloxone. Naloxone competes with narcotics at the opioid receptors in the brain and spinal cord to quickly reverse Ms. C's lethargy. Unfortunately, the half-life of naloxone, a narcotic antagonist, is shorter than the narcotics it reverses; effective amounts of naloxone are depleted while effective narcotic still isavailable. Epidural fentanyl has a relatively short duration of action compared with morphine but can produce recurrent sedation (renarcotization).

O'Hara, DA: Opioids in Anesthesia Practice in Dripps/Eckenhoff/Vandam Introduction to Anesthesia, *8th ed (Longnecker, DE & Murphy, FL, Eds). Philadelphia, Saunders, p. 108, 1992; Drain, C:* The Post Anesthesia Care Unit: A Critical Care Approach to Post Anesthesia Nursing, *3rd ed. Philadelphia, Saunders, pp. 222-223, 1994.*

5.43. Correct Answer: **d**

Reversal of narcotic depression also reverses any analgesic benefit from circulating narcotic, including Ms. C's intraoperative narcotics and any serum or cerebrospinal fentanyl. Naloxone is best administered intravenously, in minute amounts, and cautiously titrated with doses just adequate to achieve conscious awareness and adequate respiratory effort. Pulmonary edema, hypertension and dysrhythmias can result from zealous reversal or naloxone overdose.

Litwack, K: Post Anesthesia Care Nursing, *2nd ed. St. Louis, Mosby, p. 142, 1995; O'Hara, DA: Opioids in Anesthesia Practice in* Dripps/Eckenhoff/Vandam Introduction to Anesthesia, *8th ed (Longnecker, DE & Murphy, FL, Eds). Philadelphia, Saunders, p. 108, 1992.*

5.44. Correct Answer: **c**

Reduce Ms. C's epidural infusion rate and stimulate her to promote deep breathing, activity and wakefulness ("stir-up"). She is increasingly drowsy, comfortable and still rousable but shows evidence of hypoventilation. Naloxone and mechanical ventilation are excessive responses now. Though epidurally placed narcotics generally require 2 hours to achieve adequate pain relief, Ms. C still benefits from some of her intraoperative dose of fentanyl. The hospital's protocol for nurse-monitored epidural analgesia and Ms. C's physician orders establish the fentanyl dosing parametersfor titration and how her response will be managed. Catheter migration from the epidural space is always possible, though Ms. C's clinical signs do not indicate either partial pain relief or total spinal anesthesia.

Drain, C: The Post Anesthesia Care Unit: A Critical Care Approach to Post Anesthesia Nursing, *3rd ed. Philadelphia, Saunders, pp. 222-223, 1994; Litwack, K:* Post Anesthesia Care Nursing, *2nd ed. St. Louis, Mosby, pp. 169-172, 1995.*

5.45. Correct Answer: **b**

The analgesic effect of a single 0.1 mg (100 mcg) intravenous fentanyl dose is approximately equivalent, or equipotent, to 10 mg morphine sulfate. Fentanyl is 100 times more potent than morphine, which is the "gold standard" against which narcotic doses and effects are compared. Most narcotic comparisons are derived from reported effects of intramuscular doses. When applying these comparisons, the cumulative effects of multiple intravenous doses over time and the pharmacologic uniqueness of each medication must be considered. Intravenous butorphanol (Stadol) 2 mg, hydromorphone (Dilaudid) 1.5 mg, morphine 10 mg, meperidine 100 mg, and methadone 10 mg are all considered equipotent.

Baer, CL & Williams, BR: Clinical Pharmacology and Nursing, *2nd ed. Springhouse, PA, Springhouse Corp, pp. 349-351, 1992.*

5.46. Correct Answer: **c**

A decision to extubate a patient must be determined in each clinical situation using criteria to guide assessment of adequate ventilation and predict lack of respiratory fatigue. Clinicians generally agree that a vital capacity of >15 ml/kg with inspiratory force >-20 cm H_20, ability to maintain head lift, acid-base and electrolyte balance, intact airway reflexes and wakefulness indicate readiness for extubation.

Sauer, D: Post Anesthesia Respiratory Care in ASPAN's Core Curriculum for Post Anesthesia Nusing Practice, *3rd ed (Litwack, K, Ed). Philadelphia, Saunders, pp. 140-141, 1994; Geer, RT: Critical Care of the Surgical Patient in* Dripps/Eckenhoff/Vandam Introduction to Anesthesia, *8th ed (Longnecker, DE & Murphy, FL, Eds). Philadelphia, Saunders, pp. 463-469, 1992.*

5.47. Correct Answer: **a**

Assuring oxygenation and regularly stimulating her to awaken, deep breathe and move are most likely adequate interventions. Unless she develops symptoms of decreased cardiac output like profound hypotension, ventricular escape beats, vertigo or nausea, Ms. K's heart rate probably requires no treatment despite the low rate. Postoperatively, sinus bradycardia, defined as a heart rate of less than 60 beats/minute, is associated with increased vagal tone, hypoxia, significant hypothermia, or total spinal blockade. When determining a correct response in this situation, the nurse must recognize that neostigmine increases bradycardia, pseudocholinesterase effect requires encouraging, not inhibiting, conditions, and a 4 mg dose of atropine far exceeds the recommended 0.5-1.0 mg dose. In addition, bradycardia is a normal phenomenon when a patient uses beta blocking medications or is athletically fit.

Drain, C: The Post Anesthesia Care Unit: A Critical Care Approach to Post Anesthesia Nursing, *3rd ed. Philadelphia, Saunders, pp. 233-237 & 274, 1994; Tremblay, DR, Fischer, RL, Caouette, CJ, et al: Arrhythmias in the PACU.* Crit Care Clin North Am *3(1): 95-99, 1991.*

5.48. Correct Answer: **c**

The underlying cause of postanesthesia shaking/shivering is not known. Research has not demonstrated a cause-effect relationship between hypothermia and postanesthesia shaking, though shivering occurs in 22-50% of patients after general anesthesia. Many clinicians believe shivering is associated with interoperative temperature decreases. Shaking occurs in both men and women with several potential consequences but few adverse clinical outcomes. Shivering incidence is not consistently affected by anesthetic medications or type of surgery but does decrease with age.

Vogelsang, J: Patients Who Develop Postanesthesia Shaking Show No Difference in Postoperative Temperature From Those Who Do Not Develop Shaking. Post Anesth Nurs *6(4): 231-128, 1991; Belatti, R: Common Post Anesthetic Problems in* J Post Anesthesia Care *(Vender, JS & Speiss, BD, Eds). Philadelphia, Saunders, pp. 18-20, 1992.*

5.49. Correct Answer: **a**

Oxygen is a required intervention until shivering ends. Shivering greatly increases oxygen consumption and can stress the cardiovascular and respiratory reserves of elderly or marginally healthy patients. One researcher-observed that postanesthesia shivering/shaking activity develops during emergence when a patient enters a light plane of anesthesia (Stage II) and responds to verbal or pain stimuli. At Stage II, a patient is hyperreflexic, with potentially harmful uncontrolled movements. Resedation to this anesthetic level is therefore inappropriate; relaxation therapy is unlikely to adequately suppress involuntary activity in sedated patients.

Burden, N: Ambulatory Surgical Nursing. *Philadelphia, Saunders, pp. 289-290, 1993; Vogelsang, J: The Treatment of Postanesthesia Shaking.* AORN *J 57(6): 1449-1456, 1993; Murphy, FL: Conduct of General Anesthesia in* Dripps/Eckenhoff/Vandam Introduction to Anesthesia *(Longnecker, DE & Murphy, FL, Eds). Philadelphia, Saunders, p. 159, 1993.*

5.50. Correct Answer: **d**

Gloves, gown, and face and eye protection, the usual personal protective equipment required to comply with universal precautions requirements mandated by the Occupational Safety and Health Administration (OSHA), are sufficient to protect against hepatitis C. Hepatitis C (formerly non-A, non-B) is spread to health care workers through direct contact with blood or blood products.

Odom, J: Management and Policies in The Post Anesthesia Care Unit: A Critical Care Approach to Post Anesthesia Care Nursing, *3rd ed (Drain, C, Ed). Philadelphia, Saunders, p. 26, 1994; Long, M & Miller, MD: Infection Control in* Basic Nursing: Theory and Practice, *3rd ed (Potter, PA & Perry, AG, Eds). St Louis, Mosby Year Book, pp. 623-628, 1994.*

5.51. Correct Answer: **d**

The opioid-antagonist effects of naloxone (Narcan) titrated in small increments relieve dose-related itching from morphine. Morphine's histamine release produces no visible rash or wheals and usually varies with dose. Treatment options include diphenhydramine (Benadryl), nalbuphine (Nubain), a narcotic agonist/antagonist, or lotions and cool compresses.

McShane, FJ: Epidural Narcotics: Mechanism of Action and Nursing Implications. J Post Anesth Nurs *7(3): 155-162, 1992; Wild, L & Coyne, C: The Basics and Beyond:*

Epidural Analgesia. Am J Nurs *92(4): 26-36, 1992.*

5.52. Correct Answer: **b**

During block infiltration, the patient often feels *transient* paresthesias, which are sensations like tingling or prickling. Pain or unrelenting burning or numbness may mean nerve irritation; the physician may redirect the needle or reattempt the block. Interscalene injection of local anesthetic medications blocks nerves in the brachial plexus sheath to reduce shoulder and upper arm pain. The patient's head and neck must be secure and not move to minimize complications like pneumothorax, which could require ventilatory support.

Burden, N: Ambulatory Surgical Nursing. *Philadelphia, Saunders, pp. 94-98, 1993; Brown, DL:* Atlas of Regional Anesthesia. *Philadelphia, Saunders, pp. 23-29, 1992.*

5.53. Correct Answer: **a**

Horner's syndrome is an expected result of interscalene block; signs include ptosis of the eyelid and constriction of the pupil on the side of the block. Extremity vasodilation also occurs, increasing skin temperature.

Shpritz, DW: The Neurosurgical Patient in ASPAN's Core Curriculum for Post Anesthesia Nursing Practice, *3rd ed (Litwack, K, Ed). Philadelphia, Saunders, p. 384, 1994; Burden, N:* Ambulatory Surgical Nursing. *Philadelphia, Saunders, pp. 96-98 & 566, 1993.*

5.54. Correct Answer: **a**

After a local anesthetic block for analgesia, the now-numbed extremity requires guidance to maintain alignment and protect from injury—to self and others. An effective brachial plexus block can produce motor and sensory blockade that disrupts normal muscular control and awareness of injuries. Limit wide and flowing arm movements but do determine adequate blood flow and the patient's level of comfort and sedation. A patient who knows to report a nonreceding block and has stable vital signs can leave PACU or, when surgically appropriate, leave for home. Additional analgesic support is likely—pain will return as the block recedes.

Drain, C: The Post Anesthesia Care Unit: A Critical Care Approach to Post Anesthesia Care Nursing, *3rd ed. Philadelphia, Saunders, p. 256, 1994; Litwack, K:* Post Anesthesia Care Nursing, *2nd ed. St. Louis, Mosby, pp. 162-164, 1995.*

5.55. Correct Answer: **c**

Prevention is the best latex sensitivity treatment. Use glass or vinyl products; eliminate contact with blood pressure tubing, rubber-stoppered syringes or vials and IV injection ports. Pretreatment with histamine-blocking medications is often recommended for identified latex reactivity. Clearly identify and treat at-risk patients with written communication and focused planning. Reactions occur when latex-containing products touch exposed intestinal or airway tissues of previously sensitized patients.

Benner, SD: Latex Allergy. CPANewsletter, *pp. 3-4, 8 Nov, 1994; Markey, J: Latex Allergy.* J Intravenous Nurs *17(1): 35-39, 1994.*

5.56. Correct Answer: **b**

When administered to a patient with no circulating narcotic, nalbuphine has potent analagesic, or agonist, effects that resemble those of morphine. Nalbuphine (Nubain) is classified as a mixed narcotic agonist-antagonist. Nalbuphine does antagonize the analgesia produced by other opioids.

Drain, C: The Post Anesthesia Care Unit: A Critical Care Approach to Post Anesthesia Nursing, *3rd ed. Philadelphia, Saunders, p. 220, 1994; Burden, N:* Ambulatory Surgical Nursing. *Philadelphia, Saunders, p. 297, 1993.*

5.57. Correct Answer: **d**

Meperidine may exaggerate the response to sympathetic stimulation and generally is not given to a patient who takes monoamine oxidase inhibitors (MAOI). The neurologic and vascular excitation can be fatal. Hypertensive crisis, hyperthermia, seizures, and rigidity have resulted when *meperidine* interacts with a circulating MAOI. Reactions with other narcotics are not as severe; when morphine sulfate is used, a dose reduction is considered sufficient. MAOI levels remain in the system for 3-4 weeks even after discontinuance.

McHenry, LM & Salerno, E: Mosby's Pharmacology in Nursing. *St. Louis, Mosby Year Book, p. 347, 1992; Skoog, RE: Monoamine Oxidase Inhibitors: Pharmacology and Implications in the Perioperative Period.* J Post Anesth Nurs *4(4): 264-267, 1989; Morgan, GE & Mikhail:* Clinical Anesthesiology. *Norwalk, CT, Appleton & Lange, p. 449, 1992.*

5.58. Correct Answer: **b**

As tuberculosis (TB) is spread through airborne droplets, minimizing transmission focuses on avoiding inhalation of infected bacilli. Universal precautions are not enough. The Centers for Disease Control (CDC) now recommend that care providers wear a snugly fitting, high-filtration, particulate respirator when caring for coughing patients who are suspected of having TB. Patient care should occur in a room with *negative* pressure ventilation that provides at least 6 air exchanges per hour. To protect patient confidentiality, avoid any door label that specifies the patient's disease.

Long, M & Miller, MD: Infection Control in Basic Nursing: Theory and Practice, *3rd ed (Potter, PA & Perry, AG, Eds). St Louis, Mosby Year Book, pp. 623-628, 1994; Litwack, K:* Post Anesthesia Care Practice, *2nd ed. St. Louis, Mosby Year Book, pp. 37-39, 1995.*

5.59. Correct Answer: **c**

Studies consistently indicate intravenous meperidine effectively decreases postanesthesia shivering/shaking in up to 83% of patients. Unless given in high, respiratory-depressing doses, morphine sulfate appears to have no effect on shivering. Responses to intravenous fluid or airway warming and surface rewarming with lamps and blankets are inconsistently effective interventions to decrease shaking. Some literature suggests rewarming peripheral (skin) surfaces rather than central (core) areas is key toshivering suppression.

Vogelsang, J: Butorphanol Tartrate (Stadol) Relieves Postanesthesia Shaking More Effectively than Meperidine (Demerol) or Morphine. J Post Anesth Nurs *7(2): 94-100, 1992; Belatti, R: Common Post Anesthetic Prob-*

lems in Post Anesthesia Care *(Vender, JS & Speiss, BD, Eds). Philadelphia, Saunders, pp. 18-20, 1992.*

5.60. Correct Answer: **c**

The seizure activity produced during electroconvulsive therapy stimulates the sympathetic nervous system and increases catecholamine release. Until these subside, the patient often is hypertensive and tachycardic. Most patients have no consequences, but the occasional patient has cardiovasuclar or cerebral damage from additional oxygen demand.

O'Brien, D & Burden, N: The ASC as a Special Procedures Unit in Ambulatory Surgical Nursing *(Burden, N, Ed.) Philadelphia, Saunders, pp. 580-581, 1993; Castro, AD: Management of Anesthesia for Specialty Procedures in* Dripps/Eckenhoff/Vandam Introduction to Anesthesia, *8th ed (Longnecker, DE & Murphy, FL, Eds). Philadelphia, Saunders, pp. 402-403, 1992.*

SET III

Answer Key

5.61. b
5.62. b
5.63. d
5.64. d
5.65. c
5.66. a
5.67. d
5.68. d
5.69. b
5.70. b
5.71. b
5.72. c
5.73. a
5.74. c
5.75. c

Set III

Rationales and References

5.61. Correct Answer: **b**

Tetracaine provides a block for $1\frac{1}{2}$-4 hours (approximately 90-240 minutes of anesthesia); this woman's block was placed $2\frac{1}{2}$ hours ago. Predicting a specific time when effects from a regional block will resolve is difficult; individual and environmental factors affect metabolism of the drug. For spinal anesthesia, the local anesthetic tetracaine provides a long-acting motor and sensory block. Adding epinephrine vasoconstricts the spinal vasculature and further slows absorption to extend the duration of action.

Drain, C: The Post Anesthesia Care Unit: A Critical Care Approach to Post Anesthesia Nursing, *3rd ed. Philadelphia, Saunders, p. 249, 1994; Brown, DL:* Atlas of Regional Anesthesia. *Philadelphia, Saunders, pp. 3-11 & 269-281, 1992.*

5.62. Correct Answer: **b**

Headache that decreases in intensity with a head-flat, recumbent position, abdominal pressure and decreased stimulation may be due to postdural puncture headache (PDPH). Though small gauge needles to inject intraspinal medications significantly decrease the incidence of postspinal headache, PDPH is still a potential. Headache is most often frontal or occipital. One study of 10,000 patients indicated PDPH is affected by age and sex. Women more often develop headache than men, as do younger adults 20-40 years of age. This woman's hip pain may herald early return of her sensation.

Burden, N: Ambulatory Surgical Nursing. *Philadelphia, Saunders, pp. 310-311, 1993; Morgan, GE & Mikhail, MS:* Clinical Anesthesiology. *Norwalk, CT, Appleton & Lange, pp. 209-210, 1992.*

5.63. Correct Answer: **d**

Bracheal plexus nerve damage is the most common peripheral nerve injury associated with the supine position. Whenever a patient's arm is extended more than 90 degrees, nerve damage is a potential outcome. Damage will likely be detected in PACU, perhaps when the patient mentions paresthesias or numbness or notes a motion deficit.

Walsh, J: Postop Effects of OR Positioning. RN *56(2): 50-57, 1993; Litwack, K:* Post Anesthesia Care Nursing, *2nd ed. St. Louis, Mosby, pp. 482-485, 1995.*

5.64. Correct Answer: **d**

An increase in heart and respiratory rates may be the only symptoms to signal aspiration, particularly if the incident was unwitnessed or silent. Hypoxemia, decreased or normal pCO_2, tachycardia, wheezing and pulmonary edema are associated with aspiration. Clinical evidence of aspiration can vary with the substance taken into the lung. Acutely occurring Mobitz II block is a delay in intracardiac electrical conduction most often caused by acute myocardial infarction.

Litwack, K: Post Anesthesia Care Nursing, *2nd ed. Philadelphia, Saunders, pp. 404-405, 1995; Chomka Leya, CM & Bandala, LC: Respiratory Complications in* Post Anesthesia Care *(Vender, JS & Speiss, BD, Eds). Philadelphia, Saunders, pp. 83-86, 1992.*

5.65. Correct Answer: **c**

The nurse's clinical assessment revealed this patient is *pulseless,* even though electrical activity appears on the cardiac monitor. Rely on clinical cues—this is a dire emergency!! Absent effective mechanical cardiac events, namely no palpable pulse or detectable blood pressure, despite a display of cardiac electrical activity (an EKG pattern), characterize pulseless electrical activity (PEA), once known as electromechanical dissociation (EMD). Research indicates that the heart may indeed produce weak, though non-life-sustaining and nonmeasureable, mechanical quivers during PEA.

American Heart Association: Textbook of Advanced Cardiac Life Support *(Cummins, RO, Ed). Dallas, American Heart Association, pp. 1.21-1.23, 1992; American Heart Association: Adult Cardiac Advanced Life Support.* JAMA *268(16): 219-220, 1992.*

5.66. Correct Answer: **a**

A patient with PEA *must* receive cardiopulmonary resuscitation (CPR). Simultaneously, the underlying cause of PEA (or electromechanical dissociation) is identified and treated. Blood and oxygen must be propelled through the body until cardiac output is restored. In addition, the patient with PEA should receive epinephrine in a 1:10,000 concentration every 5 minutes to improve myocardial oxygenation. The unintubated patient should be intubated to assure adequate, high-flow oxygenation. Rhythms associated with PEA may include idioventricular or ventricular escape rhythms as well as "some type of electrical activity," though not ventricular tachycardia or fibrillation.

Litwack, K: ASPAN's Core Curriculum for Post Anesthesia Nursing Practice, *3rd ed. Philadelphia, Saunders, p. 213, 1994; American Heart Association: Adult Cardiac Advanced Life Support.* JAMA *268(16): 219-220, 1992.*

5.67. Correct Answer: **d**

Layrngeal obstruction is the least likely cause of PEA. The significantly elevated ST segment of *this* patient's EKG complex should signal the nurse to consider *acute myocardial infarction* as the underlying reason for this patient's PEA—even though his surgery was an abdominal aneurysmectomy. CPR continues, but the underlying cause of PEA determines the intervention. Hemorrhage and hypovolemia, cardiac tamponade, tension pneumothorax, massive myocardial infarction, ischemia, pulmonary embolism, hypoxia, and acid-base or electrolyte imbalances are possible causes of PEA.

American Heart Association: Adult Cardiac Advanced Life Support. JAMA *268(16): 219-220, 1992; Litwack, K:* ASPAN's Core Curriculum for Post Anesthesia Nursing Practice, *3rd ed. Philadelphia, Saunders, p. 213, 1994.*

5.68. Correct Answer: **d**

Patients with high spinal blockade may perceive an inability to breathe. Sensation at the chest wall is blocked and the patient cannot feel deep breaths. Coughing and inspiratory capacity are imparied, though clinical signs like ventilatory effort, respiratory rate, muscle strength, and oxygen saturation with pulse oximeter may appear adequate.

Drain, C: The Post Anesthesia Care Unit: A Critical Care Approach to Post Anesthesia Nursing, *3rd ed. Philadelphia, Saunders, pp. 253-254, 1994; Brown, DL:* Atlas of Regional Anesthesia. *Philadelphia, Saunders, pp. 280-281, 1992.*

5.69. Correct Answer: **b**

Despite adherence to principles of universal precautions, handwashing remains a mandatory practice to prevent spread of disease-producing microorganisms. Gloves may have minute holes that allow bacteria to escape; tiny skin cracks or lesions then permit entry. Washing with unirritating antiseptic skin cleansers for 10-15 seconds and a warm water rinse effectively eliminate skin microorganisms.

Pfaff, S: Infection Prevention and Control in Ambulatory Surgical Nursing *(Burden, N, Ed). Philadelphia, Saunders, pp. 627-628, 1993; Long, M & Miller, MD: Infection Control in* Basic Nursing: Theory and Practice, *3rd ed (Potter, PA & Perry, AG, Eds). St. Louis, Mosby Year Book, pp. 620-623, 1994.*

5.70. Correct Answer: **b**

Nearly all anesthetic medications and techniques can produce postanesthesia shivering. Patients shiver after receiving halothane, enflurane, or isoflurane inhalation agents and also after narcotic–nitrous oxide combinations, and even after epidural techniques, especially in obstetrics. Conditions hypothetically linked with shivering include decreased sympathetic activity, respiratory alkalosis or decreased adrenal secretion. Though some clinicians presume that shivering always indicates significant heat loss, a patient can be severely hypothermic and not shiver. Others shiver actively at nearly normothermic temperatures.

Vogelsang, J: Butorphanol Tartrate (Stadol) Relieves Postanesthesia Shaking More Effectively Than Meperidine (Demerol) or Morphine. J Post Anesth Nurs *7(2): 94-100, 1992; Belatti, R: Common Post Anesthetic Problems in* Post Anesthesia Care *(Vender, JS & Speiss, BD, Eds). Philadelphia, Saunders, pp. 18-20, 1992.*

5.71. Correct Answer: **b**

Epidural blood patch repairs a dural leak over 90% of the time. Young female patients whose spinal anesthetic was introduced with a larger bore needle or who had repeated attempts to puncture the dura have greater likelihood of developing headache after spinal anesthesia.

Brown, DL: Atlas of Regional Anesthesia. *Philadelphia, Saunders, p. 280, 1992; Litwack, K:* Post Anesthesia Care Nursing, *2nd ed. St. Louis, Mosby, p. 175, 1995.*

5.72. Correct Answer: **c**

Bradycardia of sinus, junctional or ventricular origins most commonly heralds cardiopulmonary failure and arrest in the pediatric patient. Hypotension and hypoxemia with acidosis usually precede the bradycardia. Unresolved sinus tachycardia is a common cardiac response to injury, fever or low circulating volume and signals that the underlying cause needs correction.

American Heart Association Emergency Cardiac Care Committee: Pediatric Advanced Life Support. JAMA *268(16): 2262-2275, 1992; American Heart Association:* Textbook of Advanced Cardiac Life Support *(Cummins, RO, Ed). Dallas, American Heart Association, p. 1 & 60, 1994.*

5.73. Correct Answer: **a**

While glucose homeostasis is an essential goal for any diabetic patient, intraoperative hypoglycemia is a significant risk for children. NPO status, a young child's high calorie expenditure, potential that the child cannot recognize hypoglycemic symptoms, and surgical stress influence glucose requirements. Ideally, surgery is scheduled in the early morning. After the serum glucose is determined to be >100 mg/dl, a 5% dextrose infusion at a slow rate determined by individual fluid requirements generally is sufficient for a brief surgery.

Kirschner, RM: Diabetes in Pediatric Ambulatory Surgical Patients. J Post Anesth Nurs *8: 322-326, 1993; Steward, DJ:* Manual of Pediatric Anesthesia, *3rd ed. New York, Churchill-Livingstone, pp. 124-126, 1990.*

5.74. Correct Answer: **c**

Though criteria for discharge after anesthesia or sedation may vary among facilities, policies often include a statement that *any* postanesthesia patient must be escorted home by a responsible adult who can also provide care as needed at home. Unless specifically excluded, this policy likely applies to *any* postprocedural patient, whether afterconscious sedation or general anesthesia. The nurse must know the facility's patient discharge policy and arrange for a responsible adult with the physician, patient and hospital resources. To comply with policy and assure patient safety, hospital admission may occur.

American Society of Post Anesthesia Nurses: Standards of Perianesthesia Nursing Practice, *Resource 7. Thorofare, NJ, ASPAN, pp. 42-44, 1995; Litwack, K:* Post Anesthesia Nursing Practice, *2nd ed. St. Louis, Mosby, pp. 360-371, 1995.*

5.75. Correct Answer: **c**

Infection, dehydrating gastrointestinal vomiting and diarrhea, and stress increase the likelihood of hyperglycemia and increase insulin requirements. Even non-insulin-dependent diabetic patients may need small doses of insulin. Administration of corticosteroids and hyperalimentation increase glucose production. Cimetidine, calcium channel blockers, and thiazide diuretics are among insulin-depleting medications.

Gervasio, BA: The Endocrine Surgical Patient in ASPAN's Core Curriculum for Post Anesthesia Nursing Practice, *3rd ed (Litwack, K, Ed). Philadelphia, Saunders, pp. 553-558 1993; Loriaux, TC & Drass, JA: Endocrine and Diabetic Disorders in* AACN's Clinical Reference For Critical-Care Nursing *(Kinney, MR, Packa, DR & Dunbar, SB, Eds). St. Louis, Mosby, pp. 942-958, 1993.*

Section 6

Cardiac, Vascular and Pulmonary Systems

Scenarios and items in this section focus on the *cardiovascular, peripheral vascular,* and *pulmonary* systems. These concepts are considered together because:

- the functions of these organ systems are intricately intertwined.
- tissue oxygenation depends on adequate function of cardiac, ventilatory *and* circulatory organs.

ESSENTIAL CORE CONCEPTS	AFFILIATED CORE CURRICULUM CHAPTERS
Nursing Process	**Chapters 2, 17 & 18**
Assessment	
Planning and Implementation	
Evaluation	
Cardiac and Vascular Systems	**Chapters 17 & 18**
Cardiac and Vascular Anatomy	
Chambers, Vessels and Valves	
Cardiac Cycle and Circulation	
Electrical Conduction	
Palpation, Auscultation & Pulses	
Cardiac and Vascular Physiology	
Hemodynamic Concepts	
Afterload	
Cardiac Output	
Oxygen Delivery and Consumption	
Preload	
Cardiac and Vascular Pathophysiology	
Anesthesia Effects	
Diagnostic	
Disease and Risk	
Infarcts, Shunts and Obstructions	
Metabolic, Diet and Smoking	
Electrocardiography and Rhythms	
Hemodynamic Monitoring	Chapter 32

Life Support Concepts — Chapter 15
Pharmacology
  Pressors, Dilators and Blockers
Surgical Interventions
  Valves, Bypasses, and Revascularizations
Technology
  Balloons and Ventricular Assists
  Defibrillators and Cardioverters — Chapter 15
  Oximeters and Capnographs — Chapter 10
  Pacemakers — Chapter 17

Organ System Interrelationships

Preanesthesia and Postanesthesia Priorities

Pulmonary System — **Chapter 19**

Anatomy
Structures and Functions
  Muscles and Vessels
  Trachea to Alveolus

Physiology
Receptors and Nerves
Feedback
Ventilation Concepts
  Compliance and Resistance
  Oxygenation and Carbon Dioxide
  Pressures and Volumes
  Diffusion, Perfusion and Transport

Pathophysiology
Diseases and Risks
  Obstructions and Restrictions
  Mucous and Wheezes
Surgical Repairs: -scopes, -plasties, -ectomies

Preanasthesia and Postanesthesia Priorities
Gas Exchange and Breathing Patterns
Organ System Interrelationships
Pharmacology
  Anesthetic Effects
  Oxygen, Humidity and Aerosols — Chapter 10
  Pain Management
Technology
  Mechanincal Ventilation — Chapter 10
  Chest Tubes and Water Seals
  Ventilation
    Hyperventilation- and Hypoventilation-
    Intubation and Extubation

SET I

Items 6.1-6.50

NOTE: Consider scenario and items 6.1-6.2 together.

A 60 year old man with chronic renal failure received ketamine hydrochloride during surgery to create a pericardial window.

6.1. The PACU nurse's interventions include a plan to:

a. speak at a volume audible to a patient wearing earplugs
b. infuse crystalloid at 200 ml per hour to clear ketamine
c. frequently stimulate the patient to avoid apneic events
d. provide a quiet, calm atmosphere to observe the patient

6.2. Thirty minutes after this patient's admission to the PACU, the nurse is most concerned to discover:

a. a grating sound along the sternum during auscultation
b. 40 ml of thin red drainage in the mediastinal chest tube
c. sinus rhythm at 130 beats per minute with small QRS size
d. a laboratory report stating BUN = 74 mg/dl

6.3. The *initial* compensatory response to renal ischemia after hypotension prompts increased secretion of:

a. renin
b. erythropoietin I
c. aldosterone II
d. antidiuretic hormone

6.4. Systemic responses specifically related to renin stimulation include:

a. vasodilation and sodium retention
b. diuresis and hypertension
c. tachycardia and hyperventilation
d. fluid absorption and vasoconstriction

6.5. At the cellular level, magnesium sulfate affects cardiac conduction by altering:

a. action potential voltage height
b. sodium pump speed
c. norepinephrine effect at alpha receptors
d. calcium movement across the cell membrane

NOTE: Consider scenario and items 6.6-6.8 together.

Ms Z is a 50 kg woman with a documented 52 pack per year smoking history. Following her right shoulder reconstruction, she is admitted to PACU sitting on a stretcher in high-Fowler's position, complaining of severe shoulder pain, restless and gasping between paroxysms of coughing that produce thick mucus. She received 60 mg of lidocaine in the OR prior to extubation. SpO_2 is 91% with oxygen delivered by humidified face tent at 98%. Wheezes are scattered through her upper lungs.

6.6. The anesthesiologist orders an aerosolized albuterol inhalation. Albuterol's bronchodilating effects occur due to:

a. alpha adrenergic stimulation
b. beta and alpha adrenergic blockade
c. selective beta-2 adrenergic stimulation
d. selective beta-1 adrenergic blockade

6.7. The nurse anticipates albuterol's bronchodilating effects to occur within:

a. 60 seconds
b. 90 seconds
c. 3 minutes
d. 7 minutes

6.8. During albuterol inhalation, Ms Z is observed for:

a. angina and tachycardia
b. bradycardia and muscle weakness
c. heart block and headache
d. hypotension and nausea

6.9. After 45 minutes in PACU, the patient who is *least* likely to show signs of hypoventilation has a:

a. fading response to ulnar nerve stimulation
b. tympanic temperature of 35.4° C
c. spinal anesthetic block at T-10 dermatome
d. pain level reduced to "2" by 10 mg morphine

NOTE: Consider scenario and items 6.10-6.11 together.

General anesthesia for a 75 year old man's left carotid endarterectomy included isoflurane, midazolam, atracurium, fentaryl, and propofol. Upon admission to PACU, hemodynamic parameters are within surgeon-ordered limits, he weakly moves all extremities when asked, pupils are equal, and his face has symmetry. He cannot state his name or identify place without prompting.

6.10. This patient assessment guides the nurse to:

a. vigorously shake the patient and shout "Wake up!"
b. immediately advise the surgeon of neurologic deficit
c. observe and anticipate improved orientation
d. increase cerebral perfusion with phenylephrine

NOTE: The scenario continues.

Thirty minutes later, he is difficult to rouse, moves his right arm weakly and now requires nitroprusside to maintain systolic blood pressure at less than 160 mm Hg.

6.11. These symptoms may be associated with:

a. persistent midazolam effect
b. recurrent carotid thrombosis
c. resultant carotid artery hematoma
d. transient nitroprusside overdose

NOTE: Consider scenario and items 6.12-6.13 together.

A 78 year old woman has been in PACU for 45 minutes following open reduction to insert plates and pins to stabilize a traumatic ulnar fracture. Her cast extends from midpalm to midhumerus.

6.12. The nurse assesses *early* compartment syndrome by noting:

a. extreme pain and fingertip paresthesia
b. local hyperthermia and absent radial pulse
c. pitting edema and delayed capillary refill
d. limited motion and fingertip hypothermia

6.13. A patient with compartment syndrome has the greatest risk to develop:

a. hyperkinetic cardiomyopathy
b. fat embolism syndrome
c. acute tubular necrosis
d. mesenteric artery thrombosis

NOTE: Consider scenario and items 6.14-6.15 together.

Three months ago, a football player sustained a C-5 cervical transection. Today he develops flushed skin, diaphoresis and blood pressure of 248/126 in PACU following cystectomy and creation of an ileal conduit.

6.14. The most likely explanation for these signs is:

a. rhabdomyolysis
b. autonomic dysreflexia
c. malignant hyperthermia
d. posterior cord syndrome

6.15. Medical and nursing interventions for this patient in PACU focus on:

a. inducing hypothermia
b. sedating awareness

c. relaxing bladder spasm
d. reducing afterload

6.16. An arousable patient suddenly develops respiratory distress after right neck dissection and exploration. The nurse palpates leftward shift of larynx which *most likely* indicates:

a. carotid artery hemorrhage
b. glossopharyngeal nerve weakness
c. left vocal cord paralysis
d. brain stem herniation

NOTE: Consider scenario and items 6.17-6.18 together.

Ms W's left elbow joint was surgically replaced to treat joint degeneration resulting from her rheumatoid arthritis. The anesthesiologist provided a left brachial plexus nerve block using a supraclavicular approach. Ms W denies dyspnea, though now states sharp, localized, ipsilateral chest pain that radiates to her neck and increases with each deep breath. Vital signs are within 10% of preanesthesia values and stable.

6.17. The nurse observes that Ms W's left chest expands later than her right during inspiration, most likely due to:

a. irregularly receding local anesthetic blockade
b. left intrapulmonary volume alteration
c. incomplete pain management by local anesthetic block
d. pleural irritation from left pulmonary embolus

6.18. A chest x-ray indicates that approximately 15% of Ms W's lung is unexpanded. The PACU nurse's plan for Ms W's immediate care includes frequent monitoring of hemodynamic stability, physician collaboration and:

a. positive pressure ventilation with PEEP
b. insertion of a pleural chest tube with water seal
c. supplemental oxygen with continued observation
d. immediate needle insertion at the second intercostal space

NOTE: Consider scenario and items 6.19-6.21 together.

An actively bleeding male patient had an exploratory laparotomy following a gunshot wound to the abdomen. The anesthesiologist reports ketamine was used for rapid sequence anesthesia. Preoperative blood pressure was 80/42, with heart rate 102 beats per minute and sinus rhythm.

6.19. For this 40 year old patient, ketamine likely:

a. is an inappropriate medication choice
b. allows surgery with hypotensive technique
c. stimulates the sympathetic nervous system
d. suppresses circulating catecholamines

6.20. Rapid sequence induction of this patient's general anesthetic may have reduced his risk for:

a. postoperative nausea and vomiting (PONV)
b. intraoperative aspiration
c. coronary artery spasm
d. acute tubular necrosis (ATN)

6.21. After the first hour in PACU, the nurse notes this patient's urine is amber colored with volume of 35 ml/hour and deduces:

a. renal perfusion is adequate
b. renin release is inappropriate
c. acute tubular necrosis is likely
d. antidiuretic hormone secretion is suppressed

6.22. The most likely intraoperative cause of improper sensing by an implanted pacemaker is:

a. pulse generator battery failure
b. increased pacing threshold
c. systemic electrochemical imbalance
d. electromagnetic interference

6.23. The patient who is *most* predisposed to postoperative small airway collapse:

a. smokes heavily
b. weighs 50 kg
c. has blood pressure of 210/90
d. wheezes and states asthma

6.24. Essential respiratory support for 285 pound Ms O after her gastric stapling requires:

a. mechanical ventilation
b. liberal intravenous fluid volume
c. head and shoulder elevation
d. anxiolytic medications

6.25. Vital capacity measures:

a. productive life expectancy
b. maximal volume of air inhaled and exhaled
c. lung volume essential to life support
d. volume of air moved during each respiratory cycle

6.26. Pulmonary shunt refers to:

a. alveolar ventilation without capillary perfusion
b. surgical anastomosis of a pulmonary vein and artery
c. congenital externalization of pulmonary vasculature
d. capillary perfusion of alveoli without air exchange

NOTE: Consider scenario and items 6.27-6.28 together.

Twenty minutes after arrival in PACU, a middle-aged male patient is diaphoretic and complains of chest pain and dyspnea. A double lumen catheter was placed into the right internal jugular vein prior to transverse colon resection. Intraoperatively the catheter was used to monitor central venous pressure and administer fluid; the monitoring tubing was discontinued at the end of surgery and the catheter port was capped.

6.27. The patient is clearly dyspneic and diaphoretic and complains of dizziness and anxiety. During thoracic auscultation, the nurse hears a churning noise and suspects:

a. aortic stenosis
b. pulmonary thrombus
c. venous air embolism
d. papillary muscle rupture

6.28. The nurse *immediately* shifts the patient to:

a. left side, Trendelenburg's position
b. left side, semi-Fowler's position
c. right side, semi-Fowler's position
d. right side, Trendelenburg's position

NOTE: Consider scenario and items 6.29-6.30 together.

After 1 hour in PACU, a mechanical ventilator in the assist-control mode supports a patient's ventilations. The patient initiates some spontaneous respirations, wakens to voice, then grimaces and dozes. Blood pressure and pulse are adequate and stable; arterial blood gasses are within normal limits. Ulnar nerve stimulation elicits a slight muscle twitch. The ventilator mode is changed to the continuous positive airway pressure (CPAP) mode; the patient's minute volume is 2100 ml.

6.29. The PACU nurse's primary intervention is to:

a. remind the patient to frequently move his extremities
b. initiate protocols to wean from the ventilator
c. sedate the patient to prevent fighting the ventilator
d. resume the assist-control mode and reassure

6.30. Minimum predictors of successful weaning from ventilatory support include normal arterial blood gasses, wakefulness, and:

a. respiratory rate >8/minute, minute volume = 1600 ml
b. tital volume >7 ml/kg, able to lift head for 6 seconds

c. NIF –5 cm H_2O, strong and equal hand grasps
d. SaO_2 >92%, vital capacity >10 ml/kg

NOTE: Consider scenario and items 6.31-6.32 together.

At 6 PM, a 56 year old man is admitted to PACU following bupivacaine spinal anesthesia for open reduction and internal fixation (ORIF) of a fractured right tibia, the only apparent injury in an early morning skiing accident. Estimated intraoperative blood loss was 250 ml. Two hours postoperatively while preparing him for transfer from PACU, the PACU nurse observes a respiratory rate of 30 breaths per minute. EKG shows sinus tachycardia at 140 beats per minute, a Q wave in Lead-III and inverted T wave. Blood pressure is 100/52, a decrease from his PACU measures of 120-140/70-84, and his temperature is 38.1° C.

6.31. A prudent nursing intervention for this patient is to:

a. continue transfer preparations
b. administer midazolam 1 mg
c. increase oxygen delivery
d. request immediate echocardiogram

NOTE: The scenario continues.

During further assessment, the PACU nurse observes petechiae on the patient's left lateral chest, anxiety, and left leg weakness with toe flexion. Lab reports indicate PaO_2 of 68 mm Hg, platelets 98,000, and hemoglobin 8.8 g/dl.

6.32. A relevant nursing diagnosis is altered cardiopulmonary tissue perfusion related to:

a. posttrauma fat embolism
b. lateral myocardial infarction
c. pain from deep vein thrombosis
d. noncardiac pulmonary edema

6.33. The ratio of a suction catheter's diameter to the artificial airway's inner diameter should not exceed:

a. two-thirds
b. one-half
c. one-fourth
d. three-fourths

NOTE: Consider scenario and items 6.34-6.36 together.

During PACU admission activities, a minimally responsive, postemergency laparoscopic appendectomy patient vomits. Other than a history of esophageal reflux, the patient is healthy.

6.34. The nurse's *immediate* interventions are to suction, inform the anesthesiologist, and:

a. sweep debris from mouth and lavage with saline
b. place in high-Fowler's position with oxygen and observe
c. prepare to intubate and instill sodium bicarbonate
d. reposition in Trendelenburg's position and administer 100% oxygen

NOTE: The scenario continues.

After being suctioned, the patient is more aware and coughs frequently, and his respiratory rate increases to 35 breaths per minute while he is breathing oxygen through a low flow system. Oxygen saturations decrease from 96% to 92%. Chest x-ray interpretation is pending. pCO_2 is 34 mm Hg, pO_2 is 50 mm Hg.

6.35. While a colleague notifies the anesthesiologist, the PACU nurse's *most* appropriate intervention is to:

a. increase humidified oxygen delivery to 100%
b. administer the postoperative antibiotic
c. encourage 24 long and deep respirations per minute
d. infuse a histamine H_2 receptor antagonist

6.36. This patient must be monitored for all of the following *except:*

a. expiratory wheezes
b. inspiratory stridor
c. inspiratory crackles
d. shortened expiratory phase

6.37. During the early postoperative period, the *most appropriate* nursing intervention to reduce potential for circulatory compromise and compartment syndrome in the patient with a long arm cast is:

a. extremity heat to promote blood flow
b. epidural fentanyl infusion for analgesia
c. high arm elevation to reduce venous congestion
d. hourly reobservation of absent thumb hyperextension

6.38. The most effective way to prevent hypoventilation in a young, healthy but minimally responsive postanesthesia patient is to:

a. flush residual intravenous anesthetic with lactated Ringer's solution
b. provide humidified oxygen at FiO_2 of 60%
c. stimulate the patient every 5-10 minutes
d. suction the oropharynx to encourage deep breaths

6.39. Preload indicates the ventricular blood volume and length of cardiac muscle fiber length:

a. during coronary artery filling
b. after contraction
c. during aortic valve closure
d. before contraction

6.40. A typical healthy adult's resting cardiac output is:

a. 1-3 liters per minute
b. 4-6 liters per minute
c. 7-9 liters per minute
d. 10-12 liters per minute

6.41. By definition, cardiac output varies with changes in:

a. stroke volume and coronary perfusion pressure
b. heart rate and mean arterial pressure
c. heart rate or stroke volume
d. stroke volume or ejection fraction

6.42. Relevant observations following right carotid endarterectomy include all of the following *except:*

a. right carotid bruit
b. cranial nerve II and III symmetry
c. voice quality
d. baroreceptor response

6.43. Bedside technology used to monitor evolving respiratory acidosis or increasing respiratory dead space in a neurologically compromised patient is:

a. pulse oximetry
b. mixed venous oxygenation
c. capnography
d. negative inspiratory force

6.44. Type II heart block most likely would progress to:

a. atrial fibrillation and ventricular ectopy
b. vagal nerve overstimulaton
c. first degree block with juctional reentry
d. complete heart block

6.45. After observing second degree heart block in a drowsy, postanesthesia patient, the nurse's most appropriate responses are to stimulate the patient, reassess and:

a. deliver a precordial thump
b. locate the external pacemaker
c. massage the carotid artery
d. infuse isoproterenol at 3 mg/kg

NOTE: Consider scenario and items 6.46-6.48 together.

During the preanesthesia interview, the nurse learns an 82 year old patient has a pacemaker set in the VVI mode.

6.46. The nurse expects the EKG will show that a pacemaker artifact:

a. initiates every ventricular depolarization
b. coincides with each repolarization wave
c. follows each QRS complex
d. occurs after a delayed QRS

6.47. During this interview, the nurse inquires about symptoms of dizziness, chest pain, and congestion, primarily to ascertain:

a. adequate pacemaker function
b. impending myocardial infarction
c. pacemaker's programmed code
d. pacemaker-induced valvular stenosis

6.48. Intraoperative electromagnetic interference may affect this patient's pacemaker performance by:

a. increasing the frequency of impulse discharge
b. altering the ability to sense cardiac events
c. decreasing the cardiac resting membrane potential
d. converting a bipolar system to unipolar function

6.49. Dopamine's effect is potentiated when administered with:

a. Class I antiarrhythmics
b. monoamine oxidase inhibitors
c. beta adrenergic blockers
d. calcium channel blockers

6.50. To maximize renal perfusion, dopamine is best infused at:

a. 1-3 mcg/kg/min
b. 5-7 mcg/kg/min
c. 8-10 mcg/kg/min
d. 10-12 mcg/kg/min

SET II

Items 6.51-6.100

NOTE: Consider scenario and item 6.51 together.

While admitting a patient with a flow-directed pulmonary artery catheter to PACU, the nurse observes bursts of rapid ventricular tachycardia on the cardiac monitor. The pulmonary artery waveform is tall and spiked with pressure measured at 48/2.

6.51. A colleague informs the anesthesiologist who is in the preanesthesia area while the PACU nurse prepares to:
- a. administer a lidocaine 200 mg bolus
- b. apply synchronized countershock at 200 joules
- c. deliver a precoridal thump
- d. inflate the balloon to advance the catheter

6.52. Weaning a patient from mechanical ventilation using the intermittent mandatory ventilation (IMV) mode:
- a. delivers every breath but at a lower tidal volume
- b. allows progressive spontaneous patient respirations
- c. must incorporate positive end-expiratory pressure
- d. usually results in significant hypoventilation

6.53. An appropriate *initial* intervention to improve a partial spasm of laryngeal muscle tissue is:
- a. reassurance and humidified oxygenation by mask
- b. endotracheal intubation and ventilator support
- c. succinylcholine 25 mg and jaw support
- d. naloxone 0.2 mg and high humidity

6.54. A patient whose cardiac index is 3 L/min/m^2 following exploratory laparotomy likely has:
- a. impending myocardial infarction
- b. increased intraabdominal pressure
- c. fluid volume excess with low cardiac output
- d. adequate cardiac output for body size

6.55. Nitroprusside becomes pharmacologically unstable when exposed to:
- a. ambient light
- b. dextrose
- c. sodium chloride
- d. photosynthesis

NOTE: Consider scenario and item 6.56 together.

When nitroprusside is titrated to a patient's hemodynamic response, her blood pressure measures 70/30; cardiac rhythm is sinus without ectopy at 68 beats per minute.

6.56. The PACU nurse's *most appropriate* immediate intervention is to:
- a. infuse 500 ml hetastarch to support blood pressure
- b. begin a concurrent infusion of dopamine at 6 mcg/kg/min
- c. discontinue nitroprusside due to patient sensitivity
- d. slow nitroprusside rate to observe blood pressure rise

6.57. An environmental factor associated with occurrence of noncardiac pulmonary edema is fluctuation of:
- a. barometer
- b. altitude
- c. humidity
- d. temperature

6.58. An essential initial nursing intervention to support a patient with suspected noncardiogenic pulmonary edema is:

a. vigorous endotracheal suction
b. prompt digitalization
c. humidified oxygenation
d. recumbent, leg-elevated position

6.59. General anesthesia affects functional residual capacity (FRC) by:

a. decreasing airway closing capacity
b. relaxing chest muscles and increasing ventilatory capacity
c. inhibiting alveolar surfactant
d. decreasing diaphragmatic tone and shifting abdominal contents

NOTE: Consider scenario and items 6.60-6.62 together.

After extubation in PACU, a patient developed inspiratory stridor and received 60 mg lidocaine. The airway irritation decreased, then recurred 15 minutes later. This patient smokes, has a short, obese neck, has had prior neck surgery, and required three intubation attempts to secure a patent airway for today's bilateral bunionectomy. SpO_2 now measures 89% with delivery of 100% oxygen by humidified open face tent.

6.60. The anesthesiologist orders racemic epinephrine by aerosolized inhalation for the:

a. selective effects of alpha receptor stimulation
b. global beta-1, beta-2 and alpha receptor depression
c. combined alpha-beta cholinergic bronchodilation
d. beta-2 stimulation despite alpha adrenergic effect

6.61. Before administering the racemic epinephrine treatment, the PACU nurse verifies that the patient has no documented:

a. coagulopathy
b. angina
c. oliguria
d. cirrhosis

6.62. The anesthesiologist orders a nonrebreathing system to increase the concentration of oxygen delivered to this patient. Effective use of this high-flow method in PACU requires:

a. high oxygen flow to maintain inflation of the reservoir bag
b. the patient to be reintubated and sedated
c. astute monitoring for symptoms of oxygen toxicity
d. a Venturi valve to direct exhaled carbon dioxide to an attached collecton bag

6.63. Left tension pneumothorax is caused by:

a. accumulated air in the pleural space
b. excessive inspiratory tracheal tug
c. lung puncture by right rib fracture
d. inadequate left chest tube length

NOTE: Consider scenario and items 6.64-6.71 together.

Following repair of abdominal aortic aneurysm, Mr. S is nonresponsive, with ventilator-assisted respirations of 12 breaths per minute and positive end-expiratory pressure (PEEP) at +5 cm H_2O. Mr. S is healthy and weighs 75 kg. Nitroprusside infuses at 2 mcg/kg/min; dopamine infuses at 4 mcg/kg/min; lidocaine infuses at 2 mg/min. Intraoperative blood loss of 1800 ml was replaced with 2 units packed blood cells, 500 ml hetastarch and 3750 ml crystalloid. Urine volume is 55 ml per hour.

6.64. Positive pressure ventilation and end-expiratory airway pressure potentially alter cardiovascular function by:

a. decreasing venous return and cardiac output
b. increasing venous return and cardiac output
c. decreasing pulmonary vascular resistance
d. increasing systemic vascular resistance

6.65. Mr. S's pulmonary artery pressure measures are pulmonary artery systolic/diastolic (PAS/PAD) 20/6 mm Hg and pulmonary artery occlusion pressure (PAOP) 4 mm Hg. In the absense of increased pulmonary vascular resistance, pulmonary artery pressure reflects:

a. intrapulmonary vascular volume
b. left ventricular end-diastolic pressure
c. left ventricular end-systolic pressure
d. systemic vascular resistance resistance

6.66. Mr. S's pulmonary artery occlusion pressure (PAOP) likely indicates:

a. pulmonary edema
b. pulmonary embolus
c. cardiac tamponade
d. hypovolemia

6.67. When caring for Mr. S, the PACU nurse assures a continuous display of the pulmonary artery waveform, *primarily* to observe evidence of:

a. catheter migration
b. catheter thrombosis
c. inadvertent decannulation
d. leakage from the catheter's balloon

NOTE: The scenario continues.

During surgery, Mr. S received three bolus doses of intravenous lidocaine 100 mg to suppress ventricular tachycardia and recurrent premature ventricular contractions (PVCs). The lidocaine infusion was initiated at 4 mg/min for the final 2 hours of surgery, then decreased to 2 mg/min during reversal of muscle relaxant.

6.68. As a Class I antidysrhythmic, lidocaine alters the arrhythmia threshold and impulse conduction in the ventricles by:

a. slowing automaticity in Purkinje fibers
b. blocking sodium channels
c. slowing repolarization
d. blocking intracardiac calcium channels

6.69. During initial PACU admission, the nurse observes that Mr. S's lidocaine infusion pump is set to deliver 20 mg/min; she adjusts the infusion rate. Related to his lidocaine infusion, Mr. S has increased risk to develop:

a. right heart failure
b. acute tubular necrosis
c. convulsions
d. hypertension

6.70. Mr. S's anesthesiologist probably chose to administer a combination of sodium nitroprusside and dopamine:

a. to increase blood pressure and reduce afterload
b. in error; nitroprusside's effects oppose dopamine's
c. to counteract adverse effects of lidocaine
d. to reduce alveolar shunt and promote renal flow

6.71. When evaluating Mr S's most probable cardiovascular responses to positive airway pressure by PEEP, the PACU nurse anticipates increasing Mr. S's:

a. lidocaine infusion rate to decrease arrhythmias
b. nitroprusside titration to decrease preload
c. fluid volume rate to increase preload
d. dopamine titration to induce diuresis

6.72. The PACU nurse judiciously administers only small doses of narcotic following bilateral carotid endarterectomy, *primarily* because:

a. carotid body stimulation exaggerates hemodynamic responses to morphine
b. baroreceptor function is obliterated by narcotics

c. carotid body dysfunction alters respiratory response to hypercarbia
d. baroreceptor sensitivity to carbon dioxide is extinguished by surgery

6.73. After observing a dampened waveform while monitoring blood pressure at the radial artery, the PACU nurse's *first* action is to:
a. hyperextend the patient's wrist
b. withdraw the catheter 2 cm
c. assess transducer level, then recalibrate
d. activate the heparinized flush system

NOTE: Consider scenario and items 6.74-6.82 together.

Mr. T, a 70 kg man, had a myocardial infarction 24 weeks ago. He maintained an NPO status for 8 hours prior to today's radical prostatectomy. An estimated intraoperative blood loss of 750 ml was replaced with crystalloid infusion of 2500 ml. Preoperative hemoglobin was 11.7 g/dl. Thirty minutes after admission to PACU, Mr. T's blood pressure was 80-90 systolic/40-50 mm Hg diastolic. Heart rate is regular at 104 beats per minute and temperature 37.1° C. Oxygen saturation measures 98%. Pain is described as burning abdominal pressure and rated as 7 on a pain scale of 0-10.

6.74. Mr. T's clinical signs most suggest:
a. sepsis
b. hypovolemia
c. cardiomegaly
d. anaphylaxis

6.75. After assessing Mr. T, the PACU nurse determines Mr. T's parenteral fluid volume was probably:
a. adequately replaced; he requires cardiac evaluation
b. deficient; he requires 600 ml of whole blood
c. overestimated; he requires osmotic diuresis
d. deficient; he requires 750-1200 ml of crystalloid

NOTE: The scenario continues.

Mr. T receives oxygen at 40% open face tent; respiratory rate is 20 breaths per minute. He is drowsy, responsive and denies dyspnea. The PACU nurse observes that oxygen saturations stabilized at 90% for 5 minutes.

6.76. The PACU nurse adjusts the fit of the oxygen face tent, increases the oxygen flow, encourages Mr. T to deep breathe and move about, then consults the anesthesiologist to:
a. obtain chest x-ray
b. reintubate
c. measure hemoglobin
d. administer naloxone

6.77. When evaluating Mr. T's oxygen status, the nurse considers factors that decrease oxygen-hemoglobin affinity. These factors include all of the following *except:*
a. hyperthermia
b. alkalosis
c. decreased pH
d. increased 2,3-DPG

6.78. When interpreting Mr. T's pulse oximetry measurements, the PACU nurse considers that:
a. displayed saturations may be falsely low
b. oxygen saturation equals arterial PaO_2
c. hypotension provides falsely high saturations
d. saturation changes are best detected on the toe

6.79. While assessing Mr. T's respiratory and circulatory status, the PACU nurse asks Mr. T to describe his pain, *primarily* to assess:
a. cardiac origins
b. bladder hemorrhage
c. level of consciousness
d. pulmonary embolus

6.80. Despite drowsiness, Mr. T continues to state unrelieved incisional pain. The PACU nurse's intervention is to:

a. reassure and observe Mr. T, until he rates his pain on a numeric pain scale
b. administer morphine 10 mg IM per surgeon order
c. defer analgesia until oxygen saturation reaches 100%
d. inject doses of intravenous morphine and monitor

NOTE: The scenario continues.

Mr. T's cardiac rhythm reveals QRS complexes of 0.10 second duration that regularly occur at 130-140 beats per minute. Each QRS is preceded by an upright P wave with PR interval of 0.10-0.12 second.

6.81. The PACU nurse considers Mr. T's clinical status and interprets this rhythm as:

a. idiosynchronous ventricular tachycardia
b. accelerated junctional rhythm
c. sinus tachycardia
d. aberrant ventricular conduction

6.82. Potential nursing interventions with regard to this rhythm include reevaluating pain management and:

a. measuring serum potassium
b. verifying urine flow by gravity
c. synchronized cardioversion
d. carotid sinus massage

6.83. Decreased voltage of each QRS complex appears on the EKG monitor of a postcoronary bypass patient. Central venous pressure measures 20 mmHg. The nurse assesses this patient for additional evidence of:

a. right ventricular infarction
b. inadequate fluid volume
c. cardiac tamponade
d. digitalis effect

6.84. After insertion of a pulmonary artery catheter, a chest x-ray is used to determine occurrence of:

a. pneumothorax
b. pulmonary vasculature ligation
c. interstitial fluid
d. bronchiolar placement

6.85. Pulmonary artery pressures in healthy adults are:

a. 10/5 mm Hg
b. 25/10 mm Hg
c. 40/0 mm Hg
d. 80/40 mm Hg

6.86. Marked respiratory variation of the baseline of a pulmonary artery pressure waveform is consistent with a nursing diagnosis of:

a. fluid volume excess
b. ineffective breathing pattern
c. altered tissue perfusion
d. fluid volume deficit

6.87. A clinical situation associated with pulmonary shunt is:

a. atelectasis
b. cerebral vascular bleeding
c. congestive heart failure
d. laryngospasm

6.88. Physiologic outcomes of unsuppressed postanesthesia shivering relate to:

a. severe metabolic alkalosis
b. sustained muscle contraction
c. life-threatening hyperkalemia
d. exaggerated oxygen consumption

NOTE: Consider scenario and item 6.89 together.

Upon admission to Phase I PACU after narcotic and inhalation general anesthetic for laparoscopic tubal ligation, a healthy middle-aged woman's vital signs are blood pressure 130/76, pulse 74 beats per minute, and respirations 16 breaths per minute. Good quality breath sounds are audible bilaterally and she responds to her name. Fifteen minutes later, the patient complains of upper chest and shoulder pain and vital signs are blood pressure 110/66, pulse 66 beats per minute and respirations 12 breaths per minute.

6.89. At this time, the PACU nurse's plan of care includes:

a. reassurance and continued observation
b. sublingual nitroglycerin and cardiac monitoring
c. chest x-ray and supplemental oxygen
d. naloxone and deferred transfer to Phase II PACU

NOTE: Consider scenario and items 6.90-6.92 together.

A 72 year old man is in PACU after a balanced anesthesia technique for abdominal laparotomy to release a small bowel obstruction. Admission cardiac rhythm is sinus at 78 beats per minute with varying P wave configuration and PR interval of 0.10-0.24 seconds. After 20 minutes, the PACU nurse notes that QRS complexes occur regularly at 44 beats per minute with a PVC after every fourth QRS. P waves occur regularly at 88 waves per minute.

6.90. The primary rhythm probably originates in:

a. sinoatrial cells
b. Kent's bundle
c. junctional tissue
d. Purkinje fibers

6.91. This cardiac rhythm may evolve to:

a. Wenckebach phenomenon
b. complete heart block
c. Mobitz I block
d. Ashman's phenomenon

6.92. This patient's blood pressure is now 82/48 with this cardiac rhythm. The PACU nurse's most appropriate initial interventions are to consult with the anesthesiologist and administer:

a. crystalloid bolus of 300 ml
b. an external pacing artifact
c. atropine 0.5 mg IV
d. 2% lidocaine 70 mg IV

6.93. During PACU admission procedures for a nonresponsive and intubated patient, the nurse observes a cardiac rhythm that resembles ventricular fibrillation. The *first* action is to:

a. deliver a precordial thump
b. assess carotid pulse
c. administer 200 mg lidocaine
d. determine unconsciousness

6.94. Electrically, a PVC that occurs on the T wave may:

a. preset the electrical-mechanical cycle
b. reset sinus node automaticity
c. offset the depolarization wave
d. upset cellular repolarization

6.95. During two-person cardiopulmonary resuscitation of an adult:

a. the cardiac compression rate is 65 per minute
b. one breath is interposed after five compressions
c. fifteen compressions occur for every two ventilations
d. each compression depresses the sternum 1 inch

6.96. A patient arrives in PACU with an oral airway in place. The PACU nurse observes this patient is nonresponsive and nonbreathing. The appropriate *initial* nursing intervention in this situation is:

a. four quick breaths
b. a precordial thump
c. closed chest massage
d. mandibular lift

6.97. Poorly perfused alveoli despite adequate ventilation occur with all of the following conditions *except:*

a. mucous plug
b. pulmonary embolism
c. air embolism
d. hypovolemic shock

6.98. A potential outcome of postoperative laryngospasm is:

a. pulmonary edema
b. congestive heart failure
c. sustained vocal cord opening
d. uvular hemorrhage

6.99. Symptoms associated with noncardiac pulmonary edema (NCPE) can occur when inspiration produces large negative pressures after administration of:

a. dexamethasone
b. naloxone
c. succinylcholine
d. glycopyrrolate

6.100. The low pressure alarm of a volume-cycled ventilator sounds. To address the *most likely* cause of the alarm, the PACU nurse:

a. suctions airway secretions
b. decreases ventilator pressure limits by 20 cm H_2O
c. evaluates airway to detect air leak
d. sedates the patient

SET III

Items 6.101-6.150

6.101. The high pressure alarm on a volume ventilator alerts the caregiver to:

a. adjust the alarm limit
b. remove airway obstructions
c. withdraw the endotracheal tube 2 cm
d. administer naloxone 0.4 mg

NOTE: Consider scenario and item 6.102 together.

A healthy, 70 kg man received 250 mcg of fentanyl 2 hours ago at the end of mitral valve replacement procedure. After 1 hour in PACU, he remains mechanically ventilated in CPAP mode, rouses with touch and name call and holds his head from the pillow for 1 second; minute volume is more than 5 L/min. Arterial blood gases are within normal limits and he is surgically stable. The patient denies pain and drifts to sleep when undisturbed.

6.102. The *most appropriate* intervention at this time is to :

a. extubate and provide oxygen by face tent at FiO_2 0.40
b. continue mechanical ventilation with IMV and reassess
c. administer naloxone 0.2 mg, then extubate
d. sedate, then adjust ventilator to assist-control mode

6.103. Physiologic dead space represents airway structures that:

a. cannot exchange gases
b. are necrotic
c. have wide caverns
d. exclude nasal passages

6.104. The PACU nurse observes a sustained pulmonary artery occlusion waveform. Nursing interventions to dislodge the catheter include all of the following *except:*

a. encourage cough and deep inspiration
b. reposition the patient
c. activate the catheter's fast flush system
d. remove the syringe from balloon lumen

6.105. A therapeutic dose of nitroprusside is:

a. a total daily dose of 20-40 mg/kg
b. a renal perfusion dose of 8-16 mcg/h
c. whatever the patient requires
d. 2-7 mcg/kg/min

6.106. Nitroprusside 50 mg is diluted in 250 ml D5W and delivered to an 85 kg patient. The infusion pump is set at 40 ml. The PACU nurse *most correctly* informs the physician that this patient receives:

a. 9 mcg/min
b. 1.6 mcg/kg/min
c. 0.5 mg/h
d. 40 ml/h

6.107. The PACU nurse incorporates potential for significant hypotension into the plan of care for a 68 year old man after repair of his abdominal aneurysm. Potential causes of this hypotension might include abrupt decrease in cardiac afterload, blood loss or:

a. fluid shifts into extracellular lymphatics
b. unrecognized metabolic alkalosis
c. recirculated acid metabolites
d. mesenteric artery vasoconstriction

6.108. On EKG, a pacemaker artifact consistently appears at a rate of 70 beats per minute. The patient's intrinsic rhythm, a sinus rhythm with first degree AV block (PR = 0.28), occurs regularly at 62 beats per minute. Pacemaker artifacts vary in relationship to the patient's native rhythm. This pacemaker demonstrates failure to:

a. capture
b. sense
c. stimulate
d. compete

6.109. Following left carotid endarterectomy, Mr. J is responsive but sleepy. Speech is slurred and his tongue deviates to the left. The PACU nurse suspects:

a. motor dysfunction of cranial nerve XII
b. right-sided facial edema
c. sensory deficit of cranial nerve VII
d. inadequate reversal of muscle relaxant

6.110. Positive end-expiratory pressure (PEEP) potentially causes all of the following *except:*

a. pulmonary barotrauma
b. alveolar crenation
c. subcutaneous emphysema
d. depressed cardiac output

6.111. The PACU nurse interprets a patient's mean arterial pressure (MAP) of 75 mm Hg as indicating:

a. adequate organ perfusion
b. elevated vascular resistance
c. reduced renal blood flow
d. hyperdynamic cardiac output

6.112. The PACU nurse notes a low, faint sound at the cardiac apex following the second heart sound. The sound may reflect:

a. a normal observation among elderly adults
b. impending congestive failure
c. closure of the semilunar valves
d. papillary muscle rupture

NOTE: Consider scenario and items 6.113-6.118 together.

Five years ago, 75 year old Ms P developed congestive heart failure and atrial fibrillation; mitral valve stenosis was diagnosed. Since that time she has received digoxin 0.125 mg daily and furosemide 80 mg twice each day. During today's preanesthesia assessment, the nurse observes atrial fibrillation with ventricular response of 65 beats per minute on the cardiac monitor; premature ventricular contractions occur 5-10 times per minute. Ms P also says she's had a headache and has been nauseated for 4 days; she thinks she has the "flu."

6.113. The nurse continues to assess Ms P's cardiovascular status, suspecting:

a. digitalis toxicity
b. ventricular escape dysrhythmia
c. hyperkalemia
d. furosemide insufficiency

6.114. The preanesthesia nurse consults the anesthesiologist, sends electrolytes, hemoglobin, coagulation studies, and arterial blood gas specimens to the laboratory, and prepares to:

a. administer daily doses of digoxin and furosemide IV
b. replace serum potassium deficiency
c. obtain chest x-ray to diagnose pulmonary embolus
d. infuse 1 g calcium chloride

6.115. Hemodynamically, Ms P's mitral valve stenosis:

a. allows blood to move from the left ventricle to the atrium
b. limits blood flow to the left ventricle
c. allows blood flow to the pulmonary vasculature
d. limits blood flow into the right ventricle

6.116. The nurse further assesses Ms P for:

a. clubbing of nails
b. water-hammer pulse
c. Wenckebach phenomenon
d. jugular vein distention

6.117. Ms P's mitral valve is best auscultated when the stethoscope is placed at the:

a. fourth intercostal space, left sternal border
b. second intercostal space, right midclavicular line
c. point of minimal incursion
d. fifth intercostal space, left midclavicular line

6.118. While auscultating Ms P's heart sounds, the nurse considers all of the following characteristics *except:*

a. clicks
b. pitch
c. thrills
d. intensity

NOTE: Consider items 6.119-6.121 together.

6.119. An intraaortic balloon pump (IABP) was inserted following coronary artery bypass graft of two vessels. Physiologically, an IABP supports cardiovascular hemodynamics by:

a. increasing preload and stimulating heart rate
b. decreasing preload and oxygen demand
c. decreasing afterload and myocardial oxygen consumption
d. increasing afterload and suppressing heart rate

6.120. The balloon pump alarms to signal that the patient's systolic arterial pressure is 80 mm Hg and the augmented diastolic pressure is 70 mm Hg, a decrease from 110 mm Hg ten minutes ago. Proper intervention is to:

a. assure balloon inflation precedes the R wave on EKG
b. empty and refill the balloon
c. synchronize balloon inflation with the T wave on EKG
d. clamp the balloon catheter and titrate dopamine

6.121. Patient dysrhythmias and alarm situations caused the balloon to remain uninflated for nearly 7 minutes. The most appropriate medical and nursing intervention related to this situation is:

a. balloon removal
b. heparin instilled into balloon site
c. reset timing and resume inflations
d. antibiotic prophylaxis

6.122. Potential hazards of controlled mechanical ventilation include all of the following *except:*

a. single lung ventilation
b. accumulated mediastinal air
c. increased cardiac output
d. spontaneous extubation

6.123. A patient's right hand is cannulated with a radial artery catheter for blood pressure monitoring. The PACU nurse documents and reports specific concerns about radial artery function when neurovascular assessment indicates:

a. abduction of first and second fingers
b. pain at the tip of the fourth finger
c. capillary refill lapse of 4 seconds
d. paresthesia between thumb and index finger

6.124. A pO_2 of 70 mm Hg accompanied by pCO_2 of 25 mm Hg suggests:

a. increased physiologic dead space
b. decreased capillary perfusion
c. increased intrapulmonary shunt
d. decreased alveolar perfusion

NOTE: Consider scenario and items 6.125-6.131 together.

Following thoracotomy with left upper lobectomy, Ms L arrives in PACU with one mediastinal and one pleural chest tube. The operating room circulating nurse states that 800 ml of irrigant was used intraoperatively. The PACU nurse documents 300 ml of bloody fluid in the chest tube system now in PACU.

6.125. Initial assessment of the closed chest drainage system includes:

a. clamping the mediastinal tube to detect air leak at the skin insertion site
b. disconnecting the pleural tube to drain clots into the collection chamber
c. detecting bubbles in the water seal chamber during respiration
d. emptying fluid from the collection chamber to assure accurate PACU measurement

6.126. When the PACU nurse observes active bubbling in the water seal chamber during exhalation, the *most* appropriate intervention is to:

a. auscultate breath sounds and observe bubbling
b. apply Vaseline gauze to the skin insertion site
c. reposition the patient toward the operative side
d. reduce wall suction pressure and clamp the chest tube

6.127. After 30 minutes, the PACU nurse observes no new drainage in the collection chamber. A *most appropriate first* action is to:

a. check all system chambers for leaks
b. disconnect and hand irrigate with normal saline
c. gently squeeze the drainage tube
d. increase pressure in the suction chamber by 10 cm H_2O

6.128. Placing a clamp across the latex drainage tube increases the likelihood of:

a. pleural healing
b. tension pneumothorax
c. hemorrhage
d. pleural effusion

6.129. The preferred position for this patient is:

a. flat and supine for 24 hours
b. semi-Fowler's or turned to the operative side only
c. flat and turned only to the non-operative side
d. semi-Fowler's or turned to non-operative side

6.130. After repositioning and supporting the patient with pillows, the nurse notes 90 ml of new red drainage in the chest tube. The *most appropriate* nursing action is to:

a. measure vital signs and continue assessments
b. prepare to return the patient to surgery
c. obtain hemoglobin and request 1 unit packed cells
d. infuse 250 ml lactated Ringer's solution over 45 minutes

6.131. To prepare for transfer from PACU, safe chest tube management necessitates:

a. placing the collection system at heart level
b. providing a portable suction source
c. temporarily clamping the pleural chest tube
d. eliminating dependent loops of drainage tubing

6.132. During depolarization, the myocardial cell membrane becomes more permeable to entry of:

a. water
b. sodium
c. potassium
d. protein

NOTE: Consider scenario and items 6.133-6.134 together.

6.133. The surgeon orders infusion of low molecular weight dextran 40 for a 75 year old woman who weighs 50 kg following femoral to popliteal bypass graft primarily to augment:

a. histamine release
b. circulatory volume
c. microcirculation
d. osmotic diuresis

6.134. The patient arrives in PACU with an infusion of dextran 40 at 75 ml per hour. The PACU nurse clarifies this ordered rate with the surgeon, as the current rate may:

a. hypoperfuse the kidneys
b. prolong bleeding time
c. incite hyperpyrexia
d. decrease blood viscosity

NOTE: Consider scenario and item 6.135 together.

Thirty minutes ago a 37 year old mentally challenged patient with no preoperative medical concerns was admitted to Phase I PACU after repair of inguinal herniorrhaphy with lidocaine epidural anesthetic. Sensation is present at dermatome T-10 and he moves both feet weakly. Blood pressure is sustained at 180/100.

6.135. In addition to evaluating pain, the PACU nurse assesses this patient for:

a. overhydration by dilutional hypernatremia
b. inguinal compartment syndrome
c. suprapubic pain and bladder distention
d. hernia-related gastroesophageal reflux

6.136. Atrial fibrillation with ventricular response of 180 beats per minute was converted with synchronized cardioversion to sinus rhythm at 72 beats per minute. Nursing observation includes assessment for:

a. pulmonary embolism
b. mesenteric artery spasm
c. pulmonary edema
d. popliteal claudication

6.137. Appropriate interventions when caring for a patient immediately after left pneumonectomy include:

a. applying –90 mm Hg suction to the mediastinal chest tube
b. documenting right side-lying position as Trendelenburg's
c. managing closed drainage system for pleural chest tube
d. stimulating activity and reporting right lung crackles

6.138. The nurse observes and assesses a motor vehicle accident patient who just transferred to the preanesthesia unit from the Emergency Department. A hospitalized trauma patient's potential for airway management compromise *most commonly* occurs from:

a. flail chest
b. full stomach
c. cervical fracture
d. substance abuse

NOTE: Consider scenario and items 6.139-6.140 together.

Mr. X, an oriented and alert 69 year old, experienced visual transient ischemic attacks (TIAs) at home and sought medical attention. Angiography confirmed a high-grade (>90%) stenosis of his right carotid artery. Following right carotid endarterectomy under local anesthetic, Mr. X is admitted to PACU.

6.139. Mr. X's carotid lesion is significant because:

a. retinal TIAs predict irreversible hemiparesis
b. carotid arteries deliver 85% of cerebral blood supply
c. wild cerebral perfusion pressure increases result
d. blood flow to the posterior brain is obstructed

6.140. The PACU nurse consults Mr. X's preoperative neurologic assessment to:

a. compare assessment data
b. predict positive postoperative outcomes
c. determine risk for patch graft rupture
d. monitor progress along the critical pathway

6.141. The PACU nurse *first* suspects malignant hyperthermia when the patient develops:

a. chest skin mottling
b. unexplained hyperpyrexia
c. supraventricular tachycardia
d. leg muscle tension and shaking

6.142. After the initial malignant hyperthermia crisis passes, the nursing plan of care related to effects of dantrolene sodium includes:

a. assessing swallowing and gag reflexes
b. hemofiltration to decrease myoglobinemia
c. promoting early ambulation
d. high fluid intake to prevent infection

6.143. Sympathetic blockade:

a. increases cardiac output
b. decreases neuromuscular norepinephrine
c. decreases venous return
d. increases baroreceptor sensitivity

6.144. Mr. H's spinal anesthesia results in bilateral motor and sensory blockade at the C-4 dermatome. The nurse considers potential outcomes, which include:

a. insufficient surgical paralysis to repair Mr. H's inguinal hernia
b. descending Phase II blockade
c. likely postdural spinal headache within 48 hours
d. inadequate ventilation requiring mechanical support

NOTE: Consider scenario and items 6.145-6.146 together.

Ms T, who smokes two packs of cigarettes per day, is nonresponsive and snoring regularly upon admission to Phase I PACU. Respiratory rate is 10 shallow breaths per minute; oxygen saturation is 94% per pulse oximeter with 40% oxygen.

6.145. Ms T's airway status *most commonly* results from:

a. tongue obstruction of the upper airway
b. normal postanesthesia breathing pattern
c. subglottic edema preceding laryngospasm
d. imminent smoking-induced bronchospasm

6.146. The PACU nurse's *most* prudent intervention for Ms T is to:

a. administer racemic epinephrine stat
b. apply prompt mandibular pressure
c. monitor respiratory status every 5 minutes
d. deliver 100% oxygen with positive pressure

6.147. An adult's potential to develop pulmonary edema increases with:

a. anesthetic induction with propofol
b. nalbuphine to reverse intraoperative vecuronium
c. laryngospasm after suction of copious secretions
d. cataract extraction with intraocular lens implant

6.148. Myocardial ischemia can be detected on EKG by an inverted T wave and:

a. depression of ST segment by 1 mm
b. appearance of Q wave of 0.03 seconds in lead aVR
c. elevation of ST segment by 0.5 mm in Lead II
d. duration of QRS complex beyond 0.10 seconds

6.149. The PACU nurse is most likely to observe EKG alterations that indicate myocardial ischemia when a patient:

a. receives morphine analgesia by PCA and pO_2 = 87 mm Hg
b. shivers after receiving enflurane and temperature = 37° C
c. feels weak and potassium is 6.5 mEq/L
d. receives low-dose intravenous nitroglycerin

6.150. Following anterior and posterior decompression and fusion of C3-4 and C4-5 vertebrae for degenerative disease, 62 year old Ms Q has *greatest* potential for:

a. alteration in temperature related to vasodilation below C-5 dermatome
b. ineffective breathing pattern related to diaphragmatic muscle weakness
c. ineffective bladder function with spasm and stretch related to distention
d. altered arm sensation with paresthesia related to air embolus

SET I

Answer Key

6.1. d
6.2. c
6.3. a
6.4. d
6.5. d
6.6. c
6.7. d
6.8. a
6.9. c
6.10. c
6.11. b
6.12. a
6.13. c
6.14. b
6.15. d
6.16. a
6.17. b
6.18. c
6.19. c
6.20. b
6.21. a
6.22. d
6.23. a
6.24. c
6.25. b
6.26. d
6.27. c
6.28. a
6.29. d
6.30. b
6.31. c
6.32. a
6.33. b
6.34. b
6.35. a
6.36. d
6.37. c
6.38. c
6.39. d
6.40. b
6.41. c
6.42. a
6.43. c
6.44. d
6.45. b
6.46. d
6.47. a
6.48. b
6.49. b
6.50. a

Set I

Rationales and References

6.1. Corrrect Answer: **d**

Unpleasant dreams, delirium or hallucinations may occur during emergence from ketamine anesthesia, so an unstimulating environment is preferred. Ketamine hydrochloride is a dissociative anesthetic sometimes selected to anesthetize ill, high-risk surgical patients. The patient may feel unattached to the environment. Psychologic effects occur less often among children and elderly patients over 65 years.

Harbut, RE: Anesthetic Agents and Adjuncts in ASPAN's Core Curriculum for Post Anesthesia Nursing Practice, *3rd ed (Litwack, K, Ed). Philadelphia, Saunders, pp. 108-110, 1994; Omoigui, S:* The Anesthesia Drug Handbook. *St. Louis, Mosby, pp. 98-99, 1992.*

6.2. Correct Answer: **c**

Increasing heart rate and low amplitude complexes on EKG may indicate cardiac tamponade. Fluid or blood filling the pericardial sac surrounding the heart restricts movement of cardiac muscle. Heart rate increases compensate for falling cardiac output. The pericardial window is intended to allow accumulating fluid to escape, but a sudden decrease in the chest tube output and rising heart rate with low voltage EKG complexes signal possible reaccumulation of blood or pericardial fluid. This observation must be reported to the physician. A grating friction rub is associated with pericarditis and is no surprise. This patient's BUN of 74 mg/dl indicates significant uremia, which likely caused his pericarditis. Uremia did not cause this immediate problem, though he should be dialyzed.

Benz, JJ: Acute Myocardial Infarction and Robbins, K: Renal Transplantation in Critical Care Nursing: A Holistic Approach, *6th ed. (Hudak, GM & Gallo, BM, Eds). Phildelphia, Lippincott, pp. 341 and 600, 1994.*

6.3. Correct Answer: **a**

The kidney's juxtaglomerular cells respond to any "perceived" decrease in renal blood flow with renin release. Decreases in blood pressure, circulating blood volume or serum sodium prompt renin release to initiate a chain of chemical events through the renin-angiotensin mechanism.

Weems, J: Quick Reference to Renal Critical Care Nursing. *Gaithersburg, MD, Aspen, pp. 21-23, 1991; Morgan, GE & Mikhail, MS:* Clinical Anesthesiology. *Norwalk, CT, Appleton & Lange, p. 516, 1992.*

6.4. Correct Answer: **d**

Angiotensin I is formed in direct response to increased circulating renin, then converted to angiotensin II, which causes vascular smooth muscle to constrict and increase blood pressure. Aldosterone, also released in response to angiotensin II, increases renal reabsorption of hydrogen and sodium ions and water to reexpand plasma volumes. Renin stimulation abates when renal ischemia subsides.

Drain, C: The Post Anesthesia Care Unit: A Critical Care Approach to Post Anesthesia Nursing, *3rd ed. Philadelphia, Saunders, pp. 140-142, 1994; Morgan, GE & Mikhail, MS:* Clinical Anesthesiology. *Norwalk, CT, Appleton & Lange, p. 516, 1992.*

6.5. Correct Answer: **d**

With adenosine triphosphate (ATP), magnesium activates the sodium-potassium-ATPase pump. (This influences movement of calcium, sodium, and potassium in and out of the cells and decreases acetylcholine release. Muscle contraction depends on calcium. The cell membrane stabilizes and can reduce the likelihood of ventricular ectopy. Low magnesium levels slow return of potassium to intracellular fluid and reduce the likelihoood of successful defibrillation.

American Heart Association: Adult Advanced Cardiac Life Support. JAMA *268(16): 208, 1992; Drain, C:* The Post Anesthesia Care Unit: A Critical Care Approach to Post Anesthesia Nursing, *3rd ed. Philadelphia, Saunders, p. 237, 1994.*

6.6. Correct Answer: **c**

Albuterol stimulates beta adrenergic receptors and selectively stimulates beta-2 (bronchial) receptors more than it stimulates beta-1 (cardiac) receptors. Stimulating beta adrenergic receptors in the airways maintains bronchial smooth muscle relaxation. Hyperventilation, temperature change, and anxiety are among stimuli that produce bronchoconstriction when beta-2 receptors are unstimulated; edema and increased mucous also develop.

Ahrens, TS: Respiratory Disorders in AACN's Clinical Reference for Critical-Care Nursing *(Kinney, MR, Packa, DR & Dunbar, SB, Eds). St. Louis, Mosby, pp. 721-726, 1993; Morgan, GE & Mikhail, MS:* Clinical Anesthesiology. *Norwalk, CT, Appleton & Lange, pp. 396-398, 1992.*

6.7. Correct Answer: **d**

Specifically stimulating beta-2 receptors with albuterol produces bronchodilation that begins rapidly, within 5-30 minutes after 2-3 inhalations. Effects continue for up to 5 hours. Assessment of effect includes reauscultation of the chest to determine increased breath sounds and diminished wheezing. Bronchoconstriction may have been so severe that pulmonary wheezing and air movement were inaudible prior to respiratory intervention.

Sauer, D: Post Anesthesia Respiratory Care in ASPAN's Core Curriculum for Post Anesthesia Nursing Practice, *3rd ed (Litwack, K, Ed). Philadelphia, Saunders, pp. 133-134, 1994; Chomka Leya, CM & Bandala, LC: Respiratory Complications in* Post Anesthesia Care *(Vender, JE & Speiss, BD, Eds). Philadelphia, Saunders, pp. 79-81, 1992.*

6.8. Correct Answer: **a**

Even though albuterol selectively stimulates beta-2 adrenergic receptors, some beta-1 receptor effect occurs in cardiac vessels. Cardiac stimulation may increase heart rate, alter blood pressure and produce chest pain. Overall, albuterol is versatile and has few side effects. Prior to administering a beta-2 stimulant, or agonist, determine that the patient does not have hypertension, angina or history of cardiac disease.

Morgan, GE & Mikhail, MS: Clinical Anesthesiology. *Norwalk, CT, Appleton & Lange, pp. 296-298, 1992; Lehne, RA:* Pharmacology for Nursing Care, *Philadelphia, Saunders, pp. 755-757, 1990.*

6.9. Correct Answer: **c**

Regression of the spinal block to the T-10 level (umbilicus) is usually not associated with alteration in vital body functions. Hypoventilation and hypotension are more likely when higher dermatomes (T-5 or higher) remain blocked. A fading ulnar nerve response to "train-of-4" nerve stimulation indicates residual nondepolarizing muscle relaxant; hypothermia slows metabolism of anesthetic medications and continues their effects; minimal pain increases comfort, with potential for sedation and slowed breathing.

Saleh, KL: Practical Points in Understanding Spinal Anesthesia. J Post Anesth Nurs *6(6)L: 407-409, 1991; Burden, N:* Ambulatory Surgical Nursing. *Philadelphia, Saunders, pp. 103-104, 1993.*

6.10. Correct Answer: **c**

This patient most likely only needs continued neurologic observation and time for the effects of medications to clear his system. Though altered level of consciousness is a concern after carotid endarterectomy, *this* patient demonstrates drowsy consciousness and appropriate responses to stimuli. Midazolam's amnesic effects significantly diminish recall, his only current neurologic deficit, and will fade.

Gahart, BL: Intravenous Medications, *10th ed. St. Louis, Mosby, pp. 481-483, 1994; Holloway, NM:* Nursing the Critically Ill Adult, *4th ed. Redwood City, CA, Addison-Wesley, p. 144-148, 1993; Sphritz. DW: The Neurosurgical Patient in* ASPAN's Core Curriculum for Post Anesthesia Nursing Practice, *3rd ed (Litwack, K, Ed). Philadelphia, Saunders, p. 346, 1994.*

6.11. Correct Answer: **b**

Though stenosis and intracerebral hemorrhage can cause these symptoms, carotid artery occlusion from thrombosis must be considered. Neurologic deficit can be reversed when the carotid artery is reexplored within 12 hours. This patient's neurologic changes require astute observation of hemodynamics and ventilation, with supportive intervention as necessary. Nitroprusside overdose produces profound hypotension; the brief duration of midazolam's effects make its continued influence unlikely.

Daly, KA: Post Anesthesia Care of the Vascular Surgical Patient in The Post Anesthesia Care Unit: A Critical Care Approach to Post Anesthesia Nursing *(Drain, C, Ed). Phildadelphia, Saunders, p. 393, 1994; Holloway, NM:* Nursing the Critically Ill Adult, *4th ed. Redwood City, CA, Addison-Wesley, p. 144-148, 1993.*

6.12. Correct Answer: **a**

Severe, unresolving pain in the operative extremity with paresthesia or absent sensation and inability to move (paralysis) indicate possible compartment syndrome. Edema from biochemical changes after surgery or trauma alter microcirculation in the extremity. Increasing pressure in the arm's muscle-nerve-circulatory (osseofascial) compartment compresses nerves, muscles and blood vessels, slows cellular perfusion and causes heat and pain. Arterial blood flow typically is unobstructed. True compartment syndrome is an orthopedic emergency that requires additional surgery, a fasciotomy, to release pressure.

Childs, SA: Musculoskeletal Trauma. Crit Care Nurs Clin North Am *6(3): 487-488, 1994; Litwack, K:* Post Anesthesia Care Nursing, *2nd ed. St. Louis, Mosby, p. 255, 1995.*

6.13. Correct Answer: **c**

This patient has risk to develop acute tubular necrosis. After prolonged ischemia, necrotic muscle tissue releases myoglobin into the circulation. These large molecules can obstruct renal tubules. Serum and urine myoglobin should be monitored. Compartment inflammation promotes prostaglandin and histamine release that increases local capillary dilation and membrane leakage. Tissue pressure and edema further increase and restrict perfusion.

Kull, L: The Orthopedic Surgical Patient in ASPAN's Core Curriculum for Post Anesthesia Nursing Practice, *3rd ed (Litwack, K, Ed). Philadelphia, Saunders, pp. 515-516, 1994. Childs, SA: Musculoskeletal Trauma.* Crit Care Nurs Clin North Am *6(3): 487-488, 1994.*

6.14. Correct Answer: **b**

Patients with spinal cord injuries that transect the cord above the T-6 level often develop autonomic dysreflexia (or hyperreflexia). An unrelenting stimulus from an area below the level of injury prompts unrestrained discharge of sympathetic neurons. Bladder or bowel distention, spasm or irritation from decubitus ulcer are likely stimuli. A patient with a C-5 injury may develop sudden blood pressure elevations accompanied by profuse sweating, throbbing headache and skin redness above the C-5 injury; skin pallor and goose flesh are noted below the level of injury.

Jacobsen, WK & Isaacs, WB: Orthopedic Complications in Manual of Post Anesthesia Care *(Jacobsen, WK, Ed). Philadelphia, Saunders, p. 142, 1992; Shpritz, DW: The Neurosurgical Patient in* ASPAN's Core Curriculum for Post Anesthesia Nursing Practice, *3rd ed (Litwack, K, Ed). Philadelphia, Saunders, pp. 385-386, 1994.*

6.15. Correct Answer: **d**

Treatment of autonomic dysreflexia (hyperreflexia) focuses on relieving the triggering stimulus and aggressively by reducing blood pressure. Vasodilators to reduce afterload may be used. Hydralazine (Apresoline) may be used initially. Careful dose titration is needed to prevent deep drops in blood pressure. Eliminating the stimulus—urinary catheter patency and bowel emptying, for example—helps prevent autonomic dysreflexia. This particular patient has no bladder, though the nurse must monitor urinary drainage from the newly created ileal conduit.

Walleck, C: Patients with Spinal Cord Injury in Critical Care Nursing *(Clochesy, JM, Breu, C, Cardin, S, et al, Eds). Philadelphia, Saunders, pp. 748 & 761, 1992; Hawkins, JK & Hawkins,*

VC: Post Anesthesia Care of the Neurosurgical Patient in The Post Anesthesia Care Unit: A Critical Care Approach to Post Anesthesia Nursing, *3rd ed (Drain, C, Ed). Philadelphia, Saunders, pp. 439-440, 1994.*

6.16. Correct Answer: **a**

Tracheal deviation with respiratory distress after neck surgery suggests rapid hemorrhage into neck tissue and must be eliminated as the cause of dyspnea. Hypertensive and unreversed antiplatelet medications may contribute to artery rupture. Copious bleeding is unlikely to be removed by traditional postoperative suction systems. Microemboli to brain tissue may alter neurologic assessment, but would probably not produce a sudden increase of intracranial pressure with herniation.

Daly, KA: Post Anesthesia Care of the Vascular Surgical Patient in The Post Anesthesia Care Unit: A Critical Care Approach to Post Anesthesia Nursing, *3rd ed. (Drain, C, Ed). Phildadelphia, Saunders, p. 393, 1994; Holloway, NM:* Nursing the Critically Ill Adult, *4th ed. Redwood City, CA, Addison-Wesley, p. 144-148, 1993.*

6.17. Correct Answer: **b**

Ms W's dyspnea and sharp left-sided chest pain after an injection to place a left brachial plexus block suggest left pneumothorax. There is a small but notable 1% potential for pneumothorax associated with a supraclavicular approach to provide brachial plexus anesthesia. The small needle used to place a local anesthetic block can nick or puncture the pleural space. As air gains entry into this space, pressures inside and outside the lung equalize. The lung on the side of air entry cannot remain expanded; its volume decreases and the lung collapses. Breath sounds over the area of collapse may be decreased or absent; the patient may cough and observer may note asymmetric chest wall movement. The size of the collapsed lung tissue predicts treatment.

Drain, C: The Post Anesthesia Care Unit: A Critical Care Approach to Post Anesthesia Nursing, *3rd ed. Philadelphia, Saunders, p. 256, 1994; Chomka Leya, CM & Bandala, LC: Respiratory Complications in* Post Anesthesia Care *(Vender, JS & Speiss, BD, Eds). Philadelphia, Saunders, pp. 86-88, 1992.*

6.18. Correct Answer: **c**

Observing cardiopulmonary stability, delivering oxygen, and following resolution of the collapsed lung area with serial chest x-rays are usually adequate interventions when pneumothorax is less than 20%. Chest tubes are warranted for patients with larger areas of collapse, patients with little cardiovascular or pulmonary reserve, or patients who receive positive pressure ventilation. Ms W is currently hemodynamically stable and breathes adequately. The PACU nurse should collaborate with the anesthesiologist to mutually determine when Ms W is ready for transfer from PACU.

Drain, C: The Post Anesthesia Care Unit: A Critical Care Approach to Post Anesthesia Nursing, *3rd ed. Philadelphia, Saunders, p. 256, 1994; Chomka Leya, CM & Bandala, LC: Respiratory Complications in* Post Anesthesia Care *(Vender, JS & Speiss, BD, Eds). Philadelphia, Saunders, pp. 86-88, 1992.*

6.19. Correct Answer: **c**

Ketamine stimulates the cardiovascular system during anesthesia induction, a unique feature among anesthetic medications. For the patient in shock, such stimulation increases heart rate and sympathetic response to support blood pressure. With this desirable characteristic, ketamine earns acclaim as a safe anesthetic choice for the patient at high risk. Postshock survival may improve, perhaps due to improved capillary perfusion. Ketamine is classified as a dissociative neuroleptic and selectively alters pain perception.

Hanson, CW: Managing the Desperately Ill Patient: Trauma and Shock in Dripps/Eckenhoff/Vandam Introduction to Anesthesia, *8th ed. (Longnecker, DE & Murphy, FL, Eds). Philadelphia, Saunders, pp. 371-373, 1992; Morgan, GE & Mikhail, MS:* Clinical Anesthesiology. *Norwalk, CT, Appleton & Lange, pp. 127-139, 1992.*

6.20. Correct Answer: **b**

The trauma patient's potential to aspirate stomach contents is "presumed" to be high. The anesthesia provider may induce anesthesia using a rapid sequence technique to decrease this aspiration risk. Before induction, the patient is preoxygenated with 100% oxygen. An intravenous anesthetic like thiopental and a muscle relaxant quickly render the patient unconscious with blunted gag, swallow, and cough reflexes to allow prompt intubation. Applying simultaneous cricoid pressure collapses the esophagus to prevent regurgitation until the airway is intubated and cuff inflated. Rapid sequence induction is also used for a patient with a full stomach or one who is obese or pregnant or who has a difficult airway to intubate.

Hanson, CW: Managing the Desperately Ill Patient: Trauma and Shock in Dripps/Eckenhoff/Vandam Introduction to Anesthesia, *8th ed. (Longnecker, DE & Murphy, FL, Eds). Philadelphia, Saunders, pp. 371-373, 1992; Morgan, GE & Mikhail, MS:* Clinical Anesthesiology. *Norwalk, CT, Appleton & Lange, pp. 185-186, 1992.*

6.21. Correct Answer: **a**

Urine volume of more than 0.5 ml/kg each hour, a minimum of 30 ml, generally suggests adequate cardiac output and therefore sufficient renal perfusion. Renal blood flow consumes up to 25% of cardiac output and is maintained by autoregulation and adequate renal perfusion pressure with mean arterial blood pressure of 60-80 mmHg.

Mamaril, ME: Post Anesthesia Care of the Shock Trauma Patient in The Post Anesthesia Care Unit: A Critical Care Approach to Post Anesthesia Nursing *(Drain, C, Ed). Philadelphia, Saunders, pp. 574-575, 1994; Jacobsen, WK: Renal Complications in* Manual of Post Anesthesia Care *(Jacobsen, WK, Ed). Philadelphia, Saunders, pp. 104-105, 1992.*

6.22. Correct Answer: **d**

Electrical signals and muscle activity transmitted through an implantable pacemaker to the pulse generator are misinterpreted as "noise" and can fool the pacemaker and disrupt its sensing capability. Improperly grounded electrical equipment or surgical electrocautery can cause the pacemaker to misinterpret, or incorrectly sense, electrical energy as cardiac energy. The pacemaker either fails to deliver an impulse (spike) during the interference (oversensing), producing asystole, or reverts to a fixed rate (undersensing), producing competition.

Witherell, CL: Cardiac Rhythm Control Devices. Nurs Clin North Am *6(1): 85-95, 1994; Fetzer-Fowler, S: Caring for the Ambulatory Surgical Patient Who Has A Pacemaker: Parts I & II.* Post Anesth Nurs *8(3,4): 116-123, 1993.*

6.23. Correct Answer: **a**

Smoking decreases circulating hemoglobin by at least 10%, paralyzes cilia, increases secretion production and clearance, and closes small airways. Anesthetic medications, obesity and pain also alter lung volumes by decreasing functional residual capacity (FRC), the amount of air in the lungs at the end of a normal breath. These factors limit diaphragm movement and can, over time, promote airway closure. Hypertension and obesity increase oxygen consumption; asthma increases FRC by overdistending pulmonary structures.

Burden, N: Ambulatory Surgical Nursing. *Philadelphia, Saunders, pp. 390-391, 1993; Shekleton, ME: General Responses to Surgery in* Critical Care Nursing of the Surgical Patient *(Shekleton, ME & Litwack, K, Eds). Philadelphia, Saunders, p. 15, 1991.*

6.24. Correct Answer: **c**

The obese patient needs postoperative head and shoulder elevation and attention to body mechanics so that diaphragm movement is not limited and full lung expansion can occur. These essentials decrease aspiration risk and improve ventilation, high risks for the obese patient. Postoperative positioning affects oxygenation for up to 2 days. Ms O may be mechanically ventilated or need anxiety reduction, but just as likely not. This woman needs cautious, not liberal, fluid replacement; fat contains less than 10% water, so her total body water is reduced and she may also have vascular pathologies like hypertension.

Burden, N: Ambulatory Surgical Nursing. *Philadelphia, Saunders, pp. 388-389, 1993; Drain, C:* The Post Anesthesia Care Unit: A Critical Care Approach to Post Anesthesia Nursing, *3rd ed. Philadelphia, Saunders, pp. 525-527, 1994.*

6.25. Correct Answer: **b**

Vital capacity (VC) is the maximal volume of air that can be forcefully exhaled after a maximal inspiration. Normally, 60-70 ml/kg, VC is altered by muscle strength and lung compliance.

Morgan, GE & Mikhail, SM: Clinical Anesthesiology. *Norwalk, CT, Appleton & Lange, pp. 368-372, 1992.*

6.26. Correct Answer: **d**

An alveolar shunt is an imbalance, or mismatch, between ventilation and perfusion. Blood supply is adequate, but air exchange is impaired. Atelectatic or fluid-soaked alveoli cannot be ventilated and oxygen-carbon dioxide gas exchange between alveolus and capillary cannot occur. Unoxygenated venous blood mixes into arterial blood, producing hypoxia and respiratory acidosis. Normal anatomic shunt due to physiologic dead space is approximately 3% of cardiac output.

Brockmann, DC, Jacobsen, WK & Lobo, DP: Respiratory Management in Manual of Post Anesthesia Care *(Jacobsen, WK, Ed). Philadelphia, Saunders, p. 89, 1992; Drain, C:* The Post Anesthesia Care Unit: A Critical Care Approach to Post Anesthesia Nursing, *3rd ed. Philadelphia, Saunders, p. 127-129, 1994.*

6.27. Correct Answer: **c**

A loud, churning sound in the chest, a "mill-wheel murmur," is a classic indicator of air embolism. Check the capped catheter port. As the patient breathes, a leaking connection or frank catheter-tubing disconnection allows air to be drawn through the lumen of any catheter placed into the central venous circulation. Intrathoracic pressure increases. Air bubbles are retained at the right atrium and ventricle, eventually "bumping" the pulmonary valve. Air churns with blood in the cavities, producing foam.

Brockmann, DC, Jacobsen, WK & Lobo, DP: Respiratory Management in Manual of Post Anesthesia Care *(Jacobsen, WK, Ed). Philadelphia, Saunders, p. 88, 1992; Stoelting, RK & Dierdorf, SF:* Handbook for Anesthesia and Coexisting Diseases. *New York, Churchill-Livingstone, pp. 242-244, 1993.*

6.28. Correct Answer: **a**

Position the patient right side up and head down so air is trapped in the right heart and blood, not air, flows to the brain. Air is lighter than fluid and rises to the top of a closed system. It is possible to draw 100 ml of air into the circulatory system with each respiration. Interventions aim to impede air from traveling into the arterial circulation through the left heart and to the brain. *Any* patient with a central catheter, including pulmonary artery catheters, in a jugular or subclavian vessel has increased risk for venous air embolism.

Hudak, C & Gallo, B: Critical Care Nursing: A Holistic Approach, *6th ed. Philadelphia, Lippincott, p. 202, 1994; Stoelting, RK & Dierdorf, SF:* Handbook for Anesthesia and Coexisting Diseases. *New York, Churchill-Livingstone, pp. 242-244, 1993.*

6.29. Correct Answer: **d**

Time and continued drug metabolism will increase chances of extubation success. This patient does not yet display adequate muscle strength and wakefulness to wean from the ventilator without rapid fatigue and likely the need to reintubate. Specific tests seldom predict successful postextubation respiratory quality. Each patient's clinical status must be assessed for general improvement. Parameters might include ability to cooperate, muscle strength (including sustained respiratory rate without apnea and ability to lift head from pillow) and adequate blood gas and minute volume measures.

Schweinefus, R & Schick, L: Succinylcholine: "Good Guy, Bad Guy." J Post Anesth Nurs *6(6): 410-419, 1991; Sauer, D: Post Anesthesia Respiratory Care in* ASPAN's Core Curriculum for Post Anesthesia Care Nursing, *3rd ed (Litwack, K, Ed). Philadelphia, Saunders, pp. 140-141, 1994; Bolton, PJ & Kline, KA: Understanding Modes of Mechanical Ventilation.* Am J Nurs *94(6): 36-42, 1994.*

6.30. Correct Answer: **b**

Assessing muscle strength, particularly of respiratory muscles, helps predict whether this patient can sustain respiration without fatigue. Though any numeric criteria must be considered in the context of each patient's clinical situation, clinical measures may reflect muscle strength. Minute volume is a gauge to estimate the tidal volume a patient can generate. Ability to generate vital capacity (VC) of 15 ml/kg with tidal volumes of more than 5 ml/kg and negative inspiratory force (NIF) of -20 cm H_2O suggests adequate strength.

Schweinefus, R & Schick, L: Succinylcholine: "Good Guy, Bad Guy." J Post Anesth Nurs *6(6): 410-419, 1991; Geer, RT: Critical Care of the Surgical Patient in* Dripps/Eckenhoff/Vandam Introduction to Anesthesia, *8th ed (Longnecker, DE & Murphy, FL, Eds). Philadelphia, Saunders, pp. 468-469, 1992.*

6.31. Correct Answer: **c**

Assuring adequate oxygenation is a primary intervention when restlessness, cardiac changes and unclear clinical signs develop. Hypoxemia, with PaO_2 documented in the 60-70 mm Hg range, is likely. The patient should be held in PACU for assessment of cardiorespiratory systems, nursing and medical consultation, and any initial treatment.

Walleck, CA & Kenner, CV: Extremity Trauma in Critical Care Nursing: Body-Mind-Spirit *(Dossey, BM, Guzzetta, CE & Kenner, CV, Eds). Philadelphia, Lippincott, pp. 804-805, 1992; Kull, L: The Orthopedic Surgical Patient in* ASPAN's Core Curriculum for Post Anesthesia Nursing Care, *3rd ed. (Litwack, K, Ed). Philadelphia, Saunders, pp. 523-524, 1994.*

6.32. Correct Answer: **a**

Orthopedic patients with long bone fractures or hip surgery have high risk to develop fat embolism as early as 12 hours after fracture. Inverted T wave, Q wave in Lead III, tachycardia, dyspnea, torso petechiae, disorientation and restlessness are symptoms. Treatment includes assuring oxygenation and administering steroids. In addition to hypoxia, platelets and hemoglobin generally decrease. This patient's leg weakness likely results from residual regional anesthetic and probably is unrelated to the suspected embolus.

Walleck, CA & Kenner, CV: Extremity Trauma in Critical Care Nursing: Body-Mind-Spirit *(Dossey, BM, Guzzetta, CE & Kenner, CV, Eds). Philadelphia, Lippincott, pp. 804-805, 1992; Kull, L: The Orthopedic Surgical Patient in* ASPAN's Core Curriculum for Post Anesthesia Nursing Care, *3rd ed. (Litwack, K, Ed). Philadelphia, Saunders, pp. 523-524, 1994.*

6.33. Correct Answer: **b**

Small diameter catheters should be used to suction an endotracheal or tracheostomy tube. Technique includes preoxygenation with 100% FiO_2 for up to 5 minutes, selecting a coudé (curved) catheter that is less than one-half the inner diameter of the artificial airway, and limiting aspiration time to less than 15 seconds.

Chulay, M: Airway and Ventilatory Management in Critical Care Nursing: Body-Mind-Spirit *(Dossey, BM, Guzzetta, CE & Ken-*

ner, CV, Eds). Philadelphia, Lippincott, pp. 221, 1992.

6.34. Correct Answer: **b**

Aspiration of gastric contents or blood can occur quickly and quietly in anesthetized or sedated patients. Treatment intervention varies with the amount of aspirant and symptoms. Suction, oxygen administration, observation for hypoxia or airway obstruction, and repositioning to head-up or side-lying position are critical. Obesity, hiatal hernia, gas insufflation of the abdomen for laparoscopy, and Trendlenburg's position are among factors increasing risk of aspiration.

Brockmann, DC, Jacobsen, WK & Lobo, DP: Respiratory Management in Manual of Post Anesthesia Care *(Jacobsen, WK, Ed). Philadelphia, Saunders, pp. 90-91, 1992. Burden, N:* Ambulatory Surgical Nursing. *Philadelphia, Saunders, pp. 135-136, 1993.*

6.35. Correct Answer: **a**

Increasing the concentration of delivered oxygen is wise. Blood gases and pulse oximetry measures indicate hypoxemia. An H_2 antogonist such as cimetidine may reduce gastric acidity but will be too late, and thus ineffective, to treat this aspiration. Deep breathing may increase respiratory alkalosis. Routine administration of antibiotics is not recommended after aspiration; the antibiotic disrupts the patient's microbe balance, prompting growth of resistant strains.

Brockmann, DC, Jacobsen, WK & Lobo, DP: Respiratory Management in Manual of Post Anesthesia Care *(Jacobsen, WK, Ed). Philadelphia, Saunders, pp. 90-91, 1992; Burden, N:* Ambulatory Surgical Nursing. *Philadelphia, Saunders, pp. 135-136, 1993.*

6.36. Correct Answer: **d**

Acidic gastric contents are highly irritating to lung tissue. Bronchospasm with dyspnea, cough, diffuse wheezing and a long, sometimes forced, expiratory phase occur. Regurgitation and aspiration are most likely to occur during anesthesia induction and emergence. As little as 25 ml can prompt pulmonary symptoms, particularly when gastric pH is <2.5. Damage to capillaries and alveoli of the lung's endothelium produce varying degrees of hypoxia, pulmonary edema or airway spasm.

Brockmann, DC, Jacobsen, WK & Lobo, DP: Respiratory Management in Manual of Post Anesthesia Care *(Jacobsen, WK, Ed). Philadelphia, Saunders, pp. 90-91, 1992; Burden, N:* Ambulatory Surgical Nursing. *Philadelphia, Saunders, pp. 135-136, 1993.*

6.37. Correct Answer: **c**

Applying ice and maintaining extremity elevation to a level above the heart are recommended interventions to best promote extremity circulation. Epidurally infused narcotics are unlikely to be effective for upper extremity analgesia. Absent thumb hyperextension indicates motor compromise to the ulnar nerve and should be promptly reported, not just observed. Neurovascular reassessment occurs 3-4 times per hour during the early postoperative period.

Kull, L: The Orthopedic Surgical Patient in ASPAN's Core Curriculum for Post Anesthesia Nursing Practice, *3rd ed (Litwack, K, Ed). Philadelphia, Saunders, pp. 515-516, 1994.*

6.38. Correct Answer: **c**

Hypoventilation often occurs in tandem with sedation; drowsiness and low oxygen saturations (typically <92%) or shallow or very slow respirations are primary signals that the patient requires stimulation. Anesthetic medications depress consciousness, cardiac function and respirations. Until consciousness returns, a sedated patient depends on a nurse's vigilant observation to prevent hypoxic events. Without intervention, referred to by some as the "stir-up regimen," dangerous tissue hypoxia can result.

Burden, N: Ambulatory Surgical Nursing. *Philadelphia, Saunders, pp. 254 & 290-291, 1993; O'Brien, DD: Care of the Post Anesthesia Patient in* The Post Anesthesia Care Unit: A Critical Care Approach to Post Anesthesia Nursing, *3rd ed (Drain, C, Ed). Philadelphia, Saunders, p. 289, 1994.*

6.39. Correct Answer: **d**

Preload represents blood volume contained in the ventricles at the end of each diastole, just prior to muscle contraction. To a point ("critical volume"), cardiac output increases when preload increases and cardiac muscle fibers stretch. Ventricles fill during the diastolic portion of the cardiac cycle; if ventricles underfill, contractile force decreases and cardiac output falls. Overfilled chambers overstretch muscle fibers and also decrease force ofcontraction. The Frank-Starling Law of the heart describes the relationships between cardiac muscle fiber stretch and contractile force.

Dossey, BM, Guzzetta, CE, & Kenner, CV: Critical Care Nursing: Body-Mind-Spirit, *3rd ed. Philadelphia, Lippincott, pp. 237, 1992; Drain, C:* The Post Anesthesia Care Unit: A Critical Care Approach to Post Anesthesia Nursing, *3rd ed. Philadelphia, Saunders, pp. 82-85, 1994.*

6.40. Correct Answer: **b**

The normal range of an adult's cardiac output is 4.5-6 liters per minute.

Drain, C: The Post Anesthesia Care Unit: A Critical Care Approach to Post Anesthesia Nursing, *3rd ed. Philadelphia, Saunders, p. 84, 1994.*

6.41. Correct Answer: **c**

Cardiac output (CO) is the calculated product of heart rate (HR) and stroke volume (SV), or CO = SV × HR. Cardiac output is a measure of the volume of blood pumped by the ventricle each minuteand therefore expresses ventricular function.

Morgan, GE, & Mikhail, MS: Clinical Anesthesiology. *Norwalk, CT, Appleton & Lange, p. 290, 1992; Drain, C:* The Post Anesthesia Care Unit: A Critical Care Approach to Post Anesthesia Nursing, *3rd ed. Philadelphia, Saunders, pp. 82-85, 1994.*

6.42. Correct Answer: **a**

Plaque and obstructions to right carotid blood flow were surgically removed; evaluating an audible bruit is not necessary. Carotid endarterectomy disturbs the baroreceptors that compensate for hemodynamic and ventilatory changes. As a result, wide blood pressure swings and erratic responses to physiologic chemical changes are likely. Right-sided blood flow to the brain was interrupted; assess cranial nerve function related to vision, pupillary responses, facial symmetry and airway patency. Voice quality reveals hoarseness, inability to make sounds and laryneal nerve injury. Injury to more than one laryngeal nerve is associated with greater possibility of stridor and airway obstruction.

Mitchell, SK & Yates, RR: Cerebrovascular Disease in Critical Care Nursing: Body-Mind-Spirit, *3rd ed (Dossey, BM, Guzzetta, CE & Kenner, CV, Eds). Philadelphia, Lippincott, pp. 604-606, 1992; Morgan, GE & Mikhail, MS:* Clinical Anesthesiology. *Norwalk, CT, Appleton & Lange, p. 51, 1992.*

6.43. Correct Answer: **c**

End-tidal carbon dioxide (ET_{CO_2}) trends monitored with capnography reflect respiratory adequacy in an *intubated* patient. Increasing carbon dioxide trends or abrupt changes in the capnogram waveform signal physiologic change and alert the caregiver to reassess the patient. Carbon dioxide retention indicates respiratory acidosis, esophageal intubation, accidental extubation, or increased dead space from an acute obstruction to pulmonary blood flow. Retained carbon dioxide increases cerebral blood flow and intracranial pressure; adaption to these changes is likely altered in a neurologically compromised patient.

Sauer, D: Post Anesthesia Respiratory Care in ASPAN's Core Curriculum for Post Anesthesia Care Nursing Practice, *3rd ed (Litwack, K, Ed). Philadelphia, Saunders, p. 136, 1994; Savino, JS: Monitoring the Anesthetized Patient in* Dripps/Eckenhoff/Vandam Introduction to Anesthesia, *8th ed (Longnecker, DE & Murphy, FL, Eds). Philadelphia, Saunders, p. 61, 1992.*

6.44. Correct Answer: **d**

Particularly when associated with myocardial infarction or medications known to delay intracardiac conduction, Type II heart block may progress to complete heart block. P waves occur regularly and at a normal rate in this form of second degree AV heart block, also known as Mobitz Type II block. A QRS complex may follow only after each second, third, or fourth P wave. Ventricular conduction and cardiac output can therefore drop significantly.

Tremblay, DR, et al: Arrhythmias in the PACU: A Review. Crit Care Nurs Clin North Am *3(1): 106-108, 1991; Moungey, SJ: Patients With Sinus Node Dysfunction or Atrioventricular Blocks.* Crit Care Nurs Clin of North Amer *6(1): 55-67, 1994.*

6.45. Correct Answer: **b**

An external pacemaker supports adequate heart rate and cardiac output when AV conduction delays associated with Type II heart block produce symptoms. Some patients show no clinical symptoms. Depending upon the ventricular rate, chest pain, hypoxia, hypotension, and dizziness are possible events. Second degree heart block may progress to complete heart block (or it may not) and requires both determination of the cause of the block and close observation. Perioperative myocardial infarction, particularly with anterior wall damage, might account for significant heart block. Titrated doses of isoproterenol or atropine must beused cautiously; a 3 mg/kg isoproterenol dose is too large.

Tremblay, DR, Fischer, RL, Caouette, CJ, et al: Arrhythmias in the PACU: A Review. Crit Care Nurs

Clin North Am *3(1): 106-108, 1991; American Heart Association: Adult Advanced Cardiac Life Support.* JAMA *268(16): 2213-2214, 1992; Moungey, SJ: Patietns With Sinus Node Dysfunction or Atrioventricular Blocks.* Crit Care Nurs Clin of North Amer *6(1): 55-67, 1994.*

6.46. Correct Answer: **d**

A pacemaker programmed in the VVI mode is a demand pacemaker. This pacemaker initiates an impulse only when the patient's ventricular complex does not occur. The internationally accepted NBG pacemaker code establishes consistent, generic language to describe pacemaker functions. The VVI code designates that the ventricle (first V) is the heart chamber receiving a pacemaker impulse; the ventricle (second V) is the chamber sensed. In response to sensing a patient's ventricular impulse, the pacemaker is inhibited (I).

Fetzer-Fowler, S: Caring for the Ambulatory Surgical Patient Who Has a Pacemaker: Part I. J Post Anesth Nurs *8(2): 116-124, 1993.*

6.47. Correct Answer: **a**

Symptoms that herald pacemaker failure, whether from an exhausted power source, loss of electrode-myocardial contact or incorrect programming parameters, must be investigated prior to surgery. Light-headedness, fainting, palpitations, chest pain, and congestive failure indicate lack of adequate pacemaker function.

Fetzer-Fowler, S: Caring for the Ambulatory Surgical Patient Who Has a Pacemaker: Part I. J Post Anesth Nurs *8(2): 116-124, 1993.*

6.48. Correct Answer: **b**

Exposing a pacemaker to electromagnetic interference (EMI) may inhibit its sensing capability. Noncardiac myopotentials (muscle activity) or electrical signals from surgical cautery are sensed (misread) as cardiac electrical activity. This VVI, or demand, pacemaker typically will shut off and fail to generate an impulse. Failure to capture the ventricle may occur if electrical burns damage myocardial tissue.

Fetzer-Fowler, S: Caring for the Ambulatory Surgical Patient Who Has a Pacemaker: Part II. J Post Anesth Nurs *8(2): 174-181, 1993; Zaidan, JR: Pacemakers in* Manual of Cardiac Anesthesia, *2nd ed (Thomas, SJ & Kramer, JL, Eds). New York, Churchill-Livingstone, pp. 369-385, 1993.*

6.49. Correct Answer: **b**

The dose of dopamine must be decreased by 90% when administered to patients who take monoamine oxidase (MAO) inhibitors. Both MAO inhibitors and tricyclic antidepressants potentiate dopamine's effect on heart and blood vessels.

Whalen, DA & Izzi, G: Pharmacologic Treatment of Acute Congestive Heart Failure Resulting From Left Ventricular Systolic or Diastolic Dysfunction. Crit Care Nurs Clin North Am *5(2): 261-269, 1993; American Heart Association:* Textbook of Advanced Cardiac Life Support *(Cummins, RO, Ed). Dallas, American Heart Association, pp. 8.3-8.8, 1994.*

6.50. Correct Answer: **a**

Dopamine's effects on heart and blood vessels are dose related. Low doses (1-3 mcg/kg/min) affect dopamine receptor sites and support renal and mesenteric blood flow; moderate doses (2-10 mcg/kg/min) affect beta receptors, with peripheral vasodilating effects; highest doses (>8-10 mcg/kg/min) promote vasoconstriction that actually offsets the beneficial effects of lower doses.

Litwack, K: ASPAN's Core Curriculum for Post Anesthesia Nursing Practice, *3rd ed. Philadelphia, Saunders, pp. 222-223, 1994; American Heart Association:* Textbook of Advanced Cardiac Life Support *(Cummins, RO, Ed). Dallas, American Heart Association, pp. 8.3-8.8, 1994.*

Set II

Answer Key

6.51.	d
6.52.	b
6.53.	a
6.54.	d
6.55.	a
6.56.	d
6.57.	b
6.58.	c
6.59.	d
6.60.	d
6.61.	b
6.62.	a
6.63.	a
6.64.	a
6.65.	b
6.66.	d
6.67.	a
6.68.	a
6.69.	c
6.70.	a
6.71.	c
6.72.	c
6.73.	a
6.74.	b
6.75.	d
6.76.	c
6.77.	b
6.78.	a
6.79.	a
6.80.	d
6.81.	c
6.82.	b
6.83.	c
6.84.	a
6.85.	b
6.86.	d
6.87.	a
6.88.	d
6.89.	a
6.90.	a
6.91.	b
6.92.	c
6.93.	b
6.94.	d
6.95.	b
6.96.	d
6.97.	a
6.98.	a
6.99.	b
6.100.	c

SET II

Rationales and References

6.51. Correct Answer: **d**

Most likely, the pulmonary artery catheter slipped into the right ventricle, probably when the patient was moved from the operating table or during transport. If the catheter does not float into the pulmonary artery position with balloon inflation, the physician must reposition the catheter. After patient movement, the nurse observes the monitor for changes in measured pressures, waveform configuration or arrhythmias of ventricular origin. Lidocaine and a defibrillator are available prophylactically.

Kadota, LT: Hemodynamic Monitoring in Critical Care Nursing *(Clochesy, JM, Breu, C, Cardin, S, et al, Eds). Philadelphia, Saunders, p. 165, 1992; Biga, CD & Bethel, SA: Hemodynamic Monitoring in* ASPAN's Core Curriculum for Post Anesthesia Nursing Practice, *3rd ed (Litwack, K, Ed). Philadelphia, Saunders, pp. 662-665, 1994.*

6.52. Correct Answer: **b**

Intermittent mandatory ventilation (IMV) allows the patient to control, or "trigger," the frequency and depth of each breath during weaning from mechanical ventilation. A minimum rate and volume are preset to assure adequate ventilation and pO_2. As the patient demonstrates increasing ability to support an adequate minute volume, the frequency of ventilator-delivered breaths can be gradually decreased.

Bolton, PJ: Understanding Modes of Mechanical Ventilation. Am J Nurs *94(6): 36-42, 1994; Chulay, M: Airway and Ventilatory Management in* Critical Care Nursing: Body-Mind-Spirit, *3rd ed (Dossey, BM, Guzzetta, CE & Kenner, CV, Eds). Philadelphia, Lippincott, pp. 227, 1992.*

6.53. Correct Answer: **a**

After removing the stimulus of spasm, positive pressure ventilation by mask, oxygenation and jaw support often break the spasm. Sometimes a partial laryngeal obstruction can be reversed with jaw support, humidified oxygen, warmth to the neck, and constant attention to coach breathing and calm the patient's anxiety. Intravenous lidocaine may reduce airway irritability, thereby relaxing a spasm. Succinylcholine and reintubation are potential options if laryngospasm is prolonged or complete obstruction occurs.

Drain, C: The Post Anesthesia Care Unit: A Critical Care Approach to Post Anesthesia Nursing, *3rd ed. Philadelphia, Saunders, pp. 106-108, 1994; Berge, KH & Lanier, WL: Problems After Head, Neck, and Maxillofacial Surgery in* Post Anesthesia Care *(Vender, JS & Speiss, BD, Eds). Philadelphia, Saunders, pp. 283-288, 1992.*

6.54. Correct Answer: **d**

Cardiac index (CI) is a patient-specific calculation to indicate cardiac function. A CI of 2.7-4.3 $L/min/m^2$ indicates normal perfusion. Cardiac output is mathematically individualized to body size (CI) by dividing cardiac output (CO) by the patient's body surface area (BSA):

$$\frac{CO}{BSA} = CI.$$

Brauer, SD: Management of the Cardiac Surgery Patient in Manual of Post Anesthesia Care *(Jacobsen, WK, ED). Philadelphia, Saunders, p. 64, 1992; Dossey, BM, Guzzetta, CE & Kenner, CV:* Critical Care Nursing: Body-Mind-Spirit, *3rd ed. Philadelphia, Lippincott, pp. 470, 1992.*

6.55. Correct Answer: **a**

Exposure to light degrades a reconstituted solution of sodium nitroprusside. An opaque covering must be placed over the container.

Shannon, MT, Wilson, BA & Stang, CL: Govoni & Hayes Drugs and Nursing Implications, *8th ed. Norwalk, CT, Appleton & Lange, pp. 836-837, 1995.*

6.56. Correct Answer: **d**

Most often, blood pressure quickly returns to acceptable levels when the rate of nitroprusside infusion is reduced. The very rapid effects of sodium nitroprusside can quickly produce profound hypotension. The medication's elimination half-life is ultrashort, about 2 minutes, and metabolism is rapid.

Whalen, DA & Izzi, G: Pharmacologic Treatment of Acute Congestive Heart Failure Resulting From Left Ventricular Systolic or Diastolic Dysfunction. Crit Care Nurs Clin North Am *5(2): 265, 1993; Benowitz, NL: Antihypertensive Agents in* Basic & Clinical Pharmacology, *6th ed (Katzung, BG, Ed). Norwalk, CT, Appleton & Lange, pp. 161-162, 1995.*

6.57. Correct Answer: **b**

Altitude-related noncardiogenic pulmonary edema (NCPE), or permeability edema, evolves over 1-3 days after sudden large movement from low to high altitude. Between 9,000 and 12,000 feet above sea level, pulmonary hypertension, infiltrates, and hypoxia develop in some individuals. Reasons for this edema are unclear, but symptoms can occur in up to 15% of otherwise healthy people during abrupt change in altitude. A patient who is still acclimating to higher altitude may require emergency surgery; the physiologic changes demanded by altitude may affect the PACU nurse's intervention.

Rubenstein, EH: Physiological Adaptations to High Altitude. Sem Anesth *IX(3): 211-220, 1990; Morgan, GE & Mikhail, MS:* Clinical Anesthesiology. *Norwalk, CT, Appleton & Lange, p. 709, 1992.*

6.58. Correct Answer: **c**

Hypoxemia is extremely likely during any episode of pulmonary edema, so increasing oxygen delivery is essential. Anxiety, patient restlessness, airway excitability, and greater metabolic and cardiac work increase oxygen demand at a time when ability to adequately ventilate is limited. Suctioning only increases restlessness and secretions. A diuretic may be administered, though this is individually determined by degree of fluid infiltraton. A leg-elevated position may increase, not improve, the edema by increasing venous return. Digitalization is seldom used to treat noncardiogenic pulmonary edema (NCPE).

Hamlin, W, Schnobel, L & Smith, B: The Patient With Noncardiogenic Pulmonary Edema. J Post

Anesth Nurs *6(1): 43-49, 1991; Burden, N:* Ambulatory Surgical Nursing. *Philadelphia, Saunders, pp. 137-138, 1993.*

6.59. Correct Answer: **d**

Particularly when induced while the patient is in the supine position, general anesthesia decreases the diaphragm's muscle tone, chest and lung compliance, and functional residual capacity (FRC). Abdominal contents more easily push toward the chest. Altered lung and chest elasticity continues postoperatively. FRC is also altered by obesity, head-down positions and restrictive pulmonary diseases.

Marley, RA: Postoperative Administration of Aerosolized Medications: Part I—The Basics. J Post Anesth Nurs *8(5): 285-296, 1993; Morgan, GE & Mikhail, SM:* Clinical Anesthesiology. *Norwalk, CT, Appleton & Lange, pp. 368-372, 1992.*

6.60. Correct Answer: **d**

Stimulating adrenergic receptors dilates bronchi to relieve laryngeal edema and irritation after extubation. Racemic epinephrine is a short-acting synthetic form of epinephrine and stimulates both alpha and beta receptors. Its vascular effects are about 50% less than epinephrine. Anatomy and obesity increase intubation difficulty. Traumatic intubation, smoking and suctioning also increase reactivity of airway tissue.

McKenry, LM & Salerno, E: Pharmacology in Nursing, *18th ed. St. Louis, Mosby, pp. 631-633, 1992; Marley, RA: Postoperative Administration of Aerosolized Medications: Part I—The Basics.* J Post Anesth Nurs *8(5): 285-296, 1993.*

6.61. Correct Answer: **b**

Heart rate, vasoconstriction and cardiac contractile force increase in response to epinephrine. Avoid epinephrine in patients with coronary artery disease or hypertension. Epinephrine stimulates alpha and beta-1 receptors in the heart in addition to its beta-2 adrenergic effects that relieve airway edema.

McKenry, LM & Salerno, E: Pharmacology in Nursing, *18th ed. St. Louis, Mosby, pp. 631-633, 1992; Shannon, MT, Wilson, BA & Stang, CL:* Govoni & Hayes Drugs and Nursing Implications, *8th ed. Norwalk, CT, Appleton & Lange, pp. 464-467, 1995.*

6.62. Correct Answer: **a**

Oxygen delivery through a nonrebreathing system requires sustained inflation of the reservoir bag during inspiration and a snug fit over the mouth and nose. A flow of oxygen fills the reservoir bag and assures accurate delivery of high oxygen concentrations. Carbon dioxide does not enter the reservoir bag but leaves the system through a one-way valve. Oxygen toxicity is unlikely in PACU, as toxicity develops over several days.

Litwack, K: Post Anesthesia Care Nursing, *2nd ed. St. Louis, Mosby, pp. 411-412, 1995.*

6.63. Correct Answer: **a**

Tension pneumothorax is a clinical emergency. Air enters the pleural space and cannot escape; accumulated air compresses thoracic organs into ineffectiveness. Hypoxemia and hypercarbia, diminished breath sounds, decreased cardiac output and pulsus paradoxus are symptoms. A lung punctured by a right rib would prompt right, not left, pneumothorax. Chest tube length and respiratory effort are unrelated to pneumothorax occurrence. Nerve block techniques, central line insertions, chest trauma or spontaneous rupture of a lung bleb also produce pneumothorax.

Bernard, LM: The Pulmonary Surgical Patient in ASPAN's Core Curriculum for Post Anesthesia Nursing Care *(Litwack, K, Ed). Philadelphia, Saunders, p. 316, 1994; Geer, RT: Critical Care of the Surgical Patient in* Dripps/Eckenhoff/Vandam Introduction to Anesthesia, *8th ed (Longnecker, DE & Murphy, FL, Eds). Philadelphia, Saunders, pp. 463-465, 1992.*

6.64. Correct Answer: **a**

Positive pressure ventilation increases intrathoracic pressure. As a result, venous return into the right heart decreases and can decrease cardiac output. Mechanical ventilation and the positive end-expiratory pressure (PEEP) mode apply positive pressure in the chest cavity. Theoretically, positive airway pressures also distend the alveoli and increase intrapulmonary vascular resistance and intrapulmonary pressures. As pulmonary pressures increase, right ventricular pressure rises and can shift the intraventricular septum into the left ventricular space. The effect is less space for volume in the left ventricle, so cardiac output decreases.

Morgan, GE & Mikhail, MS: Clinical Anesthesiology. *Norwalk, CT, Appleton & Lange, p. 706, 1992; Wright, J, et al:* Advances in Mechanical Ventilation in Critical Care Nursing *(Clochesy, JM, et al, Eds). Philadelphia, Saunders, p. 604, 1993.*

6.65. Correct Answer: **b**

Pulmonary artery diastolic pressure indicates pressure in the left ventricle at the end of diastole (LVEDP) if there is no pulmonary resistance or mitral valve disease. At the end of diastolic filling, pulmonic valve closure effectively isolates the right heart from the left. The open mitral valve equalizes pressures in the left atrium, ventricle and pulmonary vessels, as if these are one chamber.

Dossey, BM, Guzzetta, CE, & Kenner, CV: Critical Care Nursing: Body-Mind-Spirit, *3rd ed. Philadelphia, Lippincott, pp. 237 & 243-246, 1992; Biga, CD & Bethel, SA: Hemodynamic Monitoring in* ASPAN's Core Curriculum for Post Anesthesia Nursing Practice, *3rd ed (Litwack, K, Ed). Philadelphia, Saunders, pp. 662-665, 1994.*

6.66. Correct Answer: **d**

A pulmonary artery occlusion pressure (PAOP) of 4 mm Hg, within the low range of normal, indicates volume deficit. Mr. S has no documented pulmonary or valve disease to distort the PAOP. Therefore, PAOP reflects left atrial filling pressure. In the normal heart, pulmonary artery pressures are 15-25 mm Hg (systolic) and 8-12 mm Hg (diastolic); occlusion pressures are 4-12 mm Hg.

Dossey, BM, Guzzetta, CE, & Kenner, CV: Critical Care Nursing: Body-Mind-Spirit, *3rd ed. Philadelphia, Lippincott, pp. 243-246, 1992; Biga, CD & Bethel, SA: Hemodynamic Monitoring in* ASPAN's Core Curriculum for Post Anesthesia Nursing Practice, *3rd ed (Litwack, K, Ed). Philadelphia, Saunders, pp. 662-665, 1994.*

6.67. Correct Answer: **a**

A flow-directed catheter can migrate forward into the pulmonary vasculature or backward into the right ventricle. Prolonged or undetected obstruction (occlusion or "wedging") of the catheter in a branch of the pulmonary artery infarcts pulmonary tissue. Slippage into the right ventricle produces arrhythmias of ventricular origin.

Kadota, LT: Hemodynamic Monitoring in Critical Care Nursing *(Clochesy, JM, et al, Eds). Philadelphia, Saunders, p. 164, 1993; Biga, CD & Bethel, SA: Hemodynamic Monitoring in* ASPAN's Core Curriculum for Post Anesthesia Nursing Practice, *3rd ed (Litwack, K, Ed). Philadelphia, Saunders, pp. 662-665, 1994.*

6.68. Correct Answer: **a**

Class I antiarrhythmics, including lidocaine, procainamide, tocainide and flecainide, slow the rate of impulse conduction. Lidocaine *only* affects ventricular arrhythmias by suppressing automaticity in the His-Purkinje system. Other than desired suppression of ventricular ectopy (PVCs), lidocaine's EKG effects are limited to shortening of the QT interval.

Shannon, MT, Wilson, BA & Stang, C: Govoni & Hayes Drugs and Nursing Implications. *Norwalk, CT, Appleton & Lange, pp. 679-681, 1995; Litwack, K:* ASPAN's Core Curriculum for Post Anesthesia Nursing Practice, *3rd ed. Philadelphia, Saunders, pp. 222-223, 1994.*

6.69. Correct Answer: **c**

Though lidocaine is a first-line choice to treat ventricular dysrhythmias, toxicity is a potential concern. Plasma levels of more than 7-8 mcg/ml or 3 mg/kg may have toxic effects and produce seizures, hypotension and cardiac arrest. Assessment in aware patients includes level of consciousness (drowsiness and confusion) and paresthesias.

Shannon, MT, Wilson, BA & Stang, C: Govoni & Hayes Drugs and Nursing Implications. *Norwalk, CT, Appleton & Lange, pp. 679-681, 1995; Dossey, BM, Guzzetta, CE & Kenner, CV:* Critical Care Nursing: Body-Mind-Spirit, *3rd ed. Philadelphia, Lippincott, p. 974, 1992.*

6.70. Correct Answer: **a**

Dopamine increases heart rate, improves cardiac output and so supports blood pressure. When used in combination with sodium nitroprusside's vasodilating and afterload reducing effects, myocardial work decreases, while efficiency improves.

Morgan, GE & Mikhail, MS: Clinical Anesthesiology. *Norwalk, CT, Appleton & Lange, p. 165, 1992; Whalen, DA & Izzi, G: Pharmacologic Treatment of Acute Congestive Heart Failure Resulting From Left Ventricular Systolic or Diastolic Dysfunction.* Crit Care Nurs Clin North Am *5(2): 261-269, 1993.*

6.71. Correct Answer: **c**

Increasing intravenous fluid volume helps support cardiac output, particularly when PEEP of more than 15 cm H_20 is needed. The objective of positive airway pressure is to maintain alveolar patency and increase oxygen delivery to tissues. Adequate renal and hepatic perfusion may require hemodynamic support with colloid, crystalloid or vasopressors during therapy with PEEP.

Morgan, GE & Mikhail, MS: Clinical Anesthesiology. *Norwalk, CT, Appleton & Lange, p. 706, 1992; Sauer, D: Post Anesthesia Respiratory Care in* ASPAN's Core Curriculum for Post Anesthesia Nursing Care, *3rd ed (Litwack, K, Ed). Philadelphia, Saunders, pp. 139-140, 1994.*

6.72. Correct Answer: **c**

Carotid bodies' ability to sense and initiate physiologic responses to hypoxia and hypercarbia is impaired during carotid endarterectomy. Unpredictable respiratory responses and potential for significant respiratory depression can be anticipated when narcotics or sedatives are administered. Baroreceptor responses to blood flow changes are also altered.

Mitchell, SK & Yates, RR: Cerebrovascular Disease in Critical Care Nursing: Body-Mind-Spirit, *3rd ed (Dossey, BM, Guzzetta, CE & Kenner, CV, Eds). Philadelphia, Lippincott, pp. 604-606, 1992.*

6.73. Correct Answer: **a**

When a hemodynamic waveform is dampened, its amplitude and characteristic markers are less distinct. Hyperextending the wrist often will reposition the arterial catheter in the artery and restore a quality waveform. Simultaneously, reassess the patient's clinical status to explain changes in waveform configuration. A blood pressure waveform is characterized by a sharp systolic upstroke, sudden decrease, and dicrotic notch. Mechanical causes of a dampened waveform include catheter malposition within the vessel wall, vessel spasms, or air, clots, kinks, or loose connections that disrupt transmission of pressures.

Dossey, BM, Guzzetta, CE & Kenner, CV: Critical Care Nursing: Body-Mind-Spirit, *3rd ed. Philadelphia, Lippincott, 1992, pp. 255; Biga, CD & Bethel, SA: Hemodynamic Monitoring in* ASPAN's Core Curriculum for Post Anesthesia Nursing Practice, *3rd ed (Litwack, K, Ed). Philadelphia, Saunders, pp. 662-665, 1994.*

6.74. Correct Answer: **b**

Hypotension, moderate blood loss with low volume replacement and borderline tachycardia suggest hypovolemia. Mr. T is neither hypothermic nor suspiciously hyperthermic and denies chest pain. While cardiac decompensation is a possibile risk 6 months after myocardial infarction, Mr. T's potential for perioperative myocardial reinfarction remains low, approximately 6%.

Morgan, GE & Mikhail, MS: Clinical Anesthesiology. *Norwalk, CT, Appleton & Lange, p. 316, 1992; Ellison, N: Managing Fluids, Electrolytes and Blood Loss in* Dripps/Eckenhoff/Vandam Introduction to Anesthesia, *8th ed. (Longnecker, DE & Murphy, FL, Eds). Philadelphia, Saunders, p. 174, 1992.*

6.75. Correct Answer: **d**

Despite his cardiac history, Mr. T most likely needs cautiously administered additional fluid. Mr. T's intraoperative fluid needs could be over 5000 ml, of which he received only 2500 ml. When calculating fluid deficit, consider his 8 hour preoperative NPO status, urinary and insensible losses, intraoperative fluid *maintenance* and replacement requirements, and intraoperative blood loss. Replacement requirements for a major abdominal procedure may be up to 12 ml/kg/h.

DeFranco, M: Fluid and Electrolyte Balance in ASPAN's Core Curriculum for Post Anesthesia Nursing Practice *(Litwack, K, Ed). Philadelphia, Saunders, pp. 170-173, 1994; Ellison, N: Managing Fluids, Electrolytes and Blood Loss in* Dripps/Eckenhoff/Vandam Introduction to Anesthesia, *8th ed (Longnecker, DE & Murphy, FL, Eds). Philadelphia, Saunders, pp. 168 & 174, 1992.*

6.76. Correct Answer: **c**

Determining hemoglobin is important, particularly when postoperative pulse oximetry measures are marginal. Blood oxygen carrying capacity depends on hemoglobin, which normally measures 15 g/dl. One gram of hemoglobin binds with 1.34 ml of oxygen. More than 95% of oxygen is carried to tissues bound to hemoglobin; only a small amount is dissolved in plasma.

Henneman, EA & Gawlinski, A: Evaluating Cardiopulmonary Instability with Continuous Monitoring of Mixed Venous Oxygen Saturation. Crit Care Nurs Clin North Am *6(4): 855-862, 1994; Sauer, D: Post Anesthesia Respiratory Care in* ASPAN's Core Curriculum for Post Anesthesia Nursing Practice, *3rd ed (Litwack, K, Ed). Philadelphia, Saunders, pp. 130-135, 1994.*

6.77. Correct Answer: **b**

Alkalosis increases oxygen's affinity for hemoglobin. Specific physiologic conditions alter oxygen-hemoglobin binding (affinity). Oxygen more readily unloads from hemoglobin and moves into the tissues with hyperthermia, increased 2,3-DPG, and acidotic (decreased pH) conditions. When plotted on the oxyhemoglobin dissociation curve, conditions that decrease affinity shift this curve to the right. Opposite physiologic conditions shift the oxyhemoglobin dissociation curve to the left, reflecting a stronger bond between oxygen and hemoglobin.

Henneman, EA & Gawlinski, A: Evaluating Cardiopulmonary Instability with Continuous Monitoring of Mixed Venous Oxygen Saturation. Crit Care Nurs Clin North Am *6(4): 855-862, 1994.*

6.78. Correct Answer: **a**

Pulse oximeter signals produce inaccurate measures at low saturations. Saturation from peripheral sites (SpO_2) do not correlate equally with oxygen saturations by blood analysis (PaO_2). Anemia, hypothermia, decreased cardiac output, and vasoconstriction contribute to poor tissue perfusion and may produce low or poor quality oximeter signals. Motion, light or electrical interference interfere with transmission of light to the oximeter's sensor and a poor pulsatile signal results.

Savino, JS: Monitoring the Anesthetized Patient in Dripps/Eckenhoff/Vandam Introduction to Anesthesia, *8th ed (Longnecker, DE & Murphy, FL, Eds). Philadelphia, Saunders, p. 62, 1992; Potter, PA & Perry, AG:* Basic Nursing: Theory and Practice, *3rd ed. St. Louis, Mosby, pp. 994-996, 1994.*

6.79. Correct Answer: **a**

Perioperative myocardial infarction is a risk for Mr. T, so discriminating chest pain from surgical pain is important. One study showed postoperative cardiac ischemia was more likely (41%) than intraoperative ischemia (25%) among patients with known coronary artery disease. In addition, the *post*operative ischemia occurred asymptomatically in that study and was associated with dire outcomes. Therefore, postoperative pain assessment must be discriminating and include documenting location, intensity and type of pain experienced. Based upon assessment, intervention and outcomes may differ vastly.

Burden, N: Ambulatory Surgical Nursing. *Philadelphia, Saunders, p. 294, 1993; Neely, CF: Cardiovascular Disease in* Dripps/Eckenhoff/Vandam Introduction to Anesthesia, *8th ed (Longnecker, DE & Murphy, FL, Eds). Philadelphia, Saunders, p. 271, 1992.*

6.80. Correct Answer: **d**

Pain assessment and intervention require the nurse's ability to balance pain relief with adequate respiratory effort and consciousness. Though objective observation may indicate a patient is pain free, the patient's subjective experience determines the significance of pain. When the respiratory rate is greater than 15 breaths per minute, a patient can generally receive morphine sulfate intravenously even *before* anesthesia emergence, according to need and tolerance.

Burden, N: Ambulatory Surgical Nursing. *Philadelphia, Saunders, p. 294, 1993; Hudak, C & Gallo, B:* Critical Care Nursing: A Holistic Approach, *6th ed. Philadelphia, Lippincott, p. 171, 1994; Greenhow, DE: Recovery From Anesthesia: The Postoperative Visit in* Dripps/Eckenhoff/Vandam Introduction to Anesthesia, *8th ed (Longnecker, DE & Murphy, FL, Eds). Philadelphia, Saunders, p. 439, 1992.*

6.81. Correct Answer: **c**

Sinus tachycardia occurs at a rate of more than 100 beats per minute, a rhythm that frequently accompanies pain, anxiety, volume shifts and acid-base disturbances. Mr. T's atria and ventricles depolarize more than 130 times each minute. The impulse originates in the sinus node; therefore rhythm is supraventricular. Atrial conduction is brief; the P wave is upright and the PR interval is only 0.12 seconds. In contrast, an accelerated junctional rhythm may have an an inverted P wave with an ultrashort PR interval and QRS complexes that occur 60-100 times per minute.

Hicks, FD: The Cardiac Surgical Patient in ASPAN's Core Curriculum for Post Anesthesia Nursing Practice, *3rd ed (Litwack, K, Ed). Philadelphia, Saunders, pp. 267-268, 1994; Potter, PA & Perry, AG:* Basic Nursing: Theory and Practice, *3rd ed. St. Louis, Mosby, pp. 988, 1994.*

6.82. Correct Answer: **b**

Sinus tachycardia is treated by eliminating the underlying cause; remembering to verify an empty bladder may eliminate one sometimes overlooked cause of tachycardia. Mr. T's bladder may be full and distended; after radical prostatectomy bleeding is likely and the catheter may be obstructed by clots or tissue.

Burden, N: Ambulatory Surgical Nursing. *Philadelphia, Saunders, p. 282 & 288, 1993; Nagle, GM: The Urologic Surgical Patient in* ASPAN's Core Curriculum for Post Anesthesia Nursing Practice,

3rd ed (Litwack, K, Ed). Philadelphia, Saunders, pp. 429-431, 1994.

6.83. Correct Answer: **c**

Cardiac tamponade, the heart's inability to pump within a fluid or blood-filled pericardium, is signified by decreased cardiac output and venous congestion. Paradoxical pulse, hypotension and electrical alternans accompany increased venous pressures due to constricted pumping.

Stoelting, RK & Dierdorf, SF: Handbook for Anesthesia and Co-existing Diseases. *New York, Churchill-Livingstone, pp. 81-82, 1993; Hicks, FD: The Cardiac Surgical Patient in* ASPAN's Core Curriculum for Post Anesthesia Nursing Practice, *3rd ed (Litwack, K, Ed). Philadelphia, Saunders, pp. 273-274, 1994.*

6.84. Correct Answer: **a**

Pneumothorax, however small in size, is a potential with any central venous cannulation. X-ray after placement of central catheters confirms bilateral lung expansion, but be aware that pneumothorax from a small puncture may not appear for hours. Regularly reassess the patient's clinical pulmonary status. Rupture of a pulmonary artery is a dire emergency complication, detected by hemoptysis, not x-ray. Elderly or anticoagulated patients or those with pulmonary hypertension have greater risk.

Morgan, GE & Mikhail, MS: Clinical Anesthesiology. *Norwalk, CT, Appleton & Lange, p. 84, 1992; Bernard, LM: The Pulmonary Surgical Patient in* ASPAN's Core Curriculum for Post Anesthesia Nursing Practice, *3rd ed (Litwack, K, Ed). Philadelphia, Saunders, p. 316, 1994.*

6.85. Correct Answer: **b**

The range of normal pressures at the pulmonary artery is 20-30 (systolic)/10-15 (diastolic).

Dossey, BM, Guzzetta, CE & Kenner, CV: Critical Care Nursing: Body-Mind-Spirit, *3rd ed. Philadelphia, Lippincott, p. 468, 1992.*

6.86. Correct Answer: **d**

Changing intrathoracic pressures produce cyclic changes in respiratory pattern. This expected variation becomes more marked with hypovolemia, pulmonary disease, heart failure, and mechanical ventilation. Measure pulmonary artery pressure at end-expiration to minimize this influence.

Kodata, LT: Hemodynamic Monitoring in Critical Care Nursing *(Clochesy, JM et al, Eds). Philadelphia, Saunders, p. 167, 1992; Taylor, C, Lillis, C & LeMone, P:* Fundamentals of Nursing: The Art and Science of Nursing Care *2nd ed. Philadelphia, Saunders, inside back cover, 1993.*

6.87. Correct Answer: **a**

Atelectasis, pulmonary obstruction, aspiration, and effusion are clinical situations that can increase the percentage of intrapulmonary shunt. Work of breathing changes when the degree of shunt reaches about 15%; when shunt reaches about 30%, significant hypoventilation may require mechanical ventilation. A shunt of more than 25%, even after efforts to improve ventilation and oxygenation, is associated with poor prognosis.

Egloff, ME: Respiratory Assessment in Critical Care Nursing: Body-Mind-Spirit, *3rd ed (Dossey, BM, Guzzetta, CE & Kenner, CV, Eds). Philadelphia, Lippincott, pp.*

307-311, 1992; Ahrens, T: Respiratory Monitoring in Critical Care Nursing *(Clochesy, JM, Breu, C, & Cardin, S, et al, Eds). Philadelphia, Saunders, pp. 200-202, 1992.*

6.88. Correct Answer: **d**

Postanesthesia shivering reportedly increases tissue oxygen consumption more than 400% and increases the risk of hypoxemia-related outcomes. Although the cause is undetermined and the occurrence is unpredictable, outcomes of shivering after surgery and anesthesia range from patient discomfort to wound dehiscence. Volatile anesthetic agents, enchanced spinal cord reflexes, intraoperative heat loss and vasodilation have been implicated.

Vogelsang, J: Patients Who Develop Postanesthesia Shaking Increase Body Temperature at the Same Rate as Those Who Do Not Develop Shaking. J Post Anesth Nurs *8(1): 3-12, 1993; Gliniecki, AM: Postanesthesia Shaking: A Review.* J Post Anesth Nurs *7(2): 89-93, 1992.*

6.89. Correct Answer: **a**

Comfort measures are most likely adequate and effective in this situation. To establish priorities and a plan of care, the nurse must weigh the patient's surgical procedures (laparoscopy) and her age and relative risk for complications of cardiac or pulmonary origin. Laparoscopic procedures require abdominal insufflation with carbon dioxide. Unpleasant abdominal discomfort and pain from forced distention frequently occur. As the gas rises in the abdomen, "shoulder girdle pain" is common.

Burden, N: Ambulatory Surgery Nursing. *Philadelphia, Saunders, p. 514, 1993.*

6.90. Correct Answer: **a**

The rhythm described is a Mobitz Type II heart block with 2:1 conduction. A conduction delay (block) occurs at the atrioventricular (AV) node. The AV node does not conduct every second sinus beat that originated in the sinoatrial node to the ventricles. Hence, two P waves occur for every QRS. Atrial rate is 88 beats per minute while ventricular rate is 44 beats per minute. The PVCs are "escape beats" that originate in the ventricle and represent the heart's attempt to generate adequate cardiac output.

Dossey, BM, Guzzetta, CE & Kenner, CV: Critical Care Nursing: Body-Mind-Spirit, *3rd ed. Philadelphia, Lippincott, p. 178-180, 1992; Purcell, JA: Cardiac Electrical Activity in* AACN's Clinical Reference for Critical-Care Nursing *(Kenney, MR, Packa, DR & Dunbar, SB, Eds). St. Louis, Mosby, pp. 255-259, 1993.*

6.91. Correct Answer: **b**

Type II second degree heart block (Mobitz II) can evolve to third degree, or complete, heart block in which the atria and ventricles generate totally independent, nonrelated rhythms. Depending on the ventricular rate, type II AV block may decrease cardiac output and close observation is warranted. Cardiac depressant medications, some physiologic imbalances and anterior myocardial infarction depress AVconduction. Pacemaker availability is recommended.

Dossey, BM, Guzzetta, CE & Kenner, CV: Critical Care Nursing: Body-Mind-Spirit, *3rd ed. Philadelphia, Lippincott, p. 178-80, 1992; Purcell, JA: Cardiac Electrical Activity in* AACN's Clinical

Reference for Critical-Care Nursing *(Kenney, MR, Packa, DR & Dunbar, SB, Eds). St. Louis, Mosby, pp. 258, 1993.*

6.92. Correct Answer: **c**

Atropine 0.5 mg to 1 mg increases conduction through the AV junction. Heart rate increases. The ventricular beats are "escape beats" and represent ventricular cell automaticity. These beats are a compensatory response to a slow heart rate and a ventriclar effort to increase cardiac output. Overriding the slow rate to improve cardiac ouput is desired. Do not eradicate the ventricular beats with lidocaine. Particularly for patients without new cardiac disease, improving intracardiac conduction usually involves medication and correcting metabolic imbalances before applying pacemaker technology.

Dossey, BM, Guzzetta, CE & Kenner, CV: Critical Care Nursing: Body-Mind-Spirit, *3rd ed. Philadelphia, Lippincott, pp. 183 & 975-6, 1992; Litwack, K: Basic and Advanced Cardiac Life Support in* ASPAN's Core Curriculum for Post Anesthesia Nursing Practice, *3rd ed (Litwack, K, Ed). Philadelphia, Saunders, pp. 216-219, 1994.*

6.93. Correct Answer: **b**

Even a witnessed electrical arrest requires clinical confirmation: verify that the patient is indeed pulseless. The presumed fibrillation may be artifact. Although a tenet of basic life support is to assess unresponsiveness, this particular patient's awareness is already suppressed by anesthetics. Hypoxia and hypotension, common precursors to cardiac decompensation, are likely in the postanesthetic patient. A precordial thump might be used when new ventricular fibrillation can be documented. Lidocaine might be administered in an individualized, weight-specific dose during resuscitation.

Craddock, LD & Krumbach B: Cardiopulmonary Resuscitation in Critical Care Nursing: A Holistic Approach, *6th ed (Hudak, CM & Gallo, BM, Eds). Philadelphia, Lippincott, 295-304, 1994; American Heart Association:* Textbook of Adult Advanced Cardiac Life Support *(Cummins, RO, Ed). Dallas, American Heart Association, pp. 1.5-1.7, 1994.*

6.94. Correct Answer: **d**

Potential for ventricular tachycardia or even fibrillation increases when a PVC strikes atop the T wave during cellular repolarization. The T wave, from peak until return to the EKG's isoelectric baseline, represents the cell membrane's relative refractory, or vulnerable, period. As sodium channels reactivate and recover from the prior depolarization, the cell actually becomes more easily receptive to electrical stimuli.

Dossey, BM, Guzzetta, CE & Kenner, CV: Critical Care Nursing: Body-Mind-Spirit, *3rd ed. Philadelphia, Lippincott, pp. 161-164, 1992; Stalheim-Smith, A & Fitch, GK:* Understanding Human Anatomy and Physiology. *Minneapolis/St. Paul, West Publishing, pp. 597-601, 1994.*

6.95. Correct Answer: **b**

Basic life support (BLS) criteria specify the ratio of cardiac compressions to ventilations. For resuscitation with two rescuers, this ratio is five compressions to one breath.

Drain, C: The Post Anesthesia Care Unit: A Critical Care Approach to Post Anesthesia Nursing, *3rd ed. Philadelphia, Saunders, pp. 584-590, 1994; American Heart Association: Adult Basic Life Support.* JAMA *268(16): 2184-2197, 1992.*

6.96. Correct Answer: **d**

Head tilt or jaw thrust often effectively opens the airway. The nurse might expect the oral airway to adequately displace the patient's tongue and maintain a patent air-passage. The still-anesthetized patient's jaw may be ultrarelaxed, perpetuating upper airway obstruction. Supporting the jaw while also stimulating the patient may sufficiently spur this patient to breathe. If not, additional assessment and respiratory support are needed.

Drain, C: The Post Anesthesia Care Unit: A Critical Care Approach to Post Anesthesia Nursing, *3rd ed. Philadelphia, Saunders, pp. 584-590, 1994; American Heart Association: Adult Basic Life Support.* JAMA *268(16): 2184-2197, 1992.*

6.97. Correct Answer: **a**

A mucous plug lies within the alveolus and thus disturbs ventilation, not perfusion. Alveolar ventilation without capillary perfusion increases physiologic dead space. The result is hypoxemia (decreased pO_2) and hypercarbia (increased pCO_2). Conditions that increase dead space, such as embolism or shock, arise from changes in blood flow.

Egloff, ME: Respiratory Assessment in Critical Care Nursing: Body-Mind-Spirit, *3rd ed (Dossey, BM, Guzzetta, CE & Kenner, CV, Eds). Philadelphia, Lippincott, pp. 307-311, 1992; Drain, C:* The Post Anesthesia Care Unit: A Critical Care Approach to Post Anesthesia Nursing, *3rd ed. Philadelphia, Saunders, p. 128, 1994.*

6.98. Correct Answer: **a**

Strong negative pressures generated during attempts to breathe through an obstructed airway can damage capillary and alveolar permeability. Hydrostatic pressure allows fluid to enter lung tissue, producing pulmonary edema of noncardiac origin (NCPE).

Hamlin, W, Schnobel, L & Smith, B: The Patient With Noncardiogenic Pulmonary Edema. J Post Anesth Nurs *6(1): 43-49, 1991; Burden, N:* Ambulatory Surgical Nursing. *Philadelphia, Saunders, pp. 267-269, 1993.*

6.99. Correct Answer: **b**

Naloxone, billed as the "prototype of opioid antagonists," has been implicated as one cause of pulmonary edema. Naloxone (Narcan) is often used to reverse the respiratory depressant effects of narcotics, thereby stimulating the central nervous system. Also termed "negative-pressure pulmonary edema (NPPE)," noncardiogenic pulmonary edema (NCPE) may occur in children and otherwise healthy adults after an anesthetic-related episode of laryngospasm or croup. Episodes may be limited to cough and respiratory distress or extend to hypoxia and "wet," congested alveoli.

Enger, E: Patients with Adult Respiratory Distress Syndrome in Critical Care Nursing *(Clochesy, J, et al, Eds). Philadelphia, Saunders, pp. 546-567, 1992; Burden, N:* Ambulatory Surgical Nursing. *Philadelphia, Saunders, pp. 137-138, 1993.*

6.100. Correct Answer: **c**

A low-pressure ventilator alarm occurs whenever the ventilator senses the set inspiratory volume is delivered too easily, without resistance. An air leak occurs with actual ventilator disconnection from the patient's endotracheal tube. This is a dire emergency. An air leak in the ventilator system or endotracheal cuff also may cause significant pressure loss, sounding the low-pressure alarm.

Bolton, PJ & Kline, KA: Understanding Modes of Mechanical Ventilation. Am J Nurs *94(6): 36-42, 1994; Hudak, C & Gallo, B:* Critical Care Nursing: A Holistic Approach, *6th ed, Philadelphia, Lippincott, pp. 463-464 & 478, 1994.*

SET III

Answer Key

6.101. b
6.102. b
6.103. a
6.104. c
6.105. d
6.106. b
6.107. c
6.108. b
6.109. a
6.110. b
6.111. a
6.112. b
6.113. a
6.114. b
6.115. b
6.116. d
6.117. d
6.118. c
6.119. c
6.120. b
6.121. a
6.122. c
6.123. d
6.124. c
6.125. c
6.126. a
6.127. c
6.128. b
6.129. b
6.130. a
6.131. d
6.132. b
6.133. c
6.134. b
6.135. c
6.136. a
6.137. d
6.138. b
6.139. b
6.140. a
6.141. c
6.142. a
6.143. c
6.144. d
6.145. a
6.146. b
6.147. c
6.148. a
6.149. b
6.150. b

SET III

Rationales and References

6.101. Correct Answer: **b**

The high pressure alarm sounds and abruptly ends the inspiratory phase whenever the ventilator system generates pressures that exceed the set pressure limit. Delivery of the preset volume of air is interrupted. Secretions, tubing kinks, patient restlessness, or patient's coughing or biting on the endotracheal tube signals airway obstruction and produces a high pressure alarm.

Bolton, PJ & Kline, KA: Understanding Modes of Mechanical Ventilation. Am J Nurs *94(6): 36-42, 1994; Hudak, C & Gallo, B:* Critical Care Nursing: A Holistic Approach, *6th ed. Philadelphia, Lippincott, pp. 463-464 & 478, 1994.*

6.102. Correct Answer: **b**

A patient's respiratory quality must be clinically adequate for extubation. Awareness, ability to communicate with head nod or hand squeeze, protect the airway with swallow and cough reflexes and a rate of more than 10 breaths per minute constitute observations that indicate readiness for extubation. If a patient can sustain respiratory rate and minute volume with ventilatory assistance in the IMV mode, even while sleeping, success after extubation is more likely.

Litwack, K: Post Anesthesia Care Nursing, *2nd ed. Phildelphia, Saunders, pp. 414-415, 1995; Bolton, PJ & Kline, KA: Understanding Modes of Mechanical Ventilation.* Am J Nurs *94 (6): 36-43, 1994.*

6.103. Correct Answer: **a**

Dead space includes any airway structures that do not participate in air exchange. Physiologic dead space includes anatomic dead space (nasal passages, trachea, bronchi) and any obstructed alveoli. Hence patients with pulmonary embolism or atelectasis have increased physiologic dead space.

Egloff, ME: Respiratory Assessment in Critical Care Nursing: Body-Mind-Spirit, *3rd ed (Dossey, BM, Guzzetta, CE & Kenner, CV, Eds). Philadelphia, Lippincott, pp. 307-11, 1992; Ahrens, T: Respiratory Monitoring in* Critical Care Nursing *(Clochesy, JM, Breu, C, Cardin, S, et al, Eds). Philadelphia, Saunders, pp. 193-207, 1992.*

6.104. Correct Answer: **c**

Activating the catheter's flush system or adding additional air to the balloon increases pressure on pulmonary capillaries. Pulmonary artery rupture is a risk with disastrous potential. However, if this inflated balloon on the pulmonary artery catheter continues to occlude a segment of the pulmonary artery, pulmonary infarction will result. Repositioning the patient, a deep inspiration, and the force of coughing may permit a mechanically "wedged" balloon to move from a branch of the pulmonary artery. Removing the syringe allows passive deflation of a partially inflated balloon.

Dossey, BM, Guzzetta, CE & Kenner, CV: Critical Care Nursing: Body-Mind-Spirit, *3rd ed. Philadelphia, Lippincott, pp. 248-250, 1992; Biga, CD & Bethel, SA: Hemodynamic Monitoring in* ASPAN's Core Curriculum for Post Anesthesia Nursing Practice, *3rd ed (Litwack, K, Ed). Philadelphia, Saunders, pp. 662-665, 1994.*

6.105. Correct Answer: **d**

The normal rate of sodium nitroprusside infusion, *always* by infusion pump to control rate, is 3-8 mcg/kg/min. Doses greater than 10 mcg/kg/min increase the risk of cyanide toxicity.

Shannon, MT, Wilson, BA & Stang, CL: Govoni & Hayes Drugs and Nursing Implications, *8th ed. Norwalk, CT, Appleton & Lange, pp. 836-837, 1995.*

6.106. Correct Answer: **b**

Expressing the nitroprusside infusion rate as 1.6 mcg/kg/min indicates an individually calculated dose, adjusted for the patient's size. While 40 ml/h is the infusion rate, stating this information does not indicate the effective dose, which will differ between a 50 kg and an 80 kg patient. One vial of 50 mg of sodium nitroprusside (or 50,000 mcg, a mathematically easier unit to express this potent medication) is diluted in 250 ml D5W. No medication should ever be infused with the nitroprusside. Dosage calculation is as follows:

concentration × infusion rate × time = dosage

A. $\frac{50{,}000\text{ mcg}}{250\text{ ml}} \; \frac{40\text{ ml}}{1\text{ h}} \; \frac{1\text{ h}}{60\text{ min}} = 133.33\text{ mcg/min}$

B. $\frac{\text{dosage (from Step A)}}{\text{patient weight}} = \text{individual dose}$

Therefore: $\frac{133.33\text{ mcg/min}}{85\text{ kg}} = 1.6\text{ mcg/kg/min}$

Taylor, C, Lillis, C, LeMone, P: Fundamentals of Nursing: The Art and Science of Nursing Care, *2nd ed. Philadelphia, Saunders, pp. 1199-1202, 1993; Shannon, MT, Wilson, BA & Stang, CL:* Govoni & Hayes Drugs and Nursing Implications, *8th ed. Norwalk, CT, Appleton & Lange, pp. 836-837, 1995.*

6.107. Correct Answer: **c**

To surgically repair an abdominal aortic aneurysm, the aorta is clamped to impede surging blood flow. After the aortic cross clamp is released, potential for profound hypotension increases. Effects of this "release hypotension" may continue into the postanesthesia period. Some believe that while the aorta is clamped, acidic metabolites accumulate below the clamped site and produce ischemia. Releasing these accumulated metabolites is thought to produce peripheral vasodilation and "release hypotension." Intraoperative blood loss and sudden decrease in resistance to cardiac output (afterload) after clamp release also may produce hypotension.

Morgan, GE & Mikhail, MS: Clinical Anesthesiology. *Norwalk, CT, Appleton & Lange, p. 357, 1992; Barash, PG, Cullen, BE & Stoelting, RK:* Handbook of Clinical Anesthesia. *Philadelphia, Lippincott, pp. 278-279, 1991.*

6.108. Correct Answer: **b**

This pacemaker has failed to sense—and so actually competes with—the patient's native cardiac activity. Pacing artifacts may occur at a regular cadence, perhaps even in the middle of a patient's own complex. When pacemaker activity coincides with the vulnerble period or T wave denoting cardiac repolarization, ventricular tachycardia or fibrillation may occur.

Witherell, CL: Cardiac Rhythm Control Devices. Crit Care Nurs Clin North Am. *6(1): 85-95, 1994; Fetzer-Fowler, S: Caring for the Ambulatory Surgical Patient Who Has a Pacemaker: Part I.* J Post Anesth Nurs *8(2): 116-124, 1993.*

6.109. Correct Answer: **a**

Cranial nerve branches are manipulated during carotid endarterectomy. Damage to cranial nerve XII, the hypoglossal, weakens the tongue. Unilateral motor damage causes the tongue to deviate to the opposite side and affects swallowing and speech. Bilateral damage can precipitate full airway obstruction. Injury to either sensory or motor function can occur, and usually resolves with time. Until then, disrupted motor function increases patient risk, particularly related to airway protection.

Kenner, CV: Neurologic Assessment in Critical Care Nursing: Body-Mind-Spirit, *3rd ed (Dossey, BM, Guzzetta, CE & Kenner, CV, Eds). Philadelphia, Lippincott, pp. 543-547, 1992; Kane, HL & Wilson, LB: Practical Points in the Care of the Patient Post-Carotid Endarterectomy.* J Post Anesth Nurs *6(6): 403-405, 1993.*

6.110. Correct Answer: **b**

Positive end-expiratory pressure (PEEP), especially at high levels (>15-20 mmHg) or when applied to noncompliant lungs, increases the potential for alveolar rupture. Tension pneumothorax or air leakage into tissues, indicated by palpable crepitus from subcutaneous emphysema, may result. Overdistention of alveoli with high PEEP pressures compresses alveolar capillaries, increasing vascular resistance. Sustained vascular changes are reflected back to baroreceptors, which, over time, adapt to new levels of vascular tone.

Morgan, GE & Mikhail, MS: Clinical Anesthesiology. *Norwalk, CT, Appleton & Lange, pp. 296-298 & 705-706, 1992; Sauer, D: Post Anesthesia Respiratory Care in* ASPAN's Core Curriculum for Post Anesthesia Nursing Practice *3rd ed (Litwack, K, Ed). Philadelphia, Saunders, pp. 138-141, 1994.*

6.111. Correct Answer: **a**

Mean arterial pressure (MAP) in the healthy person is 70-90mm Hg. MAP varies with cardiac output and the amount of vascular resistance. MAP represents the average pressure in the aortic system during the cardiac cycle. MAP can be estimated by a mathematical calculation:

$$\text{MAP} = \frac{(\text{Systolic BP}) + 2(\text{Diastolic BP})}{3}$$

Dossey, BM, Guzzetta, CE & Kenner, CV: Critical Care Nursing: Body-Mind-Spirit, *3rd ed. Philadelphia, Lippincott, p. 251, 1992; Morgan, GE & Mikhail, MS:* Clinical Anesthesiology. *Norwalk, CT, Appleton & Lange, p. 67, 1992.*

6.112. Correct Answer: **b**

Though a normal finding in children and young adults, a third heart sound (S3) that develops in an older adult may herald early congestive heart failure. This sound should be distinguished from a preexisting cardiac murmur of mitral valve stenosis. When heard at the left apex, an S_3 may indicate mitral regurgitation or ventricular failure from ischemia; at the right apex, an S_3 suggests impending embolism or pulmonary hypertension.

Hicks, FD: The Cardiac Surgical Patient in ASPAN's Core Curriculum for Post Anesthesia Nursing Practice, *3rd ed (Litwack, K, Ed). Philadelphia, Saunders, pp. 253-254 & 267-268, 1994; Dossey, BM, Guzzetta, CE & Kenner, CV:* Critical Care Nursing: Body-Mind-Spirit, *3rd ed. Philadelphia, Lippincott, pp. 398-399, 1992.*

6.113. Correct Answer: **a**

Frequent premature ventricular contractions (PVCs) are a classic indicator of digitalis toxicity in patients who take digoxin. Diuretics, both thiazide and loop, compound the risk of arrhythmia by increasing potassium excretion; dysrhythmias, particularly PVCs, are commonly associated with hypokalemia in digitalized patients. Patients with congestive heart failure use both diuretics to promote fluid excretion and digoxin to increase the heart's contractile force. Therefore these patients have increased risk for toxicity. Symptoms of digitalis toxicity are varied, but visual disturbances, arrhythmias, gastrointestinal tract upset, headaches, and confusion are strongly associated.

Litwack, K: Basic and Advanced Cardiac Life Support in ASPAN's Core Curriculum for Post Anesthesia Nursing Practice, *3rd ed. Philadelphia, Saunders, p. 221, 1994; Dennison, RD & Nappi, J: Cardiac Glycoside Agents and Bipyridines in* Clinical Pharmacology and Nursing, *2nd ed. Springhouse, PA, Springhouse Corp, pp. 471-478, 1992.*

6.114. Correct Answer: **b**

A digitalized patient with a serum potassium of less than 4 mEq/L generally receives preoperative potassium replacement to reduce cardiac risk from anesthetic medications; nondigitalized patients may not receive potassium replacement unless serum potassium is 3-3.5 mEq/L. Potassium replacement aims to correct immediately dangerous hypokalemia, not replace postassium stores in the intracellular fluid (ICF) where most potassium ions reside. Cardiac monitoring is advised when more than 20 mEq per hour are replaced. Calcium, dextrose and alkalosis only accentuate hypokalemia by driving potassium into cells.

Morgan, GE & Mikhail, MS: Clinical Anesthesiology. *Norwalk, CT, Appleton & Lange, pp. 466-468, 1992; Hicks, FD: The Cardiac Surgical Patient in* ASPAN's Core Curriculum for Post Anesthesia Nursing Practice, *3rd ed (Litwack, K, Ed). Philadelphia, Saunders, p. 255, 1994.*

6.115. Correct Answer: **b**

Anatomically, the mitral valve is located between the left atrium and ventricle. Stenosis, or a narrowed opening, obstructs forward flow and therefore the volume of blood that can be ejected from the atrium. Residual blood volume and the pressure it creates increase in the left atrium.

Abramczyk, EL & Brown, MM: Valvular Heart Disease in Comprehensive Cardiac Care, *7th ed (Kinney, MR, Packa, DR, Andreoli, KG, et al, Eds). St. Louis, Mosby, pp. 328 & 334-338, 1991; Hicks, FD: The Cardiac Surgical Patient in* ASPAN's Core Curriculum for Post Anesthesia Nursing Practice, *3rd ed (Litwack, K, Ed). Philadelphia, Saunders, pp. 253-255, 1994.*

6.116. Correct Answer: **d**

Dyspnea, cough, peripheral edema and distention of jugular neck veins are among the common symptoms of mitral valve stenosis. Pressure in a dilated left atrium eventually moves fluid back into lung tissue. As left atrial pressures increase, retrograde pressure also increases on the pulmonary vasculature. Pulmonary hypertension, lung compliance, vital capacity and oxygen diffusion at the alveoli decrease. Nail clubbing reflects chronic hypoxemia; a Wenckebach pattern signals second degree heart block; high stroke volume and wide pulse pressure produce a bounding pulse known as a water-hammer pulse.

Abramczyk, EL & Brown, MM: Valvular Heart Disease in Comprehensive Cardiac Care, *7th ed (Kinney, MR, Packa, DR, Andreoli, KG, et al, Eds). St. Louis, Mosby, pp. 328 & 334-338, 1991; Potter, PA & Perry, AG:* Basic Nursing: Theory and Practice, *3rd ed. St. Louis, Mosby, pp. 338-339, 1995.*

6.117. Correct Answer: **d**

Auscultation assesses heart sounds produced by valve closure. Mitral and tricuspid valve closure (the AV valves) produce the first heart sound (S_1). These sounds are bestheard at the heart's apex, normally located at about the fifth intercostal space and below the midclavicle.

Taylor, C, Lillis, C & LeMone, P: Fundamentals of Nursing: The Art and Science of Nursing Care, *2nd ed. Philadelphia, Saunders, p. 452, 1993; Abramczyk, EL & Brown, MM: Valvular Heart Disease in* Comprehensive Cardiac Care, *7th ed (Kinney, MR, Packa, DR, Andreoli, KG, et al, Eds). St. Louis, Mosby, pp. 34-39, 1991.*

6.118. Correct Answer: **c**

A thrill is a vibration noted during palpation. During auscultation, sounds are evaluated for intensity, pitch, quality, timing and respiratory variation. Presence of friction rubs, murmurs, clicks, splitting or extra sounds are also noted. Sounds are documented and associated with location.

Dossey, BM, Guzzetta, CE & Kenner, CV: Critical Care Nursing: Body-Mind-Spirit, *3rd ed. Philadelphia, Lippincott, p. 397, 1992.*

6.119. Correct Answer: **c**

The balloon pump uses synchronized counterpulsation to reduce myocardial work and support the unstable or failing heart. A long, narrow balloon inserted into the aorta inflates during diastole, displaces blood to fill the aortic space and propels blood back to the coronary arteries.

This increases coronary artery blood flow by 5-15%. Balloon deflation just before cardiac ejection reduces afterload and resistance on the aortic valve by 10-15% The effect decreases the heart's oxygen consumption.

Shinn, AE & Joseph, D: Concepts of Intraaortic Balloon Counterpulsation. J Cardiovasc Nurs *8(2): 45-60, 1994; Hicks, FD: The Cardiac Surgical Patient in* ASPAN's Core Curriculum for Post Anesthesia Nursing Practice, *3rd ed (Litwack, K, Ed). Philadelphia, Saunders, p. 273, 1994.*

6.120. Correct Answer: **b**

Purge and refill the catheter's balloon after first determining that balloon inflation actually occurs on the R wave of the EKG. After an alarm, emptying and refilling the balloon allows intraaortic balloon pump (IABP) counterpulsation to continue. Timing is crucial during intraaortic counterpulsation. Improper synchronization actually increases cardiac work and opposes treatment objectives. Balloon inflation *must not* occur before or during any other part of the cardiac cycle than contraction (R wave). The balloon catheter should *never* be clamped. Consider non-IABP-related reasons for hypotension; despite proper IABP timing, titrating dopamine may be appropriate to support blood pressure.

Shinn, AE & Joseph, D: Concepts of Intraaortic Balloon Counterpulsation. J Cardiovasc Nurs *8(2): 45-60. 1994; Dossey, BM, Guzzetta, CE & Kenner, CV:* Critical Care Nursing: Body-Mind-Spirit, *3rd ed. Philadelphia, Lippincott, p. 261-266, 1992.*

6.121. Correct Answer: **a**

Most likely, this balloon requires removal unless the manufacturer states the balloon can safely remain immobile for a longer period of time. A dormant, uninflated balloon promotes clotting of stagnant blood around the catheter sheath. Resuming counterpulsation increases patient risk of clot embolization; local heparin instillation is not appropriate. Infection and bleeding are considerations during IABP intervention, but are not urgently relevant to this situation.

Shinn, AE & Joseph, D: Concepts of Intraaortic Balloon Counterpulsation. J Cardiovasc Nurs *8(2): 45-60. 1994; Dossey, BM, Guzzetta, CE & Kenner, CV:* Critical Care Nursing: Body-Mind-Spirit, *3rd ed. Philadelphia, Lippincott, p. 267, 1992.*

6.122. Correct Answer: **c**

Cardiac output generally *decreases* when a mechanical ventilator forcefully distends alveoli with preset volumes of air. Airway inflation can cause pneumothorax, mediastinal, pleural, or pericardial air, or subcutaneous emphysema. With movement or improper placement the endotracheal tube can slide into one bronchus, usually the right. Only one lung receives oxygen. A restless patient can indeed spontaneously extubate himself.

Hudak, C & Gallo, B: Critical Care Nursing: A Holistic Approach, *6th ed. Philadelphia, Lippincott, pp. 478 & 506, 1994;*

Geer, RT: Critical Care of the Surgical Patient in Dripps/Eckenhoff/Vandam Introduction to Anesthesia, *8th ed (Longnecker, DE & Murphy, FL, Eds). Philadelphia, Saunders, pp. 463-465, 1992.*

6.123. Correct Answer: **d**

Sensory function of the radial nerve is assessed at the web between thumb and index finger. Paresthesia (numbness or tingling) indicates nerve compression or vascular compromise by thrombus or spasm. Ability to flex the wrist and spread (abduct) fingers can be used to evaluate motor function. Rapid capillary refill time indicates adequate palmar circulation. The ulnar nerve affects the third and fourth fingers. Adequate outcomes after invasive monitoring require full vascular and neurologic function of the cannulated extremity.

Eden-Kilgour, S & Miller, B: Understanding Neurovascular Assessment. Nursing *23(8): 56-58, 1993; Stalheim-Smith, A & Fitch, GK:* Understanding Human Anatomy and Physiology. *Minneapolis/St. Paul, West Publishing, pp. 443-446, 1994.*

6.124. Correct Answer: **c**

This patient's mild hypoxemia and decreased pCO_2 reflect increased intrapulmonary shunt, or venous admixture. This is a concern about ventilation, not perfusion. Adequate blood flows past the alveolus, but gas exchange is impaired and little or no alveolar ventilation occurs. As oxygenated blood passes obstructed alveoli, more unreleased oxygen remixes with venous blood, increasing the percentage of intrapulmonary shunt. Normally up to 10% of the cardiac output mixes or shunts from pulmonary venous circulation back into arterial circulation. Alveolar hypoventilation and increased physiologic dead space promote CO_2 retention, raising pCO_2.

Egloff, ME: Respiratory Assessment in Critical Care Nursing: Body-Mind-Spirit, *3rd ed (Dossey, BM, Guzzetta, CE & Kenner, CV, Eds). Philadelphia, Lippincott, pp. 307-311, 1992; Sauer, D: Post Anesthesia Respiratory Care in* ASPAN's Core Curriculum for Post Anesthesia Nursing Practice *3rd ed (Litwack, K, Ed). Philadelphia, Saunders, p. 130, 1992.*

6.125. Correct Answer: **c**

Surgically entering the pleural space opens a closed, negative pressure (normally -8 mm Hg) lung environment to atmospheric air pressure. As pressures inside and outside the lung equalize, the negative force maintaining lung expansion is lost and the lung collapses. The chest tube inserted into the pleural space removes air (and/or entrapped fluid), restores intrapulmonary negative pressure and expands the lung. The tube is placed under water; through a one-way valve, air can only escape into the water seal, signified by bubbling in the chamber with respiration, cough or forced expiration. All tubing connections *must* be airtight and protected from inadvertent disconnection.

Gross, SB: Current Challenges, Concepts, and Controversies in Chest Tube Management. AACN Clinical Issues in Critical Care

Nursing *4(2): 260-275, 1993; Potter, PA & Perry, AG:* Basic Nursing: Theory and Practice, *3rd ed. St. Louis, Mosby, pp. 998-999, 1994.*

6.126. Correct Answer: **a**

Ongoing observation and assessment are appropriate. An active pleural air leak is an anticipated finding after thoracotomy. The chest tube is an extension of the patient's lung. A patient with an active air leak requires a patent connection to an intact water seal—an unclamped chest tube. Clamping the tube traps air in the chest, gradually increasing potential for tension pneumothorax.

Gross, SB: Current Challenges, Concepts, and Controversies in Chest Tube Management. AACN Clinical Issues in Critical Care Nursing *4(2): 260-275, 1993; Staff: Managing Chest Drainage Problems.* Nursing *23: 8, August, 1993.*

6.127. Correct Answer: **c**

Gentle pressure on the latex drainage tube moves fluid through the chest tube system. The nurse looks for fluctuation in the tubing's fluid level during respiration (tidaling) to indicate chest tube patency. Absent drainage may mean the flow of blood from the chest is obstructed by a blood clot or tubing kink. Disconnection, hand irrigation and increasing chamber pressures are not appropriate. Hard ("power") stripping or milking the tube to promote drainage or remove clots can produce excessive negative pressures that may disrupt sutures or lung tissue. The value (or harm) of milking chest tubes, long a traditional intervention, has never been scientifically confirmed.

Gross, SB: Current Challenges, Concepts, and Controversies in Chest Tube Management. AACN Clinical Issues in Critical Care Nursing *4(2): 260-275, 1993; Potter, PA & Perry, AG:* Basic Nursing: Theory and Practice, *3rd ed. St. Louis, Mosby, pp. 998-9, 1994.*

6.128. Correct Answer: **b**

Clamping the tube traps air in the chest, gradually increasing potential for tension pneumothorax. With each breath, the volume of air trapped in the chest increases, without an avenue for escape. Intrathoracic pressure grows, collapsing the lung. Pressure eventually forces the trachea, bronchi and heart to the opposite side of the chest, compressing and deflating the other lung. Positive pressure ventilation only increases the pressure—and speeds hemodynamic catastrophe.

Gross, SB: Current Challenges, Concepts, and Controversies in Chest Tube Management. AACN Clinical Issues in Critical Care Nursing *4(2): 260-275, 1993; Dossey, BM, Guzzetta, CE & Kenner, CV:* Critical Care Nursing: Body-Mind-Spirit, *3rd ed. Philadelphia, Lippincott, pp. 345-349, 1992.*

6.129. Correct Answer: **b**

A semi- to high-Fowler's position promotes chest wall and lung tissue expansion, and movement of the diaphragm. Turning so the operative lung is dependent may improve drainage and promote alveolar exchange in the "healthy" lung.

Dossey, BM, Guzzetta, CE & Kenner, CV: Critical Care Nursing: Body-Mind-Spirit, *3rd ed. Philadelphia, Lippincott, pp. 354-365, 1992; Potter, PA & Perry, AG:* Basic Nursing: Theory and Practice, *3rd ed. St. Louis, Mosby, pp. 998-999, 1994.*

6.130. Correct Answer: **a**

An abrupt gush of fluid through the chest tube is common after repositioning. Pooled fluid shifts in the chest and appears for drainage. It is appropriate to observe for 15-30 minutes to assess whether increased amounts of drainage will continue, indicating possible hemorrhage.

Potter, PA & Perry, AG: Basic Nursing: Theory and Practice, *3rd ed. St. Louis, Mosby, pp. 998-999, 1994; Staff: Managing Chest Drainage Problems.* Nursing, *23: 8, August, 1993.*

6.131. Correct Answer: **d**

Loops of tubing draping dependently below chest level oppose drainage of fluid from the chest and potentially allow air and fluid to reenter the chest. The drainage collection system is always below the heart and never raised onto the bed or stretcher. Clamping a pleural tube, particularly one with an air leak, is not appropriate during transport. Portable suction is unnecessary for transport.

Managing Chest Drainage Problems. Nursing, *23: 8, August, 1993; Gross, SB: Current Challenges, Concepts, and Controversies in Chest Tube Management.* AACN Clinical Issues in Critical Care Nursing *4(2): 260-275, 1993.*

6.132. Correct Answer: **b**

At the resting membrane potential of –80 to –90 millivolts (mV), the myocardial cell membrane holds potassium within the cell and limits entry of sodium ions. Gradual movement of sodium into the cell raises the cell membrane potential to –50 to –60 mV, the threshold for stimulation. Rapid depolarization, or the cellular action potential, represents rapid entry of sodium into the cell.

Morgan, GE & Mikhail, MG: Clinical Anesthesiology. *Norwalk, CT, Appleton & Lange, pp. 287-88, 1992; Stalheim-Smith, A & Fitch, GK:* Understanding Human Anatomy and Physiology. *Minneapolis / St. Paul, West Publishing, pp. 261-263 & 345-352, 1994.*

6.133. Correct Answer: **c**

Dextrose starch, a synthetic colloid solution, is available in molecular weights of 70,000 and 40,000. Dextran 40, the lower molecular weight solution, is used for antiplatelet effects and to improve blood flow through microcirculation. The heavier solution, dextran 70, may be selected for volume expansion.

Morgan, GE & Mikhail, MG: Clinical Anesthesiology. *Norwalk, CT, Appleton & Lange, p. 479, 1992; Silinsky, J: The Hematologic System in* ASPAN's Core Curriculum for Post Anesthesia Nursing Practice, *3rd ed (Litwack, K, Ed). Philadelphia, Saunders, pp. 198-199, 1994.*

6.134. Correct Answer: **b**

Dextran's antiplatelet effects decrease blood viscosity by decreasing red cell aggregation and platelet adhesiveness. Infusions that exceed 20 ml/kg/day may prolong bleeding time. For this patient, approximately 40 ml per hour would be the maximum infusion rate. Dextran can alter blood cross-matching techniques, possibly promote renal failure or produce anaphylaxis.

Morgan, GE & Mikhail, MG: Clinical Anesthesiology. *Norwalk, CT, Appleton & Lange, p. 479, 1992; Silinsky, J: The Hematologic System in* ASPAN's Core Curriculum for Post Anesthesia Nursing Practice, *3rd ed (Litwack, K, Ed). Philadelphia, Saunders, pp. 198-199, 1994.*

6.135. Correct Answer: **c**

Bladder fullness is one cause of postoperative hypertension. The nurse's plan of care includes inquiry about bladder pain, observation of distention above the symphysis pubis, and verifying patency of any urinary catheters. Spinal or epidural anesthesia and surgical technique to repair inguinal hernia can disrupt bladder emptying. Sphincter release and the sensation of a full bladder may be impaired.

Burden, N: Ambulatory Surgical Nursing. *Philadelphia, Saunders, p. 288, 1993.*

6.136. Correct Answer: **a**

After cardioversion, this patient is at risk for developing pulmonary embolism. When atria fibrillate rather than contract, blood pools in the atrial chambers, stagnates and begins to clot. Conversion to sinus rhythm restores atrial contraction and can shower any clots through the circulation. Clots from the right atrium are propelled into the lungs and can obstruct smaller pulmonary vessels. Anticoagulation is often recommended prior to cardioversion to reduce this risk.

Erickson, BA: Dysrhythmias in Comprehensive Cardiac Care, *7th ed (Kinney, MR, Packa, DR & Andreoli, KG, et al, Eds). St. Louis, Mosby, pp. 152-154, 1991.*

6.137. Correct Answer: **d**

This patient lost nearly 50% of his ventilatory capacity. He now requires ongoing respiratory assessment, frequent position changes, stimulation and activity to maintain ventilation and adequate lung capacity in the remaining (right) lung. Crackles indicate fluid has moved into the right lung tissue; this finding should be reported and treated. A mediastinal chest tube might be placed for fluid drainage, though drainage may be allowed instead to accumulate in the chest. This pooled fluid occupies the empty left lung space and limits shift of the heart and right lung. There is no need for a pleural chest tube after pneumonectomy. Trendelenburg's position and positioning on the nonoperative (right) side inhibit right lung expansion and are not used.

Drain, C: The Post Anesthesia Care Unit: A Critical Care Approach to Post Anesthesia Nursing, *3rd ed. Philadelphia, Saunders, pp. 360-361, 1994; Bernard, LM: The Pulmonary Surgical Patient in* ASPAN's Core Curriculum for Post Anesthesia Nursing Practice, *3rd ed (Litwack, K, Ed). Philadelphia, Saunders, p. 321, 1994.*

6.138. Correct Answer: **b**

A newly admitted, preoperative trauma patient is presumed to have a full stomach. Anticipate the high potential for aspiration and manage the full stomach to prevent airway and pulmonary complications. Head injury may blunt protective reflexes and suppress consciousness, neck injuries prohibit hyperextension to relieve obstruction by soft tissue or foreign objects, and chest injuries impair ventilation.

Capan, SM: Airway Management in Trauma: Anesthesia and Intensive Care *(Capan, LM, Miller, SM & Turner, H, Eds). Philadelphia, Lippincott, pp. 43-83, 1991; Hanson, WC: Managing the Desperately Ill Patient: Trauma and Shock in* Dripps/Eckenhoff/Vandam Introduction to Anesthesia, *8th ed. Philadelphia, Saunders, pp. 377-381, 1992.*

6.139. Correct Answer: **b**

The carotid arteries provide 85% of the blood supply to the anterior cerebral hemispheres. Transient visual blurring or blindness (amaurosis fugax) is a classic indicator of carotid artery disease. Muscle weakness or dysphasia also suggests transient ischemic attack (TIA) and increases the risk of cerebrovascular accident (CVA). The vertebrobasilar arteries deliver approximately 15% of the brain's blood supply, primarily to the posterior system. Intracranial blood flow is provided by four branches of the internal carotid artery (ICA)—the anterior cerebral artery, middle cerebral artery, ophthalmic artery, and posterior communicating artery.

Fode, NC: Carotid Endarterectomy: Nursing Care and Controversies. J Neurosci Nurs *22(1): 25-30, 1990; Kane, HL & Wilson, LB: Practical Points in the Care of the Patient Post-Carotid Endarterectomy.* J Post Anesth Nurs *8(6): 403-405, 1993.*

6.140. Correct Answer: **a**

The baseline preoperative assessment data provide essential comparative information to detect and confirm even small changes in postoperative neurologic function. While ongoing estimates of gross neurologic function are easily documented on the Glasgow Coma Scale, detecting specific and subtlevariations that can have "devastating complications" requires detailed description.

Kane, HL & Wilson, LB: Practical Points in the Care of the Patient Post-Carotid Endarterectomy. J Post Anesth Nurs *8(6): 403-405, 1993; Johnson, SM & Anderson, B: Carotid Endarterectomy: A Review.* Crit Care Clin North Am *3(3): 499-505, 1991.*

6.141. Correct Answer: **c**

Tachycardia or ventricular arrhythmias often appear as the cardinal signs of malignant hyperthermia and precede any muscle rigidity. The nurse who monitors an intubated patient with an end-tidal carbon dioxide monitor may observe a trend of rising pCO_2, thereby detecting malignant hyperthermia even before the tachycardia develops. Temperature elevation is one of the *last* clinical signs. Skin mottling indicates significant vasoconstriction and hypoxemia and appears after the biochemical chain of events is well underway.

Wlody, GS: Malignant Hyperthermia. Crit Care Nurs Clin North Am *3: 129-134, 1991;*

Drain, C: The Post Anesthesia Care Unit: A Critical Care Approach to Post Anesthesia Nursing, *3rd ed. Philadelphia, Saunders, pp. 564-569, 1994.*

6.142. Correct Answer: **a**

Dantrolene sodium is a skeletal muscle relaxant. Adequate muscle strength to breathe, stand, and prevent aspiration is an important determination after dantrolene administration. Dantrolene is continued after a malignant hyperthermia crisis until 10 mg are given; dantrolene doses continue into the time period when unassisted respiration, ambulation and oral intake may begin.

Wlody, GS: Malignant Hyperthermia. Crit Care Nurs Clin North Am *3: 129-134, 1991; Miller, RD: Skeletal Muscle Relaxants in* Basic & Clinical Pharmacology, *6th ed. Norwalk, CT, Appleton & Lange, pp. 416-417, 1995.*

6.143. Correct Answer: **c**

The vasodilating effects of sympathetic blockade decrease venous return and preload. Cardiac output falls unless simultaneous rehydration occurs to maintain blood pressure within 20% of preoperative parameters. Decreased venous return and blockade of T-1 to T-4 cardioaccelerator fibers cause bradycardia.

Burden, N: Ambulatory Surgical Nursing. *Philadelphia, Saunders, pp. 255-256, 1993; Saleh, KL: Spinal Anesthesia.* J Post Anesth Nurs *6: 407-409, 1991.*

6.144. Correct Answer: **d**

Mr. H most likely is not breathing due to paralysis of his respiratory muscles—and is probably awake. Emergency treatment of this complication necessitates cardiorespiratory support with mechanical ventilation, vasopressors and fluid volume. Migration of local anesthetic medication ascending through cerebrospinal fluid to interfere with motor and sensory function higher than the T-3 dermatome produces a high, or total, spinal-block.

Burden, N: Ambulatory Surgical Nursing. *Philadelphia, Saunders, pp. 258, 1993; Saleh, KL: Spinal Anesthesia.* J Post Anesth Nurs *6: 407-409, 1991.*

6.145. Correct Answer: **a**

The tongue is the most common obstructor of the unconscious patient's airway. Snoring sounds indicate partial obstruction in the upper airway. A recumbent, sedated and nonalert patient is unable to prevent soft tissue (tongue) from relaxing against the posterior pharynx, limiting air passage. Procedures or situations that produce tongue swelling contribute to difficulty in managing upper airway patency.

Burden, N: Ambulatory Surgical Nursing. *Philadelphia, Saunders, pp. 263-264, 1993; Drain, C:* The Post Ansesthesia Care Unit: A Critical Care Approach to Post Anesthesia Care Nursing, *3rd ed. Philadelphia, Saunders, pp. 305-306, 1994.*

6.146. Correct Answer: **b**

If untreated, Ms T's airway obstruction may produce hypoxia and hypercarbia. Partial upper airway obstruction is generally alleviated by tilting the patient's head back and firmly pushing the jaw behind the mandibular joint to extend the mandible. In addition, manually extending the tongue and inserting a nasal, oral or (rarely) endotracheal airway and repositioning the patient to a side-lying position may decrease the obstruction.

Burden, N: Ambulatory Surgical Nursing. *Philadelphia, Saunders, pp. 263-264, 1993; Drain, C:* The Post Anesthesia Care Unit: A Critical Care Approach to Post Anesthesia Care Nursing, *3rd ed. Philadelphia, Saunders, pp. 305-306, 1994.*

6.147. Correct Answer: **c**

Long-term cigarette smokers often have copious airway mucous, coughing spells and airway irritability. Frequent suctioning of tenacious secretions can further irritate airway tissue and prompt laryngospasm. Laryngospasm may produce pulmonary edema even in healthy, noncardiac patients. Agitated attempts to breathe through an obstructed airway generate high intrapulmonary negative pressures, which start a cascade of physiologic events that can result in pulmonary edema.

Burden, N: Ambulatory Surgical Nursing. *Philadelphia, Saunders, pp. 390-391, 1993; Chomka Leya, CM & Bandala, LC: Respiratory Complications in* Post Anesthesia Care *(Vender, JS & Speiss, BD, Eds). Philadelphia, Saunders, pp. 88-90, 1992.*

6.148. Correct Answer: **a**

Medications and the stress of surgery and anesthesia can cause myocardial muscle ischemia, particluarly in a patient with coronary artery disease. Ischemic changes are represented on EKG by ST segment depression, especially in leads V4 and V5. Appearance of a new Q wave indicates infarction. When ischemic changes are noted during monitoring of the cardiac rhythm in PACU, a 12-lead EKG should be obtained to confirm these changes across several cardiac leads. Downsloping ST segment depression of more than 1 mm below baseline or ST elevation of more than 1 mm above baseline is considered diagnostic, except when digitalis effect or left bundle branch block distort the cardiac complex.

Hudak, CM & Gallo, BM: Critical Care Nursing: A Holistic Approach, *6th ed. Philadelphia, Lippincott, p. 156, 1994; Neely, CR: Cardiovascular Disease in* Dripps/Eckenhoff/Vandam Introduction to Anesthesia *(Longnecker, DE & Murphy, FL, Eds). Philadelphia, Saunders, pp. 271-272, 1992.*

6.149. Correct Answer: **b**

EKG signs of myocardial ischemia (ST depression and T wave inversion) can be seen with digitalis administration, effects of inhalation anesthetics, periods of shivering, hypothermia, cardiac dysrhythmia, and electrolyte disturbances. Hyperkalemia produces tall, peaked T waves; nitroglycerin at low doses increases collateral blood flow and improves oxygenation to ischemic muscle; morphine decreases the catecholamine surges associated with pain and physiologic stress and so should promote oxygenation and comfort.

Burden, N: Ambulatory Surgical Nursing. *Philadelphia, Saunders, pp. 281, 1993; Marymont, JH & O'Connor, BS: Postopera-*

tive Cardiovascular Complications in Post Anesthesia Care *(Vender, JS & Speiss, BD, Eds). Philadelphia, Saunders, pp. 26-37 & 40-43, 1992.*

6.150. Correct Answer: **b**

Cervical nerves 3, 4, and 5 innervate the diaphragm. Postoperative deficit in function of these nerves compromises diaphragmatic excursion. Potential for inadequate ventilation occurs, as this patient may use only intercostal and accessory muscles to breathe. Ms Q may have postoperative neck and arm discomfort or numbness, which are unrelated to any intraoperative air embolism. Analgesia and assuring alignment may increase comfort.

Barnes, SS: Post Anesthesia Care of the Orthopedic Surgical Patient in The Post Anesthesia Care Unit: A Critical Care Approach to Post Anesthesia Nursing, *3rd ed (Drain, C, Ed). Philadelphia, Saunders, pp. 406-407, 1994; McCarthy, RE : Back Pain and Intervertebral Disk Trauma in* The Clinical Practice of Neurological and Neurosurgical Nursing, *3rd ed (Hickey, JV, Ed). Philadelphia, Lippincott, 460-466, 1992.*

Section 7

Physiologic Balance

Scenarios and items in this section focus on issues of *physiologic balance* of the body's internal *chemical* (acid-base, oxygen and electrolyte), *fluid, coagulation, endocrine* and *thermal* environment. These concepts are considered together because each:

- has defined "balance" parameters (normal values)
- causes measurable outcomes related to deficit (hypo-) or excess (hyper-)
- produces pharmacokinetic and pharmacodynamic effects related to anesthetics and medications
- suggests nursing process responses to restore balance

ESSENTIAL CORE CONCEPTS	AFFILIATED CORE CURRICULUM CHAPTERS
Nursing Process	
Assessment	Chapters 2, 11,
Planning and Implementation	12, 13, 16, & 26
Evaluation	
Chemical and Electrolyte Balance	
Acid-Base Concepts	Chapter 11
Acidosis	
Respiratory	
Metabolic	
Alkalosis	
Respiratory	
Metabolic	
Compensation, Mixed Imbalances	
Buffers	
Renal	
Respiratory	
Interpreting Arterial Blood Gases	
Oxygenation	Chapter 10
Hypoventilation	
Hypoxemia	
Oxygen Delivery Systems	
Toxicity	
Restoring Balance	

Electrolyte Stability — Chapter 12

Concentration
- Anions
- Cations

Deficits and Excesses
- Causes
- Symptoms
- Nursing Assessment and Intervention

Principles
- Diffusion

Restoring Balance

Fluid Balance — **Chapter 12**

Composition: Extracellular, Intracellular

Distribution and Volumes

Fluid Regulation: Loss, Gain and Balance
- Causes
- Compartment Shifts
- Symptoms

Principles and Concepts
- Hydrostatic Pressure
- Osmosis
- Osmolality
- Tonicity: iso- hypo- and hyper-
- Volume Replacement
  - Colloid
  - Crystalloid
- Restoring Balance

Hematologic Balance — **Chapter 13**

Blood Components

Structure and Function

Antigens and Antibodies: ABO, Rh and Immunity

Platelets and Thrombin: Hemostasis and Clots

Red Cells: Anemias, Hemolysis, and Sickling

White Cells: Leukemias

Order and Disorder

Characteristics and Symptoms
- Blood Loss
- Coagulation Cascade
- Disseminated Intravascular Coagulation

Normal Values

Restoring Balance
- Transfusion Therapy
  - Blood Components
  - Hemolysis, Allergy, and Anaphylaxis
  - Infection Transmission
    - Hepatitis

HIV and AIDS
Virus
Universal Precautions

Thermal Balance **Chapter 16**

Hypothermia
Concepts of Heat Loss
Heat Generation
Postanestheisa Shivering
Active Rewarming

Hyperthermia
Malignant
Sepsis

Endocrine Balance **Chapter 26**

Glands and Hormones
Assessment and Function
Adrenal: Mineralocorticoids, Glucocorticoids
Pancreas: Glucose Balance
Parathyroid: Calcium Balance
Pituitary: "Master" Regulation
Thyroid: Metabolic Rate
Excesses and Deficits
Characteristics and Symptoms
Feedback Regulation

Restoring Balance
Anesthetic Interactions, Surgical Interventions
Nursing Responsibilities

SET I

Items 7.1-7.35

7.1. A late-developing sign of hypoxia is:
a. restless agitation
b. peripheral cyanosis
c. disoriented confusion
d. supraventricular tachycardia

7.2. A 4 week old infant has increased risk for fluid overload due to:
a. immature tubular regulation
b. low metabolic rate
c. intrinsic hypernatremia
d. high percentage of body fat

7.3. Arterial blood gas values of pH = 7.20, pCO_2 = 46 mm Hg, pO_2 = 150 mm Hg, and HCO_3^- = 15 mEq/L indicate:
a. partially compensated metabolic acidosis with respiratory alkalosis
b. mixed and uncompensated respiratory alkalosis with metabolic acidosis
c. mixed and uncompensated metabolic and respiratory acidosis
d. simultaneous and partially corrected respiratory and metabolic acidosis

7.4. A low-flow oxygen delivery system that provides oxygen at an FiO_2 of 0.4 is a:
a. T-piece at 10 L/min
b. Venturi mask at 8 L/min
c. intermittent mandatory ventilation at 6 L/min
d. nasal cannula at 5 L/min

7.5. The patient *least* likely to normally metabolize atracurium besylate has:
a. serum creatinine = 3.6 ml/min
b. tympanic temperature = 36.6° C.
c. serum pH = 7.31
d. pseudocholinesterase = 15 mg/kg

NOTE: Consider scenario and items 7.6-7.7 together.

The preanesthesia nurse observes that a patient with cirrhosis and an actively bleeding gastric ulcer received 5 units of packed red cells to stabilize for a partial gastrectomy, vagotomy and pyloroplasty. A unit of whole blood infuses now and bleeding has abated.

7.6. Following massive transfusion, this patient has increased potential for:
a. hypoglycemia related to banked packed cells
b. hyperkalemia related to respiratory alkalosis
c. hypocalcemia related to citrate preservative
d. hyponatremia related to hemodilution

7.7. The clinical nurse expects that infusing 1 unit of red blood cells will increase the patient's hemoglobin by:
a. 0.5 g/dl
b. 1.0 g/dl
c. 1.5 g/dl
d. 2.0 g/dl

7.8. Oxygen desaturation detected by a pulse oximeter may indicate any of the following situations *except:*
a. hemoglobin loss with normal oxygen-hemoglobin binding
b. vasoconstriction and greater oxygen-hemoglobin affinity
c. intraesophageal intubation with adequate oxygen-hemoglobin affinity
d. carbon dioxide retention and increasing oxygen-hemoglobin binding

NOTE: Consider items 7.9-7.11 together.

7.9. During Ms R's admission to PACU, the anesthesiologist announces that Ms R has Phase II block, which indicates:

a. readiness for outpatient discharge instructions after injection of her trigger points
b. complete recovery from Phase I nondepolarizing neuromuscular blockade
c. prolonged muscle weakness after repeated doses of a depolarizing muscle relaxant
d. sustained muscle twitching during repeated ulnar nerve stimulation

7.10. Administering neostigmine to Ms R will most likely:

a. create Phase I block
b. delay neuromuscular recovery
c. prompt supraventricular tachycardia
d. produce equal train-of-four response

7.11. The PACU nurse anticipates that Ms R's Phase II block will:

a. resolve spontaneously within 30-45 minutes
b. progress to Phase I block with pseudocholinesterase elimination
c. wane with biotransformation and Hofmann elimination
d. require overnight mechanical ventilation

7.12. A patient whose serum glucose measures 728 mg/dl is most likely to develop:

a. diabetes insipidus crisis
b. uncontrolled diabetic ketoacidosis
c. hyperglycemic hyperosmolar nonketotic coma
d. gestational glucose acidosis

7.13. Cryoprecipitate is appropriately used to reverse:

a. fluid volume deficit
b. warfarin anticoagulation
c. fibrinogen deficiency
d. factor VII, IX, and X losses

7.14. Biochemically, the enzyme 2,3-diphosphoglycerate (2,3-DPG) is important for cellular:

a. protein synthesis by mitochondria
b. oxygen release from hemoglobin
c. carbon dioxide reuptake in plasma
d. antigen-antibody bonding by leukocytes

7.15. Cortisol production occurs as a/an:

a. negative feedback response by the anterior hypophysis
b. indirect relationship with renal renin release
c. positive response to posterior pituitary stimulation
d. inverse relationship to hepatic gluconeogenesis

7.16. Body temperature is regulated in the:

a. pons
b. hypothalamus
c. medulla
d. hypophysis

NOTE: Consider scenario and items 7.17-7.19 together.

During a lumbar decompression and fusion of vertebrae L-2 to S-1, Ms B's estimated blood loss was 800 ml. Her hemoglobin in PACU is 7.2 g/dl, and the surgeon orders an infusion of 2 units of autologous blood. The blood bank technician informs the PACU nurse Ms B has "cold agglutinins."

7.17. The PACU nurse responds by:

a. informing the surgeon Ms B cannot receive blood
b. infusing blood through a blood warmer
c. diluting blood cells with fresh frozen plasma
d. applying a hypothermia blanket to cool Ms B

7.18. Ms B's blood type is A negative. She has serum antibodies to each of the following *except:*

a. type A positive whole blood
b. type AB positive platelets
c. type O negative packed red cells
d. type B negative cryoprecipitate

7.19. Ms B predonated 3 units of red blood cells. Safe infusion of autologous blood requires:

a. a 22 gauge intermediate length catheter
b. concurrent infusion with 5% dextrose in water
c. blood pressure assessment after infusing 150 ml
d. replacement of blood filter after the second unit

7.20. The nurse monitors whether Ms X develops diabetes insipidus after her pituitary surgery by transsphenoidal approach by observing:

a. copious volumes of dilute urine
b. parched lips and concentrated urine
c. large volumes of glucose-containing urine
d. hypertension and urinary ketone elevation

NOTE: Consider items 7.21-7.24 together.

Thirty minutes following open cholecystectomy, 35 year old Ms Z is difficult to waken and respirations are shallow and slow after a general anesthetic that included fentanyl 500 mcg, midazolam 3 mg, and atracurium 30 mg. Surgeon-requested laboratory results upon PACU admission indicate pH = 7.30, pCO_2 = 55 mm Hg, pO_2 = 80 mm Hg, BUN = 45 mg/dl, creatinine = 5.6 mg/dl, Na^+ = 135 mEq/L, K^+ = 4.8 mEq/L, Cl^- = 103 mEq/L, Mg^{++} = 5.1 mg/dl, Ca^{++} = 7.5 mg/dl, PO_4 = 5.6 g/dl.

7.21. A serum magnesium of 5.1 mg/dl is *most likely* associated with:

a. chronic nasogastric suction
b. diuretic-induced potassium deficiency
c. suppression of preterm labor
d. hypoventilation with respiratory acidosis

7.22. A factor in Ms Z's medical history that would *most* contribute to her current serum magnesium is:

a. chronic laxative use since age 18
b. insulin-dependent diabetes mellitus
c. 15 year smoking history
d. end-stage renal disease

7.23. The nurse anticipates Ms Z's serum magnesium may:

a. prolong intraoperative muscle relaxant effects
b. precede metabolic alkalosis
c. disrupt reabsorption of potassium by renal tubule
d. elicit muscle spasm and tetany

7.24. Pharmacologic interventions to restore Ms Z's magnesium balance include:

a. insulin and glucose
b. diuretics and saline
c. antacids and physostigmine
d. digitalis and potassium

NOTE: Consider scenario and item 7.25 together.

A middle-aged woman is admitted to PACU following emergency drainage of a hematoma at her neck. The malignant left lobe of her thyroid gland was resected yesterday and she developed dyspnea and tracheal deviation this morning while brushing her teeth.

7.25. Her primary nurse in PACU is *most* concerned when today's assessment reveals:

a. twitch of the upper lip
b. sore throat when swallowing
c. exophthalmos and bradycardia
d. 50 ml serosanguineous wound drainage

NOTE: Consider scenario and items 7.26-7.27 together.

Ms P has had non-insulin-dependent diabetes mellitus (NIDDM) for 10 years. Her glucose is well managed with diet and glyburide (Micronase).

7.26. Thirty minutes after PACU admission, her glucose measures 300 mg/dl by glucometer, likely due to the transient influence of:

a. pancreatic enzyme inhibition
b. intraoperative Somogyi phenomenon
c. hemoconcentration after presurgery fasting
d. adrenal cortisol secretion

NOTE: The scenario continues.

Ms P's endocrinologist has specified a sliding scale of regular insulin to cover serum glucose of >250 mg/dl. The PACU nurse administers 3 units of regular insulin subcutaneously.

7.27. The maximum effect of this insulin dose is anticipated within:

a. $\frac{1}{2}$-1 hour
b. 1-2 hours
c. 2-3 hours
d. 3-4 hours

NOTE: Consider scenario and items 7.28-7.30 together.

A 30 year old patient, Ms B, is in PACU after craniotomy to insert a ventriculoperitoneal shunt to treat her hydrocephalus. Two hours after admission, urine volume is 25 ml and specific gravity is 1.027.

7.28. A likely nursing diagnosis is fluid volume:

a. excess related to antidiuretic hormone secretion
b. deficit related to diabetes insipidus
c. deficit related to insufficient vasopressin
d. excess related to hypernatremia

7.29. An appropriate intervention for Ms B in PACU is:

a. vasopressin infusion
b. fluid restriction
c. osmotic diuresis
d. desmopressin replacement

7.30. While administering Ms B's newly ordered phenytoin to suppress postoperative seizure potential, the nurse observes closely for:

a. atrial flutter-fibrillation
b. increased bleeding into drain
c. extending QRS duration
d. paradoxic extrapyramidal tremors

7.31. During emergency treatment of abdominal hemorrhage, rapidly infusing 4 units of packed red cells through a blood warmer:

a. eliminates the potential for cell hemolysis
b. increases the likelihood of serum hypokalemia
c. reduces the risk of allergic reaction
d. promotes peripheral vasodilation for comfort

NOTE: Consider scenario and items 7.32-7.33 together.

After a mitral valve replacement, chest drainage from the mediastinal chest tube is 300 ml each hour for 3 hours. This PACU patient received intraoperative heparin sodium, which was neutralized with protamine sulfate.

7.32. Bleeding likely arises from:

a. action of underdeveloped platelets
b. protamine allergy
c. clotting factor I and X deficit
d. heparin rebound

NOTE: The scenario continues.

This patient's surgeon routinely orders an additional small dose of protamine sulfate to be administered in PACU. Following an intraoperative dose of protamine sulfate, the patient developed sustained hypotension.

7.33. When planning nursing interventions, the PACU nurse:

a. reduces the scheduled protamine dose by 50%
b. infuses 50 ml of 25% albumin with the protamine
c. consults with the surgeon about protamine allergy
d. doubles volume of diluent and extends infusion time

7.34. One physiologic response to correct increased pCO_2 is:

a. renal conservation of hydrogen
b. increased pulmonary ventilation
c. renal elimination of bicarbonate
d. decreased pulmonary vital capacity

7.35. Osmolality of extracellular fluid is determined by:

a. cations, anions, water and glucose
b. glucose, protein and red blood cells
c. nonelectrolyte substances only
d. hydrostatic water and cellular proteins only

SET II

Items 7.36-7.70

7.36. An example of a hypotonic intravenous solution is:

a. lactated Ringer's solution
b. 0.45% normal saline
c. 10% dextrose in water
d. 0.9% normal saline

7.37. The patient with signs that include hemolysis, elevated liver enzymes and low platelets probably also has:

a. gestational diabetes
b. glomerulonephritis
c. rhabdomyolysis
d. preeclampsia

7.38. Metabolic acidosis most significantly increases serum:

a. sodium
b. potassium
c. magnesium
d. bicarbonate

7.39. A mechanically ventilated patient's arterial blood gas measures are pH = 7.38, pCO_2 = 43 mm Hg, pO_2 = 87 mm Hg, HCO_3^- = 26 mEq/L. These blood gas results suggest that the nurse's interventions are *best* directed toward:

a. reducing carbon dioxide
b. reversing muscle relaxant
c. correcting metabolic acidosis
d. maintaining oxygen delivery

7.40. The physiologic alteration that initiates a malignant hyperthermia crisis is:

a. extreme muscle calcium
b. delayed metabolism
c. insufficient serum magnesium
d. acidotic hypercapnia

7.41. A 2 month old infant's primary compensatory response to hypothermia is:

a. muscle fasciculation
b. crying and agitation
c. increased metabolism
d. peripheral vasoconstriction

NOTE: Consider scenario and items 7.42-7.44 together.

During the admission assessment of a somnolent patient who had a transsphenoidal hypophysectomy, the PACU nurse observes that the patient breathes shallowly 32 times per minute and has nonsynchronous chest movements. He weakly extends his fingers when asked and moves the oral airway side to side. Extremity movements are intermittently "jerky."

7.42. The nurse interprets these signs as most likely indicating:

a. renarcotization
b. hypoglycemic seizure
c. hyperventilation effect
d. neuromuscular block

7.43. When planning nursing interventions related to these signs, the PACU nurse considers that this patient is most likely:

a. aware and anxious
b. hearing impaired
c. oversecreting ACTH
d. hyperreflexic and spastic

7.44. For this patient, prompt intervention is essential to reduce risk of:

a. status epilepticus
b. ataxic hyperventilation
c. intracranial hypertension
d. complete paralysis

NOTE: Consider scenario and items 7.45-7.46 together.

Derek is a 9 year old African-American with the sickle cell trait. He is now in PACU after a hypospadias repair.

7.45. Sickling of Derek's red blood cells is *more likely* to occur when his:

a. pain self-report is "2" on a scale of 0-10
b. temperature is 37.2° C after rapid active rewarming
c. breathing is 8 times per minute after shivering resolves
d. blood pressure is 102/64 with intravenous rate at 60 ml/h

7.46. To assess any erythrocyte sickling, the nurse observes Derek for:

a. bleeding from the site used for intraoperative epidural anesthesia
b. abdominal pain and neurovascular changes in his extremities
c. muscle fasciculations and decreased consciousness
d. unrelenting postoperative nausea and vomiting

7.47. Clinical signs most likely to appear in a patient whose pCO_2 measures 73 mm Hg include:

a. slow responsiveness, muscle weakness
b. shallow respirations, U waves on EKG
c. clear consciousness, oriented to place and person
d. tingling extremities, QRS duration of 0.20 second

7.48. Ms Q's postoperative intravenous infusion is 5% dextrose in lactated Ringer's solution at 125 ml/h. The osmotic effect of this solution increases:

a. active transport of sodium
b. solute movement out of blood
c. net movement of fluid into serum
d. transmembrane oncotic pressure

7.49. Ketoacidosis associated with diabetes mellitus is likely to produce:

a. pH = 7.48
b. pCO_2 = 33 mm Hg
c. pH = 7.40
d. HCO_3^- = 19 mEq/L

7.50. The posterior hypophysis secretes antidiuretic hormone in response to a:

a. hypertensive episode
b. catecholamine surge
c. convective heat loss
d. osmolarity increase

7.51. An alert patient with arterial blood gas measures of pH = 7.52, pCO_2 = 30 mm Hg, pO_2 = 96 mm Hg and HCO_3^- = 24 mEq/L is most likely to:

a. rate pain as "1" on a verbal pain scale of 0-10
b. mention arm tingling and fingertip numbness
c. become increasingly unresponsive to stimuli
d. cough weakly, shiver and develop seizures

7.52. A healthy middle-aged man's intraoperative loss of intravascular fluid volume was estimated at 650 ml. This volume is generally replaced with:

a. 1 unit of autologous red blood cells
b. equivalent volumes of hetastarch
c. 1 ml hypertonic saline for each milliliter loss
d. isotonic electrolyte solution in excess of loss

7.53. Intravascular and intrastitial fluid constitute the:

a. extracellular fluid compartment
b. body's total water
c. intracellular fluid compartment
d. capillary hydrostatic volume

7.54. The *primary* objective for a patient with arterial blood gas values of pH = 7.20, pCO_2 = 36 mm Hg, pO_2 = 150 mm Hg and HCO_3^- = 15 mEq/L is to:

a. prevent oxygen toxicity by weaning oxygen
b. correct hypercapnia by promoting deep breaths
c. reverse acidosis by providing sodium bicarbonate
d. compensate alkalosis by treating with diuretics

NOTE: Consider scenario and items 7.55-7.56 together.

A postoperative mechanically ventilated patient's blood gas values are pH = 7.43, pCO_2 = 28 mm Hg, pO_2 = 132 mm Hg, and HCO_3^- = 24 mEq/L. Ventilator settings are Vt = 600 ml, rate = 12, and FiO_2 = 0.6.

7.55. The nurse anticipates:

a. adding PEEP of +5 to the ventilator system
b. administering $NaHCO_3$ 30 mEq/L
c. maintaining existing ventilator settings
d. decreasing the set rate

7.56. Intentionally achieving the above arterial blood gas measures is *most* desirable for a/an:

a. 130 kg woman following gastric stapling
b. active 25 year old following resection of astrocytoma
c. elderly emphysemic man following left hip arthroplasty
d. premature 6 month infant following atrial septal defect

7.57. The oxyhemoglobin curve for a sedated, acidotic, hyperthermic patient with shallow respirations will "shift to the right," meaning that:

a. oxygen is easily released from hemoglobin
b. pH compensation will decrease oxygen saturation
c. oxygen is tightly bound to hemoglobin
d. pH decreases will increase oxygen saturation

7.58. For an adequately breathing, normothermic patient with adequate hemoglobin and acid-base balance, an oxygen saturation of 90% represents a pO_2 of approximately:

a. 90 mm Hg
b. 80 mm Hg
c. 60 mm Hg
d. 50 mm Hg

7.59. Heparin effect is monitored by observing trends in:

a. partial thromboplastin time
b. Ivy bleeding time
c. prothrombin time
d. thrombin time

Ms Y received 5 units of packed red blood cells and 1000 ml of 5% albumin after an unanticipated intraoperative blood loss of 2500 ml. A laboratory screen of serum electrolytes indicates a serum calcium of 7.5 mg/dl.

7.60. While preparing calcium replacement according to the anesthesiologist's order, the PACU nurse:

a. observes the cardiac rhythm for reentrant tachycardia
b. plans a 10 minute infusion through a central catheter
c. dilutes calcium chloride in sodium bicarbonate
d. recalls that calcium gluconate provides more calcium

7.61. The *most common* cause of coagulopathy in the postoperative trauma patient is:

a. cellular hypoxia
b. hypothermia
c. lactic acidosis
d. hemorrhage

7.62. One outcome of hyperglycemia in diabetic patients is:

a. metabolic alkalosis
b. volume depletion
c. peripheral edema
d. rebound hypoglycemia

7.63. A physiologic characteristic that distinguishes hyperglycemic hyperosmolar nonketotic syndrome (HNKS) from diabetic ketoacidosis (DKA) is:

a. comparatively lower serum glucose with HNKS
b. absence of mental status alteration with DKA
c. greater level of circulating insulin with HNKS
d. near-normal pH, pCO_2 and bicarbonate with DKA

NOTE: Consider scenario and item 7.64 together.

A 56 year old man is scheduled for craniotomy to clip a leaking cerebral aneurysm. He is settled into the preanesthesia area for nursing observation and to await his neurosurgeon's arrival.

7.64. The preanesthesia nurse specifically observes this patient for:
a. fever and hyperventilation
b. severe headache and neck stiffness
c. hydrocephalus and QRS duration of 0.16 seconds
d. atrial flutter with 3:1 conduction and seizures

7.65. Malignant hyperthermia is most likely to occur after exposure to:
a. vecuronium
b. thiopental
c. succinylcholine
d. nitrous oxide

7.66. Malignant hyperthermia symptoms primarily arise from:
a. aggressive active rewarming
b. defective calcium homeostasis
c. cellular oxygen deficit
d. excessive extracellular potassium

NOTE: Consider scenario and item 7.67 together.

While starting a patient's preoperative intravenous site, the PACU nurse inadvertently stabs her finger with the used needle. Hospital policy states blood samples for hepatitis and human immunodeficiency virus must be collected from the nurse and patient.

7.67. To collect patient specimens, the nurse plans to:
a. quietly draw them when obtaining arterial blood gases
b. request approval from the clinical nurse manager
c. obtain the patient's informed consent
d. agree to reveal personal results to the patient

7.68. Laser ablation of prostate tissue during transurethral resection of the prostate decreases the potential for postoperative:
a. hyperthermic sepsis
b. hyponatremic seizure
c. hyperosmolar pulmonary edema
d. hypovolemic oliguria

NOTE: Consider items 7.69-7.70 together.

7.69. Following left lower lobectomy, the pleural chest tube is generally inserted to:
a. remove intrathoracic air
b. restore intrapleural positive pressure
c. expand the contralateral lung and drain fluid
d. provide sampling access for culture and analysis

7.70. Following gradual blood pressure decreases over 30 minutes, this patient's blood pressure is 70/30. He is nonresponsive, and respiratory rate is 10 breaths per minute. Medical and nursing interventions may include all of the following *except:*
a. leg elevation
b. neosynephrine
c. Trendelenburg's position
d. fluid volume expansion

SET I

Answer Key

7.1. b
7.2. a
7.3. c
7.4. d
7.5. c
7.6. c
7.7. b
7.8. d
7.9. c
7.10. b
7.11. a
7.12. c
7.17. c
7.14. b
7.15. a
7.16. b
7.17. b
7.18. c
7.19. d
7.20. a
7.21. c
7.22. d
7.23. a
7.24. b
7.25. a
7.26. d
7.27. c
7.28. a
7.29. b
7.30. c
7.31. d
7.32. d
7.33. c
7.34. b
7.35. a

SET I

Rationales and References

7.1. Correct Answer: **b**

Cyanosis is not evident until a minimum of 5 g/dl of blood is oxygen-unsaturated. Thus blue-tinged lips, dusky nailbeds and mottled skin are late signs of hypoxia or suggest strong vasoconstriction from other causes. Room lighting and skin tones can mask the observer's discovery of cyanosis. Tachycardia is an early but nonspecific hint of hypoxemia. Insufficient oxygenation *must* be quickly eliminated as the cause of a postanesthesia patient's agitation or confusion.

Drain, C: The Post Anesthesia Care Unit: A Critical Care Approach to Post Anesthesia Nursing, *3rd ed. Philadelphia, Saunders, pp. 104 & 361-362, 1994; Belatti, RG: Common Post Anesthetic Problems in* Post Anesthesia Care *(Vender, JE & Speiss, BD, Eds). Philadelphia, Saunders, pp. 11-13, 1992.*

7.2. Correct Answer: **a**

A young infant's renal tubular reabsorption and secretion functions are immature, so ability to compensate for fluid imbalance is limited and fluid balance is precarious. Until approximately age 2 years, a large proportion of the infant's body water is contained in extracellular fluid space. Nephron function is approximately 80-90% of an adult's. These factors increase the infant's potential for hypervolemia. Infants have high metabolic rates, quickly exhaust fat stores, and are susceptible to hyponatremia. Sodium balance is tied to intake.

Drain, C: The Post Anesthesia Care Unit: A Critical Care Approach to Post Anesthesia Nursing, *3rd ed. Philadelphia, Saunders, pp. 537-538, 1994; Liu, LMP: Fluid Management in* A Practice of Anesthesia for Infants and Children, *2nd ed (Cote, CJ & Ryan, JF, Eds). Philadelphia, Saunders, pp. 171-182, 1993.*

7.3. Correct Answer: **c**

This patient's blood gas results indicate a mixed acidosis that so far is uncompensated. The pH value is decreased to 7.20, indicating *acidosis*. The pCO_2 (respiratory component) is elevated, indicating *respiratory acidosis*. A coexisting low bicarbonate (HCO_3^-) (metabolic component) indicates *metabolic acidosis*. A pH of 7.20 deviates significantly from the normal pH of 7.40; body systems have not yet compensated. The pO_2 indicates oxygenation is adequate.

Atsberger, DB: Interpretation of Acid-Base Balance in ASPAN's Core Curriculum for Post Anesthesia Nursing Practice, *3rd ed (Litwack, K, Ed). Philadelphia, Saunders, pp. 148-150, 1994; Rothenberg, DM: Postoperative Acid-Base Disorders: Recognition and Management in* Post Anesthesia Care *(Vender, JS & Speiss, BD, Eds). Saunders, Philadelphia, pp. 94-106, 1992.*

7.4. Correct Answer: **d**

Nasal cannulae, simple face masks, and face tents are low-flow oxygen systems. Oxygen concentration varies with the patient's inspiratory rate and depth. High-flow oxygen delivery systems increase the accuracy of oxygen delivery. Venturi and nonrebreathing masks, a T-piece, or mechanical ventilators are examples of high-flow oxygen systems.

O'Brien, DD: Care of the Post Anesthesia Patient in The Post Anesthesia Care Unit: A Critical Care Approach to Post Anesthesia Nursing, *3rd ed (Drain, C, Ed). Philadelphia, Saunders, pp. 295-298, 1994.*

7.5. Correct Answer: **c**

Normal temperature and very slight alkalinity most favor metabolism of atracurium besylate (Tracrium). This nondepolarizing muscle relaxant "self-destructs" (biotransforms) by Hofmann elimination and ester hydrolysis. These processes are independent of any liver and renal failure and do not require reversal or pseudocholinesterase. Low pH and hypothermia delay biotransformation.

Harbut, RE: Anesthetic Agents and Adjuncts in ASPAN's Core Curriculum for Post Anesthesia Nursing Practice, *3rd ed (Litwack, K, Ed). Philadelphia, Saunders, pp. 90-91, 1994; Drain, C:* The Post Anesthesia Care Unit: A Critical Care Approach to Post Anesthesia Nursing, *3rd ed. Philadelphia, Saunders, pp. 232-233, 1994.*

7.6. Correct Answer: **c**

Hypocalcemia may develop after large volumes of stored blood are rapidly infused. Citrate from the preservative citrate phosphate dextrose (CPD) used in banked blood binds ionized calcium, thereby reducing circulating, unbound calcium. Notice evidence of neuromuscular irritability like muscle tremors, extremity paresthesias, tingling, or cramps and cardiac arrhythmias. Potassium shifts among body fluid compartments restore any possible transient hypokalemia related to transfusion. Hyperkalemia is associated with acidosis, not alkalosis.

Coffland, FI & Shelton, DM: Blood Component Replacement Therapy. Nurs Clin North Am *5(3): 543-556, 1993; O'Brien, D: Care of the Post Anesthesia Patient in* The Post Anesthesia Care Unit: A Critical Care Approach to Post Anesthesia Nursing, *3rd ed (Drain, C, Ed). Philadelphia, Saunders, p. 294, 1994.*

7.7. Correct Answer: **b**

Hemoglobin promptly increases approximately 1 g/dl for each unit of red blood cells infused. The 2-3% per unit increase in hematocrit occurs sooner than if whole blood were transfused. The need to transfuse is individually determined according to a patient's physiologic tolerance and anticipated blood loss of 10-20% of total blood volume. For most patients, when hemoglobin dips to between 7-9 g/dl, transfusion is recommended.

Litwack, K: Post Anesthesia Care Nursing, *2nd ed. St. Louis, Mosby, p. 436, 1995; Vonfrolio, LG & Moore, J:* Emergency Nursing Examination Review, *2nd ed. Springhouse, PA, Springhouse Corp, p. 173, 1991.*

7.8. Correct Answer: **d**

A pulse oximeter only monitors trends of oxygenation saturation (SpO_2) and does not alert the nurse to hypercarbia; despite adequate SpO_2 values, the patient may hypoventilate and retain carbon dioxide. SpO_2 is not equivalent to arterial p_aO_2 measures. Hyperthermia, acidosis, and hypercarbia decrease hemoglobin-oxygen affinity so that hemoglobin more easily releases oxygen to tissues. The quality of the signal transmitted to the pulse oximeter and accuracy of the displayed SpO_2 depend on adequate peripheral circulation. Even though each molecule of circulating hemoglobin is adequately saturated, the oximeter displays low oxygen saturation when hemoglobin is low. Though not used to detect improper intubation, low oxygen saturations displayed on the oximeter can alert the nurse to consider causes of hypoxemia, including esophageal or single lung intubation. Hypothermia, vasoconstriction, and movement artifact are among physiologic conditions and environmental factors that can distort the oximeter's signal.

Hudak, C & Gallo, B: Critical Care Nursing: A Holistic Approach, *6th ed. Philadelphia, Lippincott, p. 398, 1994; Stalheim-Smith, A & Fitch, GK:* Understanding Human Anatomy and Physiology. *Minneapolis/St. Paul, West Publishing, pp. 973-976, 1993.*

7.9. Correct Answer: **c**

Phase II block, also called dual or open channel block, may occur after continuous infusion of succinylcholine. Muscle relaxation persists even after the succinylcholine effect ends; receptors in the neuromuscular junction fail to respond to acetylcholine. Muscles stimulated with a nerve stimulator "fade" and show decreasing strength; they behave as if a nondepolarizing muscle relaxant was used instead of a depolarizing muscle relaxant.

Harbut, RE: Anesthetic Agents and Adjuncts in ASPAN's Core Curriculum for Post Anesthesia Nursing Practice, *3rd ed (Litwack, K, Ed). Philadelphia, Saunders, pp. 97-98, 1994; Drain, C:* The Post Anesthesia Care Unit: A Critical Care Approach to Post Anesthesia Nursing, *3rd ed. Philadelphia, Saunders, pp. 240-243, 1994.*

7.10. Correct Answer: **b**

Administering a muscle relaxant reversal medication like neostigmine to a patient who has Phase II block might further delay return of neuromuscular function if Phase I block is also still present. Neostigmine can slow elimination of any still-circulating succinylcholine by inhibiting pseudocholinesterase.

Fischer, DM: Muscle Relaxants in Dripps/Eckenhoff/Vandam Introduction to Anesthesia, *8th ed (Longnecker, DE & Murphy, FL, Eds). Philadelphia, Saunders, pp. 114-115, 1992; Harbut, RE: Anesthetic Agents and Adjuncts in* ASPAN's Core Curriculum for Post Anesthesia Nursing Practice, *3rd ed (Litwack, K, Ed). Philadelphia, Saunders, p. 97, & 102-103, 1994.*

7.11. Correct Answer: **a**

Phase II blockade is a self-limiting situation. Adequate nerve conduction and muscular strength typically return within 30 minutes. Providing temporary respiratory support with a mechanical ventilator and observing for recovered function usually are adequate intervention.

Drain, C: The Post Anesthesia Care Unit: A Critical Care Approach to Post Anesthesia Nursing, *3rd ed. Philadelphia, Saunders, pp. 234 & 240-243, 1994.*

7.12. Correct Answer: **c**

Hyperglycemic hyperosmolar nonketotic coma primarily affects non-insulin-dependent diabetic patients; these patients are usually older patients who still produce some insulin. Serum glucose rises significantly above 600 mg/dl due to stress, illness, infection, or poor glucose control by diet or oral antihyperglycemic medications. Rising serum glucose levels eventually increase serum osmolarity; the osmotic effect results in severe dehydration. Ketoacidosis seldom occurs. Treatment is geared toward volume replacement and electrolyte balance.

Kraft, SA, Mihm, FG & Feeley, TW: Postoperative Endocrine Problems in Post Anesthesia Care *(Vender, JS & Speiss, BD, Eds). Philadelphia, Saunders, pp. 216-221, 1992; Gervasio, BA: The Endocrine Surgical Patient in* ASPAN's Core Curriculum for Post Anesthesia Nursing Practice, *3rd ed (Litwack, K, Ed). Philadelphia, Saunders, pp. 554-555, 1994.*

7.13. Correct Answer: **c**

Cryoprecipitate is concentrated fibrinogen and is extracted from fresh frozen plasma. Clotting factor VIII to treat hemophilia and the von Willebrand factor, an intrinsic clotting factor that mediates platelet aggregation, are also contained in cryoprecipitate. Fresh frozen plasma (plasma infused within 6 hours of collection) is the blood product that contains still-effective, labile clotting factors and reverses the effect of warfarin (Coumadin).

Silinsky, J: The Hematologic System in ASPAN's Core Curriculum for Post Anesthesia Nursing Practice, *3rd ed (Litwack, K, Ed). Philadelphia, Saunders, p. 194, 1994; Coffland, FI & Shellton, DM: Blood Component Replacement Therapy.* Nurs Clin North Am *6(3): 544-549, 1993.*

7.14. Correct Answer: **b**

The enzyme 2,3-diphosphoglycerate (2,3-DPG) affects hemoglobin's ability to release oxygen. Oxygen is more readily released at higher 2,3-DPG levels. Acidosis, hyperthermia and increased 2,3-DPG shift the oxyhemoglobin curve to the right, increasing the availability of oxygen to tissues.

Coffland, FI & Shelton, DM: Blood Component Replacement Therapy. Nurs Clin North Am *5(3): 543-556, 1993. Drain, C:* The Post Anesthesia Care Unit: A Critical Care Approach to Post Anesthesia Nursing, *3rd ed. Philadelphia, Saunders, pp. 122-123, 1994.*

7.15. Correct Answer: **a**

A negative feedback loop between the anterior pituitary and the adrenal glands control cortisol release. When the anterior pituitary senses adequate circulating corticosteroid levels, it releases less adrenocorticotropic hormone (ACTH); the adrenals do not secrete cortisol. When the anterior pituitary senses inadequate cortisol, ACTH relays an adrenal message to increase production and release of cortisol.

Genuth, SM: The Endocrine System in Physiology, *3rd ed (Berne, RM & Levy, MN, Eds). St. Louis, Mosby, pp. 955-966 & 977, 1993; Gervasio, BA: The Endocrine Surgical Patient in* ASPAN's Core Curriculum for Post Anesthesia Nursing Practice, *3rd ed (Litwack, K, Ed). Philadelphia, Saunders, pp. 547-550, 1994.*

7.16. Correct Answer: **b**

Several autonomic controls, including thermoregulation, are based in the hypothalamus. Feedback relays between thermoreceptors in the hypothalamus and skin detect thermal variations and alter metabolism, blood vessel size, sweat production and muscular movements (shivering) to balance heating and cooling. The medulla oblongata joins the spinal cord and pons to form the brain stem; motor and sensory relays and involuntary cardiopulmonary regulation occur here. The hypophysis refers to pituitary, glandular activity.

Stalheim-Smith, A & Fitch, GK: Understanding Human Anatomy and Physiology. *St. Paul, MN, West Publishing, pp. 135-140, 1993; Hudak, CM, & Gallo, BM:* Critical Care Nursing: A Holistic Approach. *Philadelphia, Lippincott, pp. 635, 1994.*

7.17. Correct Answer: **b**

Ms B's blood must be warmed to at least her body temperature during administration. Ms B has a specific protein antibody (cold agglutinin) that becomes active when blood cells are chilled, as in blood stored for future transfusion. Transfusion of the cold blood cells into Ms B's body causes clumping or agglutination. Warming the blood prevents blood cells from adhering to each other.

Alspach, JG: AACN's Core Review for Critical Care Nursing, *2nd ed. Philadelphia, Saunders, p. 44, 1991; O'Brien, D: Care of the Post Anesthesia Patient in* The Post Anesthesia Care Unit: A Critical Care Approach to Post Anesthesia Nursing, *3rd ed (Drain, C, Ed). Philadelphia, Saunders, p. 294, 1994.*

7.18. Correct Answer: **c**

Ms B can receive either type A negative or type O negative blood. A patient with type A blood forms serum antibodies to antigens of type B and type AB blood but not to type A or type O cells. Rh antigens are either positive (have the antigen) or negative (no Rh antigen); Rh negative patients receive Rh negative cells. Blood type is identified by the surface antigen (agglutinogen) on the red blood cell. When antibodies in the serum do not recognize the antigens on the infused red blood cell, the cells either agglutinate (clump) or hemolyze.

Silinsky, J: The Hematologic System in ASPAN's Core Curriculum for Post Anesthesia Nursing Practice, *3rd ed (Litwack, K, Ed). Philadelphia, Saunders, pp.190-194, 1994; Stalheim-Smith, A & Fitch, GK:* Understanding Human Anatomy and Physiology. *St. Paul, MN, West Publishing, pp. 688-691, 1994.*

7.19. Correct Answer: **d**

Recommended transfusion practice includes replacing blood tubing and filter after every 2 units of cells. The filter of a blood administration set can clog. A large gauge needle (16-18 gauge) and normal saline, never water, are used to prevent hemolysis. Ms B predonated her own blood, so compatability reactions are unlikely unless identification errors mismatch blood or patient. Monitor vital signs and temperature after the first 50 ml of each unit of blood has infused to detect blood reactions. Autologous blood is subject to the same administration requirements as any other banked blood.

Silinsky, J: The Hematologic System in ASPAN's Core Curriculum for Post Anesthesia Nursing Practice, *3rd ed (Litwack, K, Ed). Philadelphia, Saunders, pp. 199-200, 1994; O'Brien, D: Care of the Post Anesthesia Patient in* The Post Anesthesia Care Unit: A Critical Care Approach to Post Anesthesia Nursing, *3rd ed (Drain, C, Ed). Philadelphia, Saunders, pp. 292-293, 1994.*

7.20. Correct Answer: **a**

High volume, low specific gravity (dilute) urine characterize diabetes insipidus (DI). Insufficient amounts of antidiuretic hormone (ADH) are secreted by thepituitary, so fluid pours from the body, unrestrained at the kidney. Other evidence of DI includes hypotension when renal fluid loss is not replaced, increased serum osmolarity (hemoconcentration), and serum sodium elevation. DI, common after pituitary surgery, is the horomonal opposite of the syndrome of inappropriate antidiuretic horomone (SIADH).

Hawkins, JK & Hawkins, VD: Post Anesthesia Care of the Neurosurgical Patient in The Post Anesthesia Care Unit: A Critical Care Approach to Post Anesthesia Nursing, *3rd ed (Drain, C, Ed). Philadelphia, Saunders, pp. 427-428, 1994; Kay, J: Endocrine Disorders in* Manual of Anesthesia and the Medically Compromised Patient *(Cheng, EY & Kay, J Eds). Philadelphia, Lippincott, p. 390, 1990.*

7.21. Correct Answer: **c**

Iatrogenic administration or consumption of magnesium-containing products is most associated with magnesium excess. Treating pregnancy-related eclampsia or premature labor with magnesium sulfate infusions, overconsuming laxatives or antacids that contain magnesium, and parenteral nutrition are routes to hypermagnesemia. Ms Z's magnesium is elevated; normal values are 1.7-4.2 mg/dl (1.4-2 mEq/L). Observe for evidence of altered neuromuscular transmission such as muscle weakness, decreased respiratory quality, or sedation that indicate suppressed muscle contraction.

Toto, KH & Yucha, CB: Magnesium: Homeostasis, Imbalances, and Therapeutic Uses. Crit Care Clin North Am *6(4): 767-783, 1994.*

7.22. Correct Answer: **d**

When at least 75% of nephron function is destroyed and glomerular filtration is less than 30 ml/min, magnesium excretion and serum elevations are likely. Laxative abuse and diabetes mellitus are associated with low serum magnesium.

Toto, KH & Yucha, CB: Magnesium: Homeostasis, Imbalances, and Therapeutic Uses. Crit Care Clin North Am *6(4): 767-783, 1994; Morgan, GE & Mikhail, MS:* Clinical Anesthesiology. *Norwalk, CT, Appleton & Lange, pp. 474-475, 1992.*

7.23. Correct Answer: **a**

Hypermagnesemia can extend the effects of depolarizing and nondepolarizing muscle relaxants. Both acetylcholine release and sensitivity of the neuron's motor end plate to acetylcholine are suppressed. Muscle relaxant doses may be reduced up to 50% to accommodate this magnesium-induced influence on neurofunction. The tolerable range of magnesium excess before symptoms develop is wide:

deep tendon reflexes decrease when magnesium reaches levels of 4-5 mEq/L; paralysis occurs at levels of 10-15 mEq/L.

Clement, JM: Assessment: Renal System in Critical Care Nursing: A Holistic Approach, *6th ed (Hudak, CM & Gallo, BM, Eds.). Philadelphia, Lippincott, pp. 536-539, 1994; Morgan, GE & Mikhail, MS:* Clinical Anesthesiology. *Norwalk, CT, Appleton & Lange, pp. 474-475, 1992;*

7.24. Correct Answer: **b**

Diuretics and saline infusion may improve renal elimination of magnesium if Ms Z's kidneys still produce urine. Patients with significant oliguria and end-stage renal failure may require dialysis to remove excess magnesium. Discontinuing magnesium-containing substances may reverse magnesium excess when a patient has no renal disease. Acidosis and fluid deficits compound symptoms of hypermagnesemia. Calcium chloride infusion may improve symptoms but only temporarily.

Clement, JM: Assessment: Renal System in Critical Care Nursing: A Holistic Approach, *6th ed (Hudak, CM & Gallo, BM, Eds). Philadelphia, Lippincott, pp. 536-539, 1994.*

7.25. Correct Answer: **a**

Following thyroidectomy, a twitch of lip or cheek indicates hypocalcemia that likely requires intervention. Resecting thyroid tissue could produce hypocalcemia by disturbing the calcium-regulating parathyroid glands that lie beneath the thyroid. A sore throat is a likely consequence of intubation and surgery; rebleeding would likely produce copious drainage volume that may accumulate in neck tissue and compress airway structures. Exopthalmos and bradycardia are related to hypothyroidism.

Alspach, JG: AACN's Core Review for Critical Care Nursing, *2nd ed. Philadelphia, Saunders, p. 21, 1991; Gervasio, BA: The Endocrine Surgical Patient in* ASPAN's Core Curriculum for Post Anesthesia Nursing Practice, *3rd ed (Litwack, K, Ed). Philadelphia, Saunders, pp. 539-542, 1994.*

7.26. Correct Answer: **d**

Stressful physiologic events like infection or surgery promote epinephrine, growth hormone, and cortisol secretion that increases serum glucose. Insulin, a pancreatic protein, may be needed during the postanesthetic period. Successful management of any postoperative diabetic patient requires periodic assessment of glucose status and monitoring ability to tolerate food and fluids, if surgical procedure permits.

Morgan, GE & Mikhail, MS: Clinical Anesthesiology. *Norwalk, CT, Appleton & Lange, pp. 565-568, 1992; Macheca, MK: Diabetic Hypoglycemia: How to Keep the Threat at Bay.* Am J Nurs *93(4): 26-30, 1993.*

7.27. Correct Answer: **c**

Regular insulin peaks at 2-3 hours, with duration of 5-7 hours. To prevent overresponse and sudden hypoglycemia in a patient like Ms P who does not normally require insulin, only small amounts of regular insulin are administered and serum glucose is monitored often.

Kestel, F: Are You Up to Date on Diabetes Medication? Am J Nurs *94(7): 48-52, 1994; Morgan, GE &*

Mikhail, MS: Clinical Anesthesiology. *Norwalk, CT, Appleton & Lange, pp. 565-568, 1992.*

7.28. Correct Answer: **a**

Low-volume, concentrated urine in a patient with a condition that increases intracranial pressure suggests syndrome of inappropriate antidiuretic hormone (SIADH). Oversecretion of ADH occurs and water is not excreted by the kidney. Fluid volume increases and dilutes solute in the blood; serum osmolality and sodium both decrease. Insufficient amounts of posterior pituitary horomones (vasporessin) and ADH-like medications (desmopressin) also cause fluid volume *excess,* not a deficit. Many factors increase ADH secretion and potential for SIADH, including stress, narcotics, pain, pulmonary pathology and hypovolemia.

Loriaux, TC & Drass, JA: Endocrine and Diabetic Disorders in AACN's Clinical Reference for Critical-Care Nursing, *3rd ed (Kinney, MR, Packa, DR & Dunbar, SB, Eds). St. Louis, Mosby, pp. 929-930, 1993; Alspach, JG:* AACN's Core Review for Critical Care Nursing, *2nd ed. Philadelphia, Saunders, p. 59, 1991.*

7.29. Correct Answer: **b**

Syndrome of "inappropriate," or oversecretion of, antidiuretic hormone (SIADH) is typically treated with fluid restriction, monitoring sodium to maintain greater than 135 mEq/L, and observing urine and serum osmolality.

Loriaux, TC & Drass, JA: Endocrine and Diabetic Disorders in AACN's Clinical Reference for Critical-Care Nursing, *3rd ed (Kinney, MR, Packa, DR & Dunbar, SB, Eds). St. Louis, Mosby, pp. 929-930, 1993.*

7.30. Correct Answer: **c**

Phenytoin (Dilantin) is an anticonvulsant with cardiac suppressant effects. Widened QRS, prolonged PR or QT intervals, or T wave depression signal the need to stop this medication. A safe infusion is slow, less than 50 mg/min. Dilantin must be diluted in normal saline to prevent precipitation.

Alspach, JG: AACN's Core Review for Critical Care Nursing, *2nd ed. Philadelphia, Saunders, p. 96, 1991; Mitchell, PH: Neurological Disorders in* AACN's Clinical Reference for Critical-Care Nursing, *3rd ed (Kinney, MR, Packa, DR & Dunbar, SB, Eds). St. Louis, Mosby, pp. 825-826, 1993.*

7.31. Correct Answer: **d**

Using a blood warmer to quickly deliver multiple units of blood maintains body temperature, decreases vasoconstriction and acidosis, and may facilitate movement of potassium into cells. Rapid infusion of cold, stored red blood cells both vasoconstricts and promotes hypothermia. Blood must not be overheated as cells can hemolyze. Warming blood has no effect on occurrence of febrile reactions to blood.

Silinsky, J: The Hematologic System in ASPAN's Core Curriculum for Post Anesthesia Nursing Practice, *3rd ed (Litwack, K, Ed). Philadelphia, Saunders, p. 197, 1994; O'Brien, D: Care of the Post Anesthesia Patient in* The Post Anesthesia Care Unit: A Critical Care Approach to Post Anesthesia Nursing, *3rd ed (Drain, C, Ed). Philadelphia, Saunders, pp. 292-293, 1994.*

7.32. Correct Answer: **d**

Anticoagulation effects, or rebound, reoccur when heparin is released from cellular spaces back into the bloodstream. Normothermia and improved general circulation affect this release. Positively charged protamine protein groups bond with negatively charged heparin groups to neutralize effects of heparin used during cardiopulmonary bypass. The effect lasts for about 2 hours.

Hudak, C & Gallo, B: Critical Care Nursing: A Holistic Approach, *6th ed. Phildelphia, Lippincott, p. 369, 1994; Atkins, PJ: Postoperative Coagulopathies.* Crit Care Nurs Clin North Am *5(3): 459-473, 1993.*

7.33. Correct Answer: **c**

Significant hypotension after previous administration of protamine suggests allergy; additional protamine is contraindicated. Bradycardia and a slight decrease in blood pressure commonly occur even with a slow rate of protamine infusion. Protamine is a heparin antagonist that actually combines with heparin to form a new and neutral substance. In high doses, however, protamine sulfate anticoagulates and may increase bleeding.

Herbert, DW: Manual of Drugs in Anesthesia and Critical Care. *Philadelphia, Saunders, pp. 266-267, 1993; Metz, S & Harrow, J: Protamine and Newer Heparin Antagonists.* Pharmacol Physiol Anesth Pract *1(3): 1994.*

7.34. Correct Answer: **b**

Increased carbon dioxide prompts the body to increase ventilation. Accumulating carbon dioxide molecules decreases pH in cerebrospinal fluid and blood. Chemoreceptors at the fourth ventricle and carotid bodies are stimulated to increase ventilatory rate and depth. The kidneys also conserve bicarbonate and excrete hydrogen ions.

Drain, C: The Post Anesthesia Care Unit: A Critical Care Approach to Post Anesthesia Nursing, *3rd ed. Philadelphia, Saunders, p. 131, 1994.*

7.35. Correct Answer: **a**

Osmolality of a solution or body fluid compartment includes the total of electrolytes (both positively and negatively charged ions) and nonelectrolyte particles like proteins, glucose and urea. These osmotically active particles (solute) affect movement of water across cell membranes. Highly concentrated fluids hold many particles and have high osmolality; water moves into a more highly concentrated solution to equilibrate solute, creating fluid and particle balance in each compartment.

Spies, MA: Fluid, Electrolyte and Acid-Base Balances in Basic Nursing: Theory and Practice, *3rd ed (Potter, PA & Perry, AG, Eds). St. Louis, Mosby, pp. 1025-1027, 1994; DeFranco, M: Fluid and Electrolyte Balance in* ASPAN's Core Curriculum for Post Anesthesia Nursing Practice, *3rd ed (Litwack, K, Ed). Philadelphia, Saunders, pp. 157-159, 1994.*

SET II

Answer Key

7.36. b
7.37. d
7.38. b
7.39. d
7.40. a
7.41. c
7.42. d
7.43. a
7.44. c
7.45. c
7.46. b
7.47. a
7.48. c
7.49. d
7.50. d
7.51. b
7.52. d
7.53. a
7.54. c
7.55. d
7.56. b
7.57. a
7.58. c
7.59. a
7.60. b
7.61. b
7.62. b
7.63. c
7.64. b
7.65. c
7.66. b
7.67. c
7.68. b
7.69. a
7.70. c

SET II

Rationales and References

7.36. Correct Answer: **b**

A hypotonic solution has more water than solute, creating an osmolality of less than 240 mOsm/L; normal serum osmolality is 280-295 mOsm/L. Infusing a hypotonic solution into the blood (extracellular fluid) dilutes the extracellular fluid. Solutions seek balance; fluid moves from the extracellular fluid (blood) into spaces with higher solute concentration.

Spies, MA: Fluid, Electrolyte and Acid-Base Balances in Basic Nursing: Theory and Practice, *3rd ed (Potter, PA & Perry, AG, Eds). St. Louis, Mosby, pp. 1025-1027, 1994; DeFranco, M: Fluid and Electrolyte Balance in* ASPAN's Core Curriculum for Post Anesthesia Nursing Practice, *3rd ed (Litwack, K, Ed). Philadelphia, Saunders, pp. 157-159, 1994.*

7.37. Correct Answer: **d**

The preeclamptic obstetric patient who develops hemolysis, elevated liver enzymes and low platelets (HELLP syndrome) is critically ill. This syndrome is potentially life threatening, involves multiple maternal organ systems andaffects the fetus. Tissue hypoxia, hemoconcentration, vasospasm with endothelial damage, coagulopathies, seizures and intracerebral bleeding occur.

Poole, JH & White, D: The Obstetric Surgical Patient in ASPAN's Core Curriculum for Post Anesthesia Nursing Practice, *3rd ed (Litwack, K, Ed). Philadelphia, Saunders, p. 482, 1994; Poole, J: HELLP Syndrome and Coagulopathies of Pregnancy.* Nurs Clin North Am *6(3): 475-487, 1993.*

7.38. Correct Answer: **b**

Potassium is released from cells to serum in an acidotic environment. Severely elevated potassium levels produce muscle weakness and eventual paralysis. Cardiac muscle strength also weakens; observe electrocardiographic changes. Tall, peaked T waves and widened QRS complexes indicate very high potassium; conduction delays will continue and perhaps progress to mechanical failure with cardiac arrest.

Weems, J: Quick Reference to Renal Critical Care Nursing. *Gaithersburg, MD, Aspen, pp. 56-57, 1991; Stanton, BA & Koeppen, BM: The Kidney in* Physiology, *3rd ed (Berne, RM & Levy, MN, Eds). St. Louis, Mosby, pp. 784-809, 1993.*

7.39. Correct Answer: **d**

Each component of these blood gases is within normal limits. The nurse need only to assure continued and adequate oxygenation to balance oxygen demand and consumption.

Atsberger, DB: Interpretation of Acid-Base Balance in ASPAN's Core Curriculum for Post Anesthesia Nursing Practice, *3rd ed (Litwack, K, Ed). Philadelphia, Saunders, pp. 144-152, 1994; Bolton, PJ & Kline, KA: Understanding Modes of Mechanical Ventilation.* Am J Nurs *94(6): 36-42, 1994.*

7.40. Correct Answer: **a**

When a genetically susceptible patient is exposed to one of several malignant hyperthermia (MH)–triggering agents, normal calcium activity in muscle cells is disrupted. In MH, calcium concentrations inside muscle cells progressively increase and reach extreme levels; calcium normally ebbs and flows with electrical changes of the cell membrane. Altered calcium activity sustains muscle contraction and cellular hypermetabolism results. MH symptoms include abrupt increase of end-tidal carbon dioxide, unexplained tachycardia, hypoxia, acidosis and eventual hyperthermia.

Murphy, FL: Hazards of Anesthesia in Dripps/Eckenhoff/Vandam Introduction to Anesthesia, *8th ed (Longnecker, DE & Murphy, FL, Eds). Philadelphia, Saunders, pp.420-427, 1992; Litwack, K:* Post Anesthesia Care Nursing, *2nd ed. St. Louis, Mosby, pp. 476.*

7.41. Correct Answer: **c**

The child's initial response to cold is increased norepinephrine production, which stimulates increased metabolism of brown fat, with lactic acid production. A child's insulating layer of subcutaneous fat is thinner and body surface area is greater than an adult's. Shivering is nearly absent in infants younger than 3 months of age.

Drain, C: The Post Anesthesia Care Unit: A Critical Care Approach to Post Anesthesia Nursing, *3rd ed. Philadelphia, Saunders, p. 539, 1994; Burden, N:* Ambulatory Surgical Nursing. *Philadelphia, Saunders, pp. 430-431, 1992.*

7.42. Correct Answer: **d**

Ongoing assessment of this patient distinguishes between neuromuscular and neurologic (seizure) origins for these muscle movements. Particularly immediately after surgery is completed, a drowsy patient who responds to some commands but has uncoordinated chest, head and extremities probably has residual neuromuscular blockade. Neurologic assessmentafter transsphenoidal hypophysectomy of a pituitary tumor is similar to assessment after other intracranial procedures. The nurse must also monitor signs of increased intracranial pressure and decreased consciousness. Any seizures for this patient more likely arise from neurologic than hypoglycemic causes.

Drain, C: The Post Anesthesia Care Unit: A Critical Care Approach to Post Anesthesia Nursing, *3rd ed. Philadelphia, Saunders, pp. 139-142, 1994; Litwack, K:* Post Anesthesia Care Nursing, *2nd ed. St. Louis, Mosby, pp. 147-149, 1995; Morgan, GE & Mikhail, MS:* Clinical Anesthesiology. *Norwalk, CT, Appleton & Lange, 441-442, 1992.*

7.43. Correct Answer: **a**

Despite weak, uncoordinated or absent muscle movements, this patient may be quite aware, in pain, anxious, and unable to let anyone know. His muscle activity is likely from residual neuromuscular blockade. Depolarizing and nondepolarizing muscle relaxants paralyze and have no effect on level of consciousness or analgesia. Depending upon the severity of the muscle weakness, the anesthesia provider may, or may not, choose to administer additional reversal medication. Following surgical removal of the pituitary gland, the patient may become acutely *deficient* in circulating adrenocorticotropic hormone (ACTH), prompting addisonian crisis. Corticosteroid replacement is essential.

Drain, C: The Post Anesthesia Care Unit: A Critical Care Approach to Post Anesthesia Nursing. *Philadelphia, Saunders, pp. 239-242, 1994; Litwack, K:* Post Anesthesia Care Nursing, *2nd ed. St. Louis, Mosby, pp. 147-149, 1995.*

7.44. Correct Answer: **c**

Following craniotomy, CO_2 retention and respiratory acidosis can have dire consequences. Hypercarbia is a potent vasodilator and can markedly (and rapidly) increase intracranial blood volume and pressure. Therefore an ineffective breathing pattern and decreased tidal volume prevents anyone from exhaling carbon dioxide. Rapid increases in intracranial pressure occur in the injured brain when intracranial contents can no longer compensate for brain tissue edema, tumor, or hemorrhage, increased blood flow due to hypercarbia, and hypoxia, or altered flow of cerebrospinal fluid. Adaptive autoregulation fails. Whether after a transphenoidal approach or open-craniotomy, neurologic assessment is similar.

Mitchell, PH: Neurological Disorders in AACN's Clinical Reference for Critical-Care Nursing, *3rd ed (Kinney, MR, Packa, DR & Dunbar, SB, Eds). St. Louis, Mosby, pp. 806-813, 1993; Shpritz, DW: The Neurosurgical Patient in* ASPAN's Core Curriculum for Post Anesthesia Nursing Practice, *3rd ed (Litwack, K, Ed). Philadelphia, Saunders, pp. 351-356, 1994.*

7.45. Correct Answer: **c**

Situations that encourage acidosis (↓pH), dehydration, hypoxemia (↓pO_2) infection and fever or physiologic stress (unrelieved pain, hypothermia or circulatory impairment) can precipitate cell sickling in susceptible patients. Derek is at risk for hypoxemia when he breathes only 8 times per minute; his expected rate is about 20 breaths per minute. His now-resolved postanesthetic shivering was a physiologic stressor that increased his oxygen consumption. Analgesic medications used to suppress the shivering and any pain can now contribute to his hypoventilation. If Derek's blood-pressure is 102/64, hydration is probably adequate; rating his pain as a "2" indicates reasonable analgesia.

Drain, C: The Post Anesthesia Care Unit: A Critical Care Approach to Post Anesthesia Nursing, *3rd ed. Philadelphia, Saunders, pp. 530-531, 1994; Burden, N:* Ambulatory Surgical Nursing. *Philadelphia, Saunders, p. 410, 1993.*

7.46. Correct Answer: **b**

Derek is observed for signs of tissue ischemia and organ infarction because vascular occlusion often heralds crisis. Sickling obstructs vessels and produces severe ischemic pain or disrupts function of vital organs, especially kidney. Hypoventilation with hypoxemia and potential respiratory acidosis, thermal imbalance and unrelieved pain, just the factors that prompt a sickle cell crisis, are highly possible during the immediate postanesthetic period.

Sickle cell trait is a genetic trait of an estimated 10% of the African-American population and a factor to consider during preanesthetic assessment.

Drain, C: The Post Anesthesia Care Unit: A Critical Care Approach to Post Anesthesia Nursing, *3rd ed. Philadelphia, Saunders, pp. 530-531, 1994; Burden, N:* Ambulatory Surgical Nursing. *Philadelphia, Saunders, p. 410, 1993.*

7.47. Correct Answer: **a**

A pCO_2 of 73 mm Hg indicates significant respiratory acidosis. The patient will probably be very slow to arouse, breathe poorly, and perhaps be confused or stuporous if responsive at all; headache, restlessness, dyspnea, fatigue, muscle weakness, and decreased reflexes are hints that suggest developing respiratory acidosis. U waves in EKG are associated with hypokalemia, not acidosis. *Aggressively reestablishing adequate ventilation is essential to life.* Carbon dioxide must be exhaled; anticipate that this patient will be reintubated and probably mechanically ventilated.

Litwack, K: Post Anesthesia Nursing Practice, *2nd ed. St. Louis, Mosby, pp. 414-419, 1995; Bolton, PJ & Kline, KA: Understanding Modes of Mechanical Ventilation.* Am J Nurs *94(6): 36-42, 1994.*

7.48. Correct Answer: **c**

A hypertonic solution like 5% dextrose in lactated Ringer's solution draws fluid from intracellular fluid to expand the extracellular fluid compartment. Cells become only moderately dehydrated while the desired effect of increasingcirculating blood volume is achieved.

Spies, MA: Fluid, Electrolyte and Acid-Base Balances in Basic Nursing: Theory and Practice, *3rd ed (Potter, PA & Perry, AG, Eds). St. Louis, Mosby, pp. 1025-1027, 1994; DeFranco, M: Fluid and Electrolyte Balance in* ASPAN's Core Curriculum for Post Anesthesia Nursing Practice, *3rd ed (Litwack, K, Ed). Philadelphia, Saunders, pp. 157-159, 1994.*

7.49. Correct Answer: **d**

Acidosis has a metabolic and/or respiratory origin. Diabetes mellitus is a metabolic condition; glucose imbalance with hyperglycemia and ketoacidosis causes (HCO_3^-) to decrease to less than 22 mEq/L (normal is 22-26 mEq/L). pH is the mathematic reflection of the body's hydrogen ion (H^+), or acid, concentration. Acidotic conditions produce pH of less than 7.35 (normal range is 7.35-7.40).

Stringfield, YN: Acidosis, Alkalosis and Arterial Blood Gases. Am J Nurs *93:11: 43-44, 1993; Drain, C:* The Post Anesthesia Care Unit: A Critical Care Approach to Post Anesthesia Nursing, *3rd ed. Philadelphia, Saunders, pp. 125-126 & 523-525, 1994.*

7.50. Correct Answer: **d**

Feedback from sensing increased serum osmolarity or from stretch of baroreceptors by hypotension prompts the pituitary neurohypophysis to secrete vasopressin (antidiuretic hormone). In response, the renal tubules reabsorb water.

Drain, C: The Post Anesthesia Care Unit: A Critical Care Approach to Post Anesthesia Nursing. *Philadelphia, Saunders, p. 150, 1994; Stalheim-Smith, A & Fitch, GK:* Understanding Human

Anatomy and Physiology. *Minneapolis/St. Paul, West Publishing, pp. 549-551, 1994.*

7.51. Correct Answer: **b**

This patient has respiratory alkalosis, indicated by below normal pCO_2 and reflected by the pH shift to 7.50. Hyperventilation, often due to significant pain, sepsis, nervousness, or overventilation with a mechanical ventilator, produces this acid-base imbalance. Symptoms can include circumoral tingling, light-headedness, generalized tingling, and extremity numbness.

Vazquez, M: Acid-Base Disorders in Critical Care Nursing, *2nd ed (Vazquez, M, Lazear, SE & Larson, EL, Eds). Philadelphia, Saunders, p. 371, 1992; Atsberger, DB: Interpretaion of Acid-Base Balance in* ASPAN's Core Curriculum for Post Anesthesia Nursing Practice, *3rd ed (Litwack, K, Ed). Philadelphia, Saunders, pp. 148-153, 1994.*

7.52. Correct Answer: **d**

Fluid replacement is a controversial issue among practitioners; however, for healthy patients, moderate intraoperative fluid deficits are typically restored with calculated volumes of isotonic electrolyte solutions. Volume replacement with crystalloid solution is usually triple or quadruple the actual volume lost and requires replacement of both preoperative deficit and new loss. Surgical fluid losses are isotonic; electrolyte and water loss does not alter the osmotic balance between extracellular and intracellular fluid. About 25% of total extracellular fluid volume is intravascular fluid.

DeFranco, M: Fluid and Electrolyte Balance in ASPAN's Core Curriculum for Post Anesthesia Nursing Practice, *3rd ed (Litwack, K, Ed). Philadelphia, Saunders, pp. 172-173, 1994; Morgan, GE & Mikhail, MS:* Clinical Anesthesiology. *Norwalk, CT, Appleton & Lange, pp. 477-481, 1992; Litwack, K:* Post Anesthesia Care Nursing, *2nd ed. St. Louis, Mosby, p. 435, 1995.*

7.53. Correct Answer: **a**

Extracellular fluid (ECF) contains intravascular fluid (blood volume) and intrastitial fluid (water between cells, the lymph fluid, and intraorgan fluid). The ECF holds approximately 20% of body water. Intracellular fluid comprises 40% of total body water.

Spies, MA: Fluid, Electrolyte and Acid-Base Balances in Basic Nursing: Theory and Practice, *3rd ed (Potter, PA & Perry, AG, Eds). St. Louis, Mosby, pp. 1025-1027 & 1046-1047, 1994; DeFranco, M: Fluid and Electrolyte Balance in* ASPAN's Core Curriculum for Post Anesthesia Nursing Practice, *3rd ed (Litwack, K, Ed). Philadelphia, Saunders, pp. 157-159, 1994.*

7.54. Correct Answer: **c**

These blood gas values indicate metabolic acidosis, as pH is significantly reduced and pCO_2 remains low-normal. As pH remains low, the acidosis is uncompensated by respiratory effort. Shock, hypoxia and organ failure create metabolic disturbances that produce metabolic acidosis. Correction of the acidosis involves replacing bicarbonate, treating the cause and restoring normal electrolyte balance.

Drain, C: The Post Anesthesia Care Unit: A Critical Care Approach to Post Anesthesia Nursing. *Philadelphia, Saunders, pp. 122-123, 1994; Litwack, K:* Post Anesthesia Care Nursing, *2nd ed. St. Louis, Mosby, pp. 415-419, 1995.*

7.55. Correct Answer: **d**

The low $paCO_2$ measure indicates respiratory alkalosis, a common outcome of overzealous mechanical ventilation. At the current ventilator settings, the patient hyperventilates. To allow the pCO_2 to return toward normal, either the tidal volume of each delivered breath or the number of breaths per minute (rate) should be reduced. The set tidal volume is already small, so reducing the ventilatory rate per minute will be less likely to continue the iatrogenic respiratory alkalosis.

Stringfield, YN: Acidosis, Alkalosis and Arterial Blood Gases. Am J Nurs *93:11: 43-44, 1993; Sauer, D: Post Anesthesia Respiratory Care and Atsberger, DB: Interpretation of Acid-Base Balance in* ASPAN's Core Curriculum for Post Anesthesia Nursing Practice, *3rd ed (Litwack, K, Ed). Phildelphia, Saunders, pp. 138-140 & 145-151, 1994.*

7.56. Correct Answer: **b**

Hyperventilation to intentionally produce hypocarbia (decreased $pC0_2$) is therapeutic for a patient with marginal tolerance for shifts in intracranial pressure (ICP). Hypocarbia helps decrease surges of intracranial blood flow that increase ICP. Following cranial surgery or trauma, the normal compensatory changes among CSF, blood volume and brain tissue are taxed; small changes in blood flow, for example, can markedly increase ICP and alter intracranial autoregulation.

Atsberger, DB: Interpretation of Acid-Base Balance and Shpritz, DW: The Neurosurgical Patient in ASPAN's Core Curriculum for Post Anesthesia Nursing Practice, *3rd ed (Litwack, K, Ed). Philadelphia, Saunders, pp. 145-151 & 351-354, 1994.*

7.57. Correct Answer: **a**

Oxygen is loosely attached to hemoglobin molecules when pH is low (acidosis) or when 2,3-DPG, temperature, or partial pressure of carbon dioxide (pCO_2) increase. Conditions that allow hemoglobin to readily release oxygen to tissues are represented on the oxyhemoglobin curve by lower slope, lower height and a shift of the whole curve to the right.

Drain, C: The Post Anesthesia Care Unit: A Critical Care Approach to Post Anesthesia Nursing, *3rd ed. Philadelphia, Saunders, pp. 121-124, 1994; Sauer, D: Post Anesthesia Respiratory Care in* ASPAN's Core Curriculum for Post Anesthesia Nursing Practice, *3rd ed (Litwack, K, Ed). Philadelphia, Saunders, p. 135, 1994.*

7.58. Correct Answer: **c**

An oxygen saturation of 90% correlates with a pO_2 of approximately 60 mm Hg and is a *critical* point when considering oxygen-hemoglobin affinity. A pO_2 of 90% represents clinical hypoxia. The oxyhemoglobin curve graphically displays the relationship between oxygen saturation (SaO_2) and oxygen tension in the blood (pO_2). At saturations above 90%, small increases in pO_2 have minimal effect on saturation. At oxygen saturations below 90%, less oxygen is attached to hemoglobin and small decreases in pO_2 produce huge and dangerous changes in saturation and oxygenation.

Burden, N: Ambulatory Surgical Nursing. *Philadelphia, Saunders, pp. 254 & 163, 1993; Sauer, D: Post Anesthesia Respiratory Care in* ASPAN's Core Curriculum for Post Anesthesia Nursing Practice, *3rd ed (Litwack, K, Ed). Philadelphia, Saunders, p. 135, 1994.*

7.59. Correct Answer: **a**

Partial thromboplastin time (PTT) measures heparin effect by measuring factors in the intrinsic coagulation pathway. Multiple factors contribute to coagulation and normal hemostasis. Prothrombin time (PT) is used to determine the effect of warfarin (Coumadin); thrombin time (TT) estimates fibrinogen levels. Ivy bleeding time is one test to assess platelet function.

Silinsky, J: The Hematologic System in ASPAN's Core Curriculum for Post Anesthesia Nursing Practice, *3rd ed (Litwack, K, Ed). Philadelphia, Saunders, pp. 185-188, 1994; Tribett, D: Hematological Data Acquisition in* AACN's Clinical Reference for Critical-Care Nursing, *3rd ed (Kinney, MR, Packa, DR & Dunbar, SB, Eds). St. Louis, Mosby, pp. 979-983, 1993.*

7.60. Correct Answer: **b**

Administering calcium solution through a high blood flow central line over a 5-10 minute period is advised. Calcium is a vessel irritant that can cause thrombophlebitis or tissue necrosis. Ms Y's calcium deficit probably developed after she received albumin and multiple transfusions of citrated blood from the blood bank. For replacement purposes, calcium chloride is three times more concentrated than calcium gluconate and therefore provides more calcium but also is more irritating to vessels. Do not combine calcium with bicarbonate, as they will precipitate, and do observe for cardiac conduction delays and hypotension.

Yucha, CB & Toto, KH: Calcium and Phosphorus Derangements. Crit Care Clin North Am *6(4): 747-758, 1994; Keen, ML: Patients With Fluid and Electrolyte Disturbances in* Critical Care Nursing *(Clochesy, KM, Breu, C Cardin, S, et al, Eds). Philadelphia, Saunders, p. 872, 1992.*

7.61. Correct Answer: **b**

Hypothermia, particularly to temperatures less than 34° C, is "probably the most common cause of coagulopathy" for trauma victims. Hypothermia-related hypoxia and cell injury may result in disseminated intravascular coagulation (DIC). Platelet number, shape and function are altered, extending bleeding and altering clotting mechanisms with potentially lethal consequences for critical patients. Rewarming reverses these alterations, though trauma, shock and multiple organ system failure also activate physiologic responses.

Kahn, RC: Coagulation Abnormalities and Their Management in the Injured in Trauma: Anesthesia and Intensive Care *(Capan, LM, Miller, SM & Turner, H, Eds). Philadelphia, Lippincott, pp. 207-219, 1991; Hanson, WC: Managing the Desperately Ill Patient: Trauma and Shock in* Dripps/Eckenhoff/Vandam Introduction to Anesthesia. *Philadelphia, Saunders, pp. 377-381, 1992.*

7.62. Correct Answer: **b**

Hyperglycemia increases serum osmolarity and increases the osmotic gradient in the blood. Osmotic diuresis and eventual volume depletion and dehydration are possible outcomes. Hyperglycemia represents glucose-insulin imbalance. A relative lack of insulin, increased glucose production due to emotional or physiologic stress or infection, a total parenteral nutrition (TPN) infusion, or steroid administration creates hyperglycemic states.

Jones: TL: From Diabetic Ketoacidosis to Hyperglycemic Hyperosmolar Nonketotic Syndrome. Crit Care Nurs Clin North Am *6(4): 703-708, 1994; Kraft, SA, Mihm, FG, & Feeley, TW: Postoperative Endocrine Problems in* Post Anesthesia Care *(Vender, JS & Speiss, BD, Eds). Philadelphia, Saunders, pp. 216-222, 1992.*

7.63. Correct Answer: **c**

Circulating insulin is adequate to prevent lipolysis with eventual ketone formation in patients with hyperosmolar nonketotic syndrome (HNKS). Despite severely elevated glucose levels (over 800 mg/dl) with insufficient insulin to reverse hyperglycemia, ketoacidosis does not occur in HNKS. Patients with diabetic ketoacidosis (DKA) are more severely acidotic and ketotic but less dehydrated and have comparatively lower serum glucoses than patients with HNKS.

Loriaux, TC & Drass, JA: Endocrine and Diabetic Disorders in AACN's Clinical Reference For Critical-Care Nursing, *(Kinney, MR, Packa, DR & Dunbar, SB, Eds). St. Louis, Mosby, pp. 942-958, 1993; Jones, TL: From Diabetic Ketoacidosis to Hyperglycemic Hyperosmolar Nonketotic Syndrome.* Crit Care Nurs Clin North Am *6(4): 703-708, 1994.*

7.64. Correct Answer: **b**

Sudden and intense headache, neck pain or stiffness, and nausea with vomiting are classic indicators of subarachnoid bleeding. Seizures, visual impairment, confusion, disorientation or complete loss of consciousness may coincide. This patient has high risk for a subarachnoid hemorrhage; his already leaking aneurysm can spontaneously rupture at any time, filling the subarachnoid space with blood. The brain loses its autoregulatory ability and cerebral perfusion pressure plummets as intracranial pressure rapidly increases. Hemorrhage may spread through subarachnoid fluid and compress intracranial structures, producing other neurologic deficits.

Whitney-Rainbolt, CM: Patients with Cerebral Vascular Disorders in Critical Care Nursing *(Clochesy, JM, Breu, Cardin, S, et al, Eds). Philadelphia, Saunders, pp. 718-721, 1992.*

7.65. Correct Answer: **c**

Succinylcholine, the depolarizing muscle relaxant, triggers malignant hyperthermia (MH) in genetically susceptible people. Halogenated anesthetics, particularly halothane (Fluothane), also may trigger an MH crisis.

Litwack-Saleh, K: Practical Points in the Management of Malignant Hyperthermia. J Post Anesth Nurs *7:327-329, 1992; Holtzclaw, B: Temperature Problems in the Post-Operative Period.* Crit Care Nurs Clin North Am *2:589-597, 1990.*

7.66. Correct Answer: **b**

A genetic biochemical defect disrupts normal intracellular calcium balance. Symptoms occur when skeletal muscle calcium-levels suddenly and unexpectedly skyrocket. A cascade of biochemical responses, including sustained muscle contraction, exaggerated metabolic rate, and activated adenosine triphosphate (ATP) occurs. The body overheats,greatly increasing cellular oxygen consumption and production of acid metabolic by-products.

Litwack-Saleh, K: Practical Points in the Management of Malignant Hyperthermia. J Post Anesth Nurs *7: 327-329, 1992; Wlody, GS: Malignant Hyperthermia.* Crit Care Nurs Clin North Am *3: 129-134, 1991.*

7.67. Correct Answer: **c**

Prior knowledge and informed consent are required before a patient can be tested for human immunodeficiency virus (HIV). In addition, confidentiality of the results must be assured, even when positive results are reported to the state health department. Seroconversion to HIV positivity occurs over weeks to months. Incidence of occupational transmission of HIV is low.

Burden, N: Ambulatory Surgical Nursing. *Philadelphia, Saunders, pp. 243-245, 1993; Tribett, D: The Patient with Human Immunodeficiency Virus (HIV) in* AACN's Clinical Reference for Critical-Care Nursing *(Kinney, MR, Packa, DR & Dunbar, SB, Eds). St. Louis, Mosby, pp. 1061-1062, 1993.*

7.68. Correct Answer: **b**

Laser technology reduces complications associated with more traditional methods of transurethral resection of the prostate (TURP). Hyponatremia with confusion and seizures and absorption of bladder irrigant through prostate vessels are both less likely. By necrosing prostatic tissue, a laser minimizes bleeding.

Payne, CK, Babiarz, JW & Raz, S: Genitourinary Problems in the Elderly Patient. Surg Clin North Am *74: 418-422, 1994; Nagle, GM: The Urologic Surgical Patient in* ASPAN's Core Curriculum for Post Anesthesia Nursing Practice, *3rd ed (Litwack, K, Ed). Philadelphia, Sauders, pp. 429-431, 1994.*

7.69. Correct Answer: **a**

A chest tube inserted into the pleural space of the deflated lung restores and preserves negative pressure. Removing air reexpands the lung. Chest tubes also drain fluid or accumulated blood in the thorax. Whenever the pleural space is entered, either by trauma or surgery, the normally *negative* intrapleural pressure within the chest cavity increases to equal atmospheric pressure. Lungs deflate. The closed chest tube system should not be entered for sampling.

Drain, CB: The Post Anesthesia Care Unit: A Critical Care Approach to Post Anesthesia Nursing, *3rd ed. Philadelphia, Saunders, pp. 356-361, 1994; Schneider, CC & Slatten, R: Thoracic Surgery in* Critical Care Nursing, *2nd ed (Vazquez, M, Lazear, SE & Larson, EL, Eds). Philadelphia, Saunders, pp. 233-239, 1992.*

7.70. Correct Answer: **c**

Following chest surgery, Trendelenburg's position is avoided, even with shock and hypotension, to prevent pressure from abdominal organs against the diaphragm. A slightly head-up and supine position maintains venous return and cardiac output and allows maximum expansion of the lungs.

Drain, CB: The Post Anesthesia Care Unit: A Critical Care Approach to Post Anesthesia Nursing, *3rd ed. Philadelphia, Saunders, pp. 360, 1994.*

Section 8

Neurologic, Neurovascular, and Musculoskeletal Systems

Scenarios and items in this section focus on perianesthesia concepts related to *intracranial* and *musculoskeletal* considerations of *neurologic function* and *orthopedics.* These concepts are considered together because:

- vascular and nerve functions are intricately interrelated; altered nerve function often alters local blood flow.
- intracranial vascular alterations or tissue edema produce autoregulatory and compensatory shifts and may alter neurologic and musculoskeletal function.
- musculoskeletal procedures (both orthopedic and neurologic) share common patient management concepts, including methods to treat and monitor pain, concerns about blood loss and hemostasis and circulation-promoting positions.
- postoperative nursing assessments involve monitoring neurovascular status and motor and sensory function after *both* orthopedic and spine-related surgical procedures.

ESSENTIAL CORE CONCEPTS	AFFILIATED CORE CURRICULUM CHAPTERS
Nursing Process Assessment Planning and Implementation Evaluation	**Chapters 2, 20, & 25**

Intracranial Concerns
Anatomy: Structure and Function
  Blood-Brain Barrier
  Cerebrospinal Fluid
  Cranial Nerves
  Lobes and Ventricles
  Vessels and Spaces
Physiology
  Intracranial Pressure Dynamics
    Autoregulation
    Herniation
    Hyperventilation
    Pharmacology
    Position, Ventilation and Rest
	Chapter 20

- Neuronal Excitation
- Neuromuscular Junction: Transmitters

Pathology
- Interventions and Anesthetic Consequences
- Trauma, Tumors, Shunts, and Bleeding

Perianesthesia Specifics
- Consciousness
- Glasgow Coma Scale
- Motor and Sensory Responses
- Pupil Reaction
- Reflexes and Vital Signs

Musculoskeletal: Spine and Orthopedics **Chapter 20**

Anatomy: Structure and Function Chapter 25
- Ascending Tracts
- Descending Tracts
- Primary Extremity Nerves
- Vertebrae, Discs, Bones and Nerves
- White Matter, Grey Matter and Dura Mater

Physiologic Neurotransmission
- Sympathetic: Adrenergic Response to Norepinephrine
- Parasympathetic: Cholinergic Response to Acetylcholine

Neurologic and Vascular Concerns
- Autonomic Hyperreflexia
- Circulation: Capillary Refill, Temperature, and Color
- Compartment Syndrome
- Discs, Lesions, and Fractures
- Edema, Embolism, and Ecchymosis
- Innervation: Pain, Sensation, and Motor Control

Perianesthesia Specifics
- Neurologic Function and Complications
- Neurovascular Monitoring
- Pain Management
- Position and Comfort
- Cardiorespiratory Risk Assessment

SET I

Items 8.1-8.30

8.1. To alter the course of malignant hyperthermia, dantrolene sodium *primarily:*

a. contracts vascular smooth muscle
b. reverses cellular acidosis
c. relaxes skeletal muscle
d. augments hypothalamic temperature regulation

NOTE: Consider scenario and item 8.2 together.

Ms F sustained a pelvic fracture in a motor vehicle accident 18 hours ago. She is a 48 year old, nonsmoking, conversant and healthy woman who has received meperidine by PCA, cefazolin, dexamethasone and midazolam since hospital admission.

8.2. The preanesthesia nurse considers Ms F's potential for fat embolism, closely monitors Ms F's pulmonary status and:

a. encourages active leg movement
b. reports disoriented agitation
c. releases traction 10 minutes each hour
d. limits intravenous fluid volume

8.3. The patient *most likely* to develop autonomic hyperreflexia had a/an:

a. 2-level anterior and posterior cervical fusion today
b. anterior cord syndrome from incomplete T-8 injury 3 days ago
c. reexploraton after resection of lumbar tumor 2 weeks ago
d. motor vehicle accident with cord transection at T-2 5 months ago

8.4. Documented postcraniotomy diabetes insipidus is treated with:

a. vasopressin and fluid replacement
b. long-acting antihyperglycemics and bicarbonate
c. 10% dextrose infusion and furosemide
d. fluid restriction and hypertonic saline

NOTE: Consider scenario and items 8.5-8.6 together.

After 45 minutes in PACU following her L-4 to L-5 decompression and fusion, 64 year old Ms P is quickly responsive to touch and name call, oriented to her environment, dozes when undisturbed, and has three documented blood pressures of greater than 195/106 mm Hg.

8.5. Of the following factors, the *most likely* contributor to Ms P's blood pressure measures is:

a. moderate analgesia
b. postspinal meningeal irritation
c. evolving epidural hematoma
d. preoperative hypertension

8.6. Untreated hypertension increases Ms P's potential to develop any of the following adverse outcomes *except:*

a. release of blood vessel suture
b. intrapulmonary rales
c. myocardial hypoperfusion
d. postspinal surgery headache

8.7. Ms E receives electroconvulsive therapy (ECT) 3 times weekly and regularly uses the antidepressant amitriptyline. Administering epinephrine is *most* likely to result in:

a. unpredictable responses to ECT energy
b. uncontrolled adrenergic stimulation
c. profound vagal effect
d. exaggerated agitation when wakening from ECT

NOTE: Consider scenario and items 8.8-8.9 together.

During the admission interview before her left knee arthroscopy, Ms W expresses concern about the proposed spinal anesthetic. She relates that her friend had a severe headache 10 years ago after a spinal anesthetic; Ms W hopes to be discharged home later today.

8.8. The nurse responds that the incidence of postdural puncture headache (PDPH) among ambulatory surgery patients is:

a. low; a small 27-gauge needle limits fluid leakage during local anesthetic injection
b. high; patients must sit and stand early to prepare for discharge
c. low; high molecular weight tetracaine injected through a 20-gauge needle seals any leak
d. high; ASU patients should not receive large volumes of prehydrating fluid for vascular expansion

8.9. Following spinal anesthesia, Ms W must meet the facility's discharge criteria and also should:

a. repeat each postoperative instruction
b. urinate spontaneously
c. indicate pinprick sensation at S-2 dermatome
d. stand without orthostatic hypertension

8.10. The patient with the *least* probable risk to develop an injury related to intraoperative position has:

a. Crohn's disease, treated with a 4 hour proctocolectomy and continent ileostomy
b. arthritis and a 2 year old left hip arthroplasty and is a 64 year old woman
c. non-insulin-dependent diabetes, is a 48 year old man and had a 50 minute surgery to revise an abdominal scar
d. a gastrostomy tube after gastric bypass surgery and weighs 88 kg at age 24 years

8.11. Wide blood pressure variability after carotid endarterectomy most likely occurs due to intraoperative:

a. fluid shifts and third spacing
b. vascular manipulation
c. intentional hypotensive technique
d. vagal nerve compression and trauma

8.12. Following craniotomy to remove an acoustic neuroma, the nurse asks the patient to clench his teeth to assess function of the:

a. spinal accessory nerve
b. temporomaxillary nerve
c. glossopharyngeal nerve
d. trigeminal nerve

8.13. The patient *most likely* to develop malignant hyperthermia crisis is a:

a. 65 year old woman with a fractured hip
b. 32 year old man with Down's syndrome
c. 15 year old boy with muscular dystrophy
d. 6 month old girl with cleft palate

NOTE: Consider scenario and item 8.14 together.

A 72 year old man is admitted to Phase I PACU after repair of a right inguinal hernia with IV conscious sedation and tissue infiltration of local anesthetic. Intraoperatively, he received 50 mcg of fentanyl and 2 mg of midazolam, both approximately 60 minutes ago. The patient is now restless and combative.

8.14. A senior surgical resident orders 3 mg midazolam in PACU. The PACU nurse's *most appropriate* response is to:

a. tactfully consult with a second phhysician
b. evaluate causes for behavior and question the dose
c. ignore the order and restrain the patient
d. administer midazolam as ordered

8.15. During patient assessment following spinal anesthesia, the PACU nurse considers the increased potential for both postdural puncture headache (PDPH) and:

a. fluid volume deficit with hypotension
b. euphoria and diaphoresis
c. respiratory stimulation and alkalosis
d. tachycardia with vasoconstriction

NOTE: Consider scenario and items 8.16-8.17 together.

Ms N's myasthenia gravis is treated by her neurologist with pyridostigmine. She is in PACU following an abdominal exploratory laparotomy and resection of a ruptured appendix.

8.16. While reviewing the surgeon's routine, preprinted postoperative orders, the PACU nurse questions the order for:

a. hydrocortisone 100 mg
b. ketorolac 30 mg
c. gentamicin 80 mg
d. neostigmine 10 mg

8.17. If Ms N develops myasthenic crisis, the PACU nurse would expect to observe:

a. exophthalmos and hyperventilation
b. mydriasis and dry mouth
c. bradycardia and abdominal cramps
d. ptosis and pulmonary secretions

NOTE: Consider scenario and items 8.18-8.19 together.

Mr. Y's intraoperative blood loss was 800 ml during his second right total knee replacement with spinal anesthetic. The first right knee replacement was 6 years ago. He received 2 units of packed red blood cells and 500 ml hetastarch during this surgery in addition to 2600 ml lactated Ringer's solution. In PACU, his hemoglobin is 10.3 mg/dl, blood pressure rises to 194/96, central venous pressure is 15 cm H_2O, heart rate is 96 beats per minute in normal sinus rhythm, he has an audible S_3 heart sound and states a pounding headache.

8.18. Mr. Y's symptoms are most probably related to acute:

a. intravascular hemolysis
b. circulatory overload
c. anxiety from spinal headache
d. myocardial ischemia

8.19. When assessing Mr. Y, the PACU nurse considers that a hemolytic blood reaction usually produces symptoms of:

a. chills with chest or flank pain
b. hypertension and dyspnea
c. hypothermia with headache
d. urticaria and hypotension

NOTE: Consider items 8.20-8.21 together.

8.20. Following exploration and excision of an intramedullary tumor and thoracic laminectomy, fusion and instrumentation, an essential nursing aspect of Ms L's postoperative care is:

a. 100% immobility to "seat" instruments
b. skeletal traction to prevent adhesions
c. hypotension to minimize bleeding
d. log rolling to assure alignment

NOTE: The scenario continues.

Thirty minutes later, Ms L reports new and sudden severe back pain and tingling in her left toes. Neurologic assessment reveals decreased strength with both dorsiflexion and plantar flexion. Pedal and posterior tibial pulses are strong and capillary refill normal.

8.21. Ms L's symptoms most likely result from:

a. intraspinal hematoma
b. dural tear
c. spinal muscle spasm
d. nerve entrapment

NOTE: Consider items 8.22-8.27 together.

8.22. A spinal anesthetic is planned for Mr. J's knee arthrotomy and meniscus repair. The local anesthetic medication with longest duration of anesthesia is:

a. 1% tetracaine in dextrose
b. 10% Procaine with meperidine
c. 0.75% bupivacaine in saline
d. 0.5% lidocaine with fentanyl

8.23. An anesthesia provider may add epinephrine to a spinal anesthetic solution *primarily* to:

a. increase the anesthetic duration
b. decrease duration of anesthetic effect
c. increase vascular absorption of medication
d. decrease potential for hypotension

8.24. Achieving the desired level of dermatome blockade from Mr. J's spinal anesthetic is *most* determined by his:

a. age and adding epinephrine to the solution
b. body weight and extremity position
c. anesthesiologist's experience and the needle size
d. body position and density of anesthetic solution

NOTE: The scenario continues.

Mr. J is admitted to PACU awake, alert, and slightly diaphoretic with pale color. Blood pressure is 84/52, heart rhythm sinus at a rate of 56 beats per miunute, respiratory rate 20 breaths per minute, oxygen saturation 98%. Preoperative blood pressure was 104/60, with pulse 64 beats per minute. He denies pain and complains of nausea.

8.25. The PACU nurse's intervention is directed toward minimizing:

a. potential for aspiration
b. fluid volume deficit
c. increased intrathoracic pressure
d. local anesthetic movement in CSF

8.26. Thirty minutes after PACU admission, Mr. J can raise his right knee from the bed. The nurse assesses his motor block at approximately dermatome:

a. S-1 to S-2
b. L-2 to L-3
c. T-12 to L-1
d. T-4 to T-5

8.27. With a motor block at this level, the PACU nurse anticipates Mr. J's sensory block is:

a. higher than both sympathetic and motor block
b. the same level as both motor and sympathetic block
c. higher than motor but below sympathetic block
d. equal to sympathetic block but below motor block

8.28. The primary neurotransmitter that promotes wakefulness is:

a. acetylcholine
b. epinephrine
c. norepinephrine
d. enkephalin

NOTE: Consider scenario and item 8.29 together.

A 56 year old man is scheduled for craniotomy to clip a leaking cerebral aneurysm. He is settled into the preanesthesia area for nursing observation and to await his neurosurgeon's arrival.

8.29. The preanesthesia nurse specifically observes this patient for:

a. fever and hyperventilation
b. headache and neck stiffness
c. hydrocephalus and QRS duration of 0.16 seconds
d. atrial flutter with 3:1 conduction and seizures

8.30. When applying a 100 mg transdermal fentanyl patch to a patient with severe left calf injury, the nurse should:

a. premedicate the patient with 3 ml IV fentanyl
b. rinse the skin with water
c. shave chest hair
d. scrub with povidone-iodine and apply patch below left knee

SET II

Items 8.31-8.60

NOTE: Consider scenario and items 8.31-8.40 together.

Forty minutes after evacuation of a left occipital subdural hematoma, Mr. Q is drowsy but rouses when his name is called; he follows commands to move his extremities, open his eyes and deep breathe. Pupils are equal and pinpoint. A suction drain into the cranium is compressed and draining small amounts of red fluid.

8.31. The PACU nurse documents that this patient is:

a. disoriented
b. stuporous
c. lethargic
d. awake

8.32. Adverse influences on Mr. Q's current level of consciousness could include any of the following factors *except:*

a. hypoxia
b. hypocarbia
c. hypoglycemia
d. hypothermia

NOTE: The scenario continues.

Twenty minutes later, Mr. Q requires a louder voice and a stronger tap at his shoulder to arouse. He drifts to sleep immediately unless continuously stimulated. Pupils are equal, about 2 mm in size, briskly reactive, and he slowly and weakly moves all extremities to command.

8.33. The PACU nurse's most appropriate intervention is to:

a. notify the neurosurgeon
b. reassess Mr. Q in 15 minutes
c. administer naloxone 0.8 mg per protocol
d. empty and recompress Mr. Q's intracranial drain

NOTE: The scenario continues.

The neurosurgeon requests dexamethasone 12 mg and frequent observation until she arrives in PACU. Within 20 minutes, Mr. Q is considerably more difficult to rouse; eyes occasionally open to heavy touch and he does not vocalize or move his right side when asked. His left arm moves fistlike toward his chest. The nurse applies the Glasgow Coma Scale to objectively grade Mr. Q's neurologic function.

8.34. According to three components of the Glasgow Coma Scale, Mr. Q's eye opening, best verbal and best motor response would best be described as:

a. (to) maximum arousal, incomprehensible and flaccid
b. inconsistent, mute and decerebrate
c. lethargic, inappropriate, and localizing
d. (to) pain, no response and flexion

8.35. The bedside nurse *most appropriately* elicits a pain response by:

a. twisting the nipple of Mr. Q's left breast
b. squeezing Mr. Q's right great toe firmly
c. applying pressure to Mr. Q's left eye orbit
d. pinching Mr. Q's right trapezius muscle vigorously

NOTE: The scenario continues.

Further neurologic reassessments indicate that Mr. Q consistently grimaces and flexes both arms and wrists toward his chest and extends his legs, pointing his toes downward and inward.

8.36. The nurse documents Mr. Q's current response as:

a. decerebrate rigidity
b. asynchronous reflex
c. decorticate posturing
d. withdrawal reaction

8.37. With these clinical signs, Mr. Q could imminently develop:
a. transtentorial herniation
b. cranial "blowout" with wound dehiscence
c. hydrocephalic shunting
d. compensatory cerebrospinal fluid displacement

8.38. The PACU nurse anticipates that Mr. Q's pupils would *most likely* dilate:
a. equally
b. contralaterally
c. ipsilaterally
d. bilaterally

8.39. The anesthesiologist intubates Mr. Q and the neurosurgeon requests a mannitol infusion and a stat CT scan. In this situation, Mr. Q's neurologic status is best protected when Mr. Q's:
a. respiratory rate and depth are increased
b. airway is vigorously and regularly suctioned
c. body position is flat and supine
d. consciousness is continuously raised with "stir-up" regimen

8.40. Dexamethasone was administered to Mr. Q *primarily* to:
a. support his physiologic stress responses
b. reduce intracranial volume
c. increase blood flow to cerebral cells
d. decrease seizure threshold

NOTE: Consider items 8.41-8.42 together.

8.41. A patient received nitrous oxide with a total of 750 mcg of fentanyl in divided doses during a $2\frac{1}{2}$ hour left thumb replantation due to a traumatic power saw injury. The PACU nurse *most* expects to observe fentanyl-induced:
a. dilated pupils and vomiting
b. hypoventilation and pupillary constriction
c. hypertension and hyperventilation
d. bradycardia and emergence shivering

8.42. Nursing care priorities for this patient focus on respiratory monitoring, neurovascular assessment, and providing:
a. ice to the inner midforearm to reduce posttrauma metabolic demand
b. limited analgesia for quick detection of neurovascular changes
c. a comfortable arm position that facilitates venous return
d. fluid restriction to minimize extremity edema

8.43. Awareness of sensory stimuli and degree of alertness occur through the:
a. limbic-pyramidal system
b. reticular activating system
c. corpus callosum system
d. thalamic projection system

8.44. Interrelationship between the cerebral hemispheres occurs through commissures of the:
a. corpus callosum
b. longitudinal fissure
c. lateral ventricle gyri
d. central sulcus

8.45. The *most serious* potential compromise to a diabetic surgical patient's recovery immediately after hip arthroplasty is:
a. absent responsiveness from unrecognized hypoglycemia
b. infection from zealous glucose sampling
c. hypercalcemia from citrated blood products
d. altered intestinal flora from dual antibiotic therapy

8.46. Mannitol's effectiveness occurs by:

a. hydrostatic pressure to increase renal exretion
b. diffusion pressure to decrease electrolyte shifts
c. oncotic pressure to increase solute removal
d. osmotic pressure to decrease intracellular fluid

NOTE: Consider scenario and item 8.47 together.

Three hours ago during her 2-level lumbar discectomy and fusion, Ms R's neurosurgeon injected a single epidural dose of preservative-free morphine 5 mg. Now in PACU, Ms R is drowsy, responds quickly to name call and follows commands.

8.47. When planning Ms R's care, the PACU nurse reasons that any residual respiratory effects from this morphine sulfate (Duramorph) dose:

a. will not develop after only a single dose
b. most likely will appear within 8 hours
c. will require nalbuphine to treat opioid overdose
d. probably occurred while Ms R was intubated in OR

NOTE: Consider items 8.48-8.49 together.

8.48. Following repair of a congenital arteriovenous malformation in a 25 year old man, the nurse anticipates that any inability to wiggle his toes will appear:

a. ipsilaterally
b. spinothalamically
c. contralaterally
d. extrapyramidally

8.49. Development of anisocoria in this patient most likely reflects:

a. meningeal irritation
b. undocumented cocaine use
c. previous iridectomy
d. temporal lobe displacement

8.50. Mr. P is a 46 year old healthy, smoking patient who today had fusion of thoracic vertebrae T-6 to T-7 and T-7 to T-8. The most likely consequences related to his intraoperative position include any of the following *except:*

a. corneal abrasion
b. impaired ear circulation
c. sciatic nerve stretch
d. skin redness at his ribs and ilia

NOTE: Consider scenario and items 8.51-8.54 together.

The anesthesiologist inserted an epidural catheter into Ms A's lumbar spine prior to her left total hip replacement. The anesthesiologist injected a total of 200 mcg fentanyl into the epidural catheter during surgery. Upon admission to PACU, Ms A is awake, alert and denies pain. Blood pressure is 146/88, heart rate 86 beats per minute and respiratory rate 16 breaths per minute. Fifteen minutes later, Ms A complains of moderate hip pain. The pharmacy is still preparing the fentanyl solution ordered by the anesthesiologist for continuous infusion.

8.51. In this situation, the PACU nurse's *most appropriate* intervention is to:

a. administer morphine sulfate 15 mg intramuscularly
b. sedate Ms A with midazolam for amnesia to pain
c. inject fentanyl 150 mcg intravenously
d. titrate intravenous morphine to comfort

NOTE: The scenario continues.

The PACU nurse inspects the insertion site of Ms A's epidural catheter and assures that the epidural tubing is clearly labeled and has no injection ports to mistakenly inject any other medication.

8.52. Before starting Ms A's epidural infusion, the nurse determines the catheter is located in the epidural space by:

a. aspirating less than 0.5 ml clear fluid
b. assuring 1 ml serosanguineous fluid flows from port

c. observing 2 ml clear amber fluid drips from port
d. injecting a 0.5 ml fentanyl test dose with ease

NOTE: The scenario continues.

Forty minutes later, Ms A states less pain; fentanyl 1 mg, diluted in 100 ml normal saline, infuses epidurally at 8 ml/h.

8.53. While monitoring the specific effects of epidurally injected fentanyl, the PACU nurse *least* expects to observe:

a. nausea with emesis
b. respirations 8 breaths per minute
c. blood pressure 76/40
d. strong left foot dorsiflexion

NOTE: The scenario continues.

During assessment for PACU discharge, Ms A complains of "a lot of pain in my back where that tube is," indicating the epidural catheter, and mentions right leg weakness and heaviness. Assessment reveals diminished right dorsiplantar flexion, a change from the strong and equal leg activity noted upon PACU admission.

8.54. The PACU nurse's most appropriate response is to:

a. transfer Ms A to the orthopedic unit for frequent neurovascular assessment
b. reassure Ms A that symptoms are common and recede without consequence
c. reposition Ms A's leg, then increase the epidural infusion rate to decrease back spasm
d. defer transfer from PACU for physician consultation and neurologic examination

NOTE: Consider scenario and items 8.55-8.56 together.

A healthy 22 year old college student had surgery to repair his right shoulder rotator cuff. He received succinylcholine, fentanyl, and nitrous oxide anesthesia. He is sedated and drowsy, breathes shallowly 14 times per minute, and has a weak response to ulnar nerve stimulation.

8.55. A likely explanation for this situation is:

a. unusual narcotic and muscle relaxant overdose
b. abnormal acetylcholine movement from the cell
c. atypical pseudocholinesterase effect
d. genetically inhibited glycopyrrolate response

8.56. While assessing this patient, the nurse is *most* concerned when the:

a. wound drainage is 120 ml during a 1.5 hour PACU stay
b. right arm is in a sling with shoulder adducted and internally rotated
c. patient quite easily abducts fingers and touches his right thumb to little finger
d. capillary refill occurs within 2 seconds

NOTE: Consider scenario and items 8.57-8.60 together.

The preanesthesia nurse observes 57 year old Ms D who just received a brachial plexus block prior to repair of a wrist fracture. Lidocaine with epinephrine was injected by axillary approach. Prior to injection, she received midazolam 1 mg to decrease anxiety. Five minutes later, Ms D mentions blurred vision and "not feeling right." Further assessment indicates tachycardia (heart rate 120 beats per minute) with palpitations, circumoral numbness, restlessness, dizziness, and tinnitus. Her current blood pressure is 160/72.

8.57. The perianesthesia nurse provides oxygen to Ms D, informs the anesthesia provider of these symptoms and:

a. prepares flumazenil to reverse midazolam
b. encourages relaxation to decrease hyperventilation
c. anticipates development of muscle tremors
d. obtains labetalol to oppose adrenergic stimulation

NOTE: The scenario continues.

Ms D's symptoms abate. After observation by the preanesthesia nurse and family visitation, surgery proceeded uneventfully 2 hours later. Now, 6 hours after her brachial plexus block, Ms D is alert, engaged in lively conversation with her daughter, tolerates food and fluids without nausea, and has urinated. Her vital signs have been stable since surgery. She requests to go home and receives approval from the anesthesiologist and surgeon.

8.58. To prepare for discharge, the PACU nurse in Phase II assures Ms D has:

a. return of normal motor and sensory function in her hand
b. strong train-of-four response to nerve stimulation
c. adequate palmar circulation, assessed by Allen's test
d. analgesic prescription and rapid capillary refill

8.59. Ms D learns to care for her plaster-casted arm by understanding the need for:

a. extremity elevation and resting her still-numbed arm against a table edge
b. leaving her casted arm open to the air for 24 hours and applying ice
c. preventing compression of her cast, which should be dry within 30 minutes
d. controlling skin pruritus by spreading lotion under cast edge with a covered pen

8.60. Ms D's orthopedic surgeon should be informed when any of the following occur *except:*

a. the right hand appears more purple than the left
b. body temperature is 38.5° C at home
c. her analgesic prescription slightly reduces her severe wrist pain for 2 hours
d. she thinks her cast feels "warm" when discharged from Phase II

SET III

Items 8.61-8.92

8.61. The occipital lobe receives and interprets:

a. auditory data
b. proprioception
c. emotional events
d. visual data

8.62. After Ms O's open reduction of a fracture to the left femoral neck, her spinal anesthetic continues to the T-10 dermatome. Postoperative nursing considerations include:

a. promoting hip adduction and limiting flexion to 90 degrees
b. assuring anatomic alignment and repositioning Ms O only on her left side
c. providing lateral leg supports and applying ice to the left hip
d. inspecting sheets below hip for drainage and supporting Ms O's legs behind the knee

NOTE: Consider scenario and items 8.63-8.66 together.

Ms S had a left lateral frontal lobotomy anterior to the central sulcus for placement of grids to map and control seizure activity. She opens her eyes, nods her head and breathes well.

8.63. One primary assessment after surgery in the left frontal area is to identify this patient's ability to:

a. state her name
b. hear music
c. comprehend instructions
d. focus on an object

8.64. Ms S's nurse is assessing function at:

a. Rolando's area
b. Broca's area
c. Brodmann's area
d. Wernicke's area

8.65. Ms S's cranial nerve function is considered normal when neurologic assessment reveals *ocular* responses that are:

a. nystagmic and convergent
b. nonconsensual and equal
c. constricted and exophthalmic
d. conjugate and brisk

8.66. Ms S's upper arm function is best tested by asking her to:

a. sustain outstretched arms
b. squeeze the nurse's hand
c. adduct her shoulder
d. hyperextend her hand and wrist

8.67. Daily production of cerebrospinal fluid in adults is:

a. 100 ml per day
b. 500 ml per day
c. 800-1000 ml per day
d. 2000 ml per day

8.68. A patient with intracranial changes known as Cushing's triad has:

a. systolic increase, diastolic decrease, bradycardia
b. diastolic decrease, elevated glucose, oliguria
c. diastolic increase, decreased aldosterone, polyuria
d. systolic decrease, tachycardia, hyperthermia

8.69. Contralateral crossing of corticospinal tracts occurs at the:

a. brain stem
b. dorsal horn
c. cerebellum
d. hippocampus

NOTE: Consider scenario and items 8.70-8.72 together.

8.70. Twelve year old Angela is in Phase I PACU after posterior fusion of L-1 to L-5 vertebrae and insertion of instrumentation to treat her scoliosis. The nurse determines that the *most important* immediate nursing priority for Angela is:

a. mobilizing fluid volume with low-dose furosemide to relieve accumulated facial edema
b. assisting Angela to use the bed trapeze for self-reposition and early mobility
c. encouraging lung expansion while restoring fluid and oxygen-carrying deficits
d. positioning her flat and nearly prone to drain secretions and relieve gastric distention

8.71. Some of Angela's intraoperative blood loss was returned by an autotransfusion technique. Physiologic advantages of retransfusion include reduced potential for disease and:

a. retained cell "freshness" for reinfusion 2 days later
b. immediate availability without need to filter small particles
c. normal potassium levels, preserved platelet number and function
d. risk of coagulopathy; processing reverses heparin and replaces thrombin

8.72. To safely administer an autotransfusion of washed and processed blood cells from lost intraoperative blood, nursing responsibilities include the following *except* to:

a. complete autotransfusion within 4 hours and flush tubing with saline
b. monitor temperature and infuse peripherally with morphine PCA
c. report abdominal cramping and circumoral tingling
d. observe for chills, hematuria, and increased wound drainage

NOTE: Consider scenario and item 8.73-8.74 together.

8.73. After calibration of the subarachnoid monitoring system, Ms W's intracranial pressure measures 18 mm Hg. Interventions to prevent further increases may include all the following *except:*

a. semi-Fowler's position with knees extended
b. mechanical ventilation at 10 breaths per minute and 1000 ml tidal volume
c. nitroprusside infusion to increase cerebral blood flow
d. immediate infusion of hyperosmotic solution

8.74. Nursing responsibility with regard to invasively monitoring Ms W's intracranial pressure includes:

a. administering scheduled steroid doses to suppress infection
b. flushing the catheter system to assure system patency
c. reporting C waves promptly and calculating intracranial compliance
d. recognizing plateau waves and identifying leaks at skull insertion site

8.75. The Monro-Kellie hypothesis describes intracranial volume as a relationship among:

a. cerebral perfusion, mean arterial and systolic blood pressures
b. oxygen and carbon dioxide partial pressures and cardiac inde
c. cerebrospinal fluid density, cerebral blood flow and cellular oxygenation
d. brain, cerebral blood and cerebrospinal fluid volumes

8.76. A cerebral perfusion pressure calculated at 43 mm Hg *most likely* represents:

a. inadequate brain blood flow
b. compensated autoregulation
c. normal cerebral circulation
d. ischemia with active CSF loss

NOTE: Consider items 8.77-8.80 together.

8.77. Mr. J is scheduled for a craniotomy to remove an infratentorial meningioma. Characteristics of a meningioma *most* increase Mr. J's potential for:

a. intraoperative hemorrhage
b. malignancy-related death
c. fluid volume excess
d. postoperative hypertension

NOTE: The scenario continues.

Postoperatively the PACU nurse observes yellow-tinged drainage at Mr. J's posterior dressing.

8.78. To confirm or refute a cerebrospinal fluid leak, the nurse *most appropriately:*

a. removes the dressing for incisional inspection
b. lowers the ventriculostomy to observe flow increase
c. determines presence of glucose in drainage
d. assesses patient for position-related headache

8.79. Immediate postsurgical complications following Mr. J's infratentorial surgery are *most likely* indicated by:

a. receptive aphasia
b. serosanguineous nasal drainage
c. altered respiratory pattern
d. muscle paralysis

8.80. Nursing intervention to best promote positive respiratory outcomes after Mr. J's infratentorial surgery includes:

a. mechanical ventilation with PEEP
b. log roll turns with neck support
c. regular tracheobronchial suction
d. achieving a functional Phase II block

8.81. The PACU nurse is *most* concerned when, after left supratentorial craniotomy, the patient develops:

a. dilation of the right pupil
b. weakness of the left arm
c. inability to move the right leg
d. nystagmus involving the left eye

8.82. Nursing management of a patient with a ventriculostomy drain includes:

a. securing the system's "zero" point near the eye or by physician order
b. assuring system sterility and a minimum of 30 ml per hour drainage
c. providing low, negative pressure suction to facilitate system patency
d. complying with physician-specified volumes of fluid drainage

NOTE: Consider scenario and items 8.83-8.86 together.

The PACU nurse assesses Wynona's muscle strength after her right transthoracic discectomy at T-6 to T-7. Comparative responses indicate Wynona moves each arm without drift and resists nurse's efforts to push them down or away. She easily lifts her left leg from the bed and has strong foot dorsiflexion and plantar flexion movements. She moves and lifts her right knee; the nurse moves Wynona's right foot from the dorsiflexed position with little resistance.

8.83. Based on this assessment, the nurse documents muscle activity as:

a. equal bilaterally in arms and legs, with normal strength
b. right leg moves with full range of motion against gravity and weakens to resistance
c. left leg strong; right leg moves but with severe weakness against gravity
d. arms have normal strength; legs move equally but with mild weakness to resistance

NOTE: The scenario continues.

Thirty minutes later, Wynona is much more drowsy. The nurse sufficiently stimulates her and determines that Wynona can still move her right leg but cannot lift it from the bed. Assessments of arm and left leg activity are unchanged.

8.84. The neurosurgeon requests an immediate CT scan and orders hourly doses of methylprednisolone, primarily to decrease:

a. autoimmune rejection of bone graft
b. traumatic intraspinal edema
c. intracranial pressure effects
d. sepsis and future reherniation

8.85. Following this medication, Wynona has increased risk to develop infection, adrenal suppression and:

a. gastric ulceration
b. dehydration
c. lethargy
d. thromboembolism

8.86. An important observation in PACU related to the continuous infusion of sufentanil Wynona received during surgery is:

a. relaxation of muscles, particularly in chest
b. altered consciousness and a staring, fixed gaze
c. recurrent respiratory depression
d. bradycardia and hypotension after large doses

8.87. Neurologically, the term *nystagmus* describes:

a. cerebellar dysfunction with uncoordinated, spastic extremity movements
b. coordinated eye movements away from the direction the head turns
c. parietal lobe disease with generalized skeletal muscle weakness
d. abnormally "jerky" eye movements that drift from a midline gaze

8.88. Mr. R's leg deep tendon reflexes are described as "2+", which indicates:

a. normal reflex responses
b. above-average responses in two of four limbs
c. suppression of reflexes
d. subnormal reactions and positive Babinski sign

8.89. An autologous bone graft:

a. substitutes for Luque rods during spinal fusion
b. transfers iliac bone to stabilize damaged bone
c. transplants bone acquired from an anonymous donor
d. requires high-dose steroids to prevent rejection

8.90. After Mr. C's total knee replacement, the nurse manages Mr. C's pain, monitors for infection and:

a. provides high leg elevation, ice and pillows behind his knee
b. checks regularly for accumulated drainage beneath his leg
c. limits leg movement to toe wiggling and foot flexion
d. informs the surgeon promptly that 180 ml red, clotty fluid collected in wound drain

8.91. Patients with greatest risk to develop compartment syndrome include all of the following *except* a:

a. 25 year old muscular man with a warm cast 4 hours after repair of a left Pott's fracture
b. 48 year old woman in lithotomy position for a 3 hour vaginal hysterectomy and pelvic floor repair
c. 65 year old man with a sequential compression device 2 hours after a total hip replacement
d. 72 year old obese woman with large left thigh hematoma 3 hours after removal of a femoral artery sheath

NOTE: Consider scenario and item 8.92 together.

An intramedullary rod and plates were inserted in Tom's right leg to repair his tibia with three fractures. He is alert, has a long-leg cast propped high on three pillows and describes severe, unrelenting leg pain after administration of 15 mg IV morphine sulfate.

8.92. The nurse observes for drainage "hidden" beneath his cast and considers Tom's potential to develop compartment syndrome, then observes for altered capillary refill. Assessment for compartment syndrome includes all of the following early signs *except:*

a. burning sensation in extremity
b. diminishing dorsalis pedal pulse quality
c. muscle weakness against resistance
d. cyanotic toes and brisk, "4+" tendon reflexes

SET I

Answer Key

8.1. c
8.2. b
8.3. d
8.4. a
8.5. d
8.6. d
8.7. b
8.8. a
8.9. b
8.10. c
8.11. b
8.12. d
8.13. c
8.14. b
8.15. a
8.16. c
8.17. d
8.18. b
8.19. a
8.20. d
8.21. a
8.22. c
8.23. a
8.24. d
8.25. b
8.26. b
8.27. c
8.28. a
8.29. b
8.30. b

SET I

Rationales and References

8.1. Correct Answer: **c**

Dantrolene sodium's direct effect on skeletal muscle suppresses release of intracellular calcium. Muscles relax and rate of further contraction slows. In malignant hyperthermia, unsuppressed muscle contractions produce heat and increase body temperature up to 1° C each minute. Dantrolene does not alter contractile rate or strength of cardiac and smooth muscle.

Wlody, GS: Malignant Hyperthermia. Crit Care Nurs Clin North Am *3: 129-134, 1991; Shannon, MT, Wilson, BA & Stang, CL:* Govoni & Hayes Drugs and Nursing Implications, *8th ed. Norwalk, CT, Appleton & Lange, pp. 369-371, 1995.*

8.2. Correct Answer: **b**

Newly developing agitation, confusion and disorientation in a trauma patient with orthopedic fractures should be reported and not ignored. These symptoms of hypoxemia could indicate developing fat embolism syndrome, particularly within 36 hours after fracture. Pelvic and long bone (femur) fractures are linked with high risk for fat embolism; Ms F warrants a "high index of suspicion" and close observation. Some physicians believe early fracture stabilization and *generous* fluid infusion help reduce risk of fat embolism. *Limit,* not encourage, limb motion. Frequently assess sensorium, cardiorespiratory status and relevant laboratory values and provide adequate support to splint fractures.

Childs, SA: Musculoskeletal Trauma. Crit Care Nurs Clin North Am *6(3): 483-489, 1994; Wallek, CA & Kenner, CV: Extremity Trauma in* Critical Care Nursing: Body-Mind-Spirit *(Dossey, BM, Guzzetta, CE & Kenner, CV, Eds). Philadelphia, Lippincott, pp. 804-805, 1992; Morgan, GE & Mikhail, MS:* Clinical Anesthesiology. *Norwalk, CT, Appleton & Lange, pp. 718-719, 1992.*

8.3. Correct Answer: **d**

Patients most likely to develop autonomic hyperreflexia (or dysreflexia) had complete spinal cord transection, usually above T-6, weeks, months or years ago. Evidence of autonomic hyperreflexia occurs after spinal shock from the initial injury has subsided. Spinal shock usually resolves within 10 days, but may last longer. Patients with long-term spinal cord injury often are well aware of their own signs of impending autonomic hyperreflexia.

Walleck, C: Patients with Spinal Cord Injury in Critical Care Nursing *(Clochesy, JM, Breu, C, Cardin, S, et al, Eds). Philadelphia, Saunders, pp. 748 & 761, 1992; Hawkins, JK & Hawkins, VC: Post Anesthesia Care of the Neurosurgical Patient in* The Post Anesthesia Care Unit: A Critical Care Approach to Post Anesthesia Nursing, *3rd ed (Drain, C, Ed). Philadelphia, Saunders, pp. 439-440, 1994.*

8.4. Correct Answer: **a**

Diabetes insipidus (DI) is treated by replacing the posterior pituitary hormone (antidiuretic hormone [ADH]) and fluid losses. ADH medications include vasopressin (Pitressin), or desmopressin (DDAVP), a synthetic ADH. DI represents ADH insufficiency and may transiently occur after intracranial trauma or pituitary removal (hypophysectomy).

Stock, MT: Pituitary Agents in Clinical Pharmacology and Nursing, *2nd ed (Baer, CL & Williams, BR, Eds). Springhouse, PA, Springhouse, pp. 890-895, 1992; Provenzano, SM: Head Injury in* Critical Care Nursing: A Holistic Approach, *6th ed (Hudak, CM & Gallo, BM, Eds). Philadelphia, Lippincott, pp. 710-712, 1994.*

8.5. Correct Answer: **d**

History of preoperative hypertension, whether documented or undiagnosed, is a prime contributing factor to postoperative hypertension. Hypertension is defined as a blood pressure greater than 160/90 or 20% more than baseline blood pressure. Approximately 80% of postoperative hypertensive events occur within 30 minutes of surgery and resolve within 3 hours. Postoperative hypertension may relate to increased catecholamine levels, cardiac output, or systemic vascular resistance. Unrelieved pain contributes to postoperative hypertension; providing analgesia may precede administration of antihypertensives in a patient with severe pain. Typically, hypertension abates as pain is managed and the patient relaxes; Ms P remains hypertensive despite her drowsiness.

Litwack, K: Post Anesthesia Complications: Respiratory, Cardiac, and Neurologic in ASPAN's Core Curriculum for Post Anesthesia Nursing Practice, *3rd ed (Litwack, K, Ed). Philadelphia, Saunders, pp. 206-209, 1994; Neely, CF: Cardiovascular Disease in* Dripps/Eckenhoff/Vandam Introduction to Anesthesia, *8th ed (Longnecker, DE & Murphy, FL, Eds). Philadelphia, Saunders, pp. 272-275, 1992.*

8.6. Correct Answer: **d**

Especially in patients with preexisting cardiac damage, any increased systemic vascular resistance and cardiac output associated with hypertension can produce damaging myocardial ischemia. Treat pain, anxiety, hypoxia, hypercarbia, and fluid volume excess before initiating antihypertensive therapy. Infarction, arrhythmias, congestive heart failure, cerebral hemorrhage, and bleeding or suture disruption at the surgical site are all possible consequences of untreated hypertension.

Neely, CF: Cardiovascular Disease in Dripps/Eckenhoff/Vandam Introduction to Anesthesia, *8th ed (Longnecker, DE & Murphy, FL, Eds). Philadelphia, Saunders, pp. 272-275, 1992; Marymont, JA & O'Conner, BS: Postoperative Cardiovascular Complications in* Post Anesthesia Care *(Vender, JE & Speiss, BD, Eds). Philadelphia, Saunders, pp. 25-29, 1992.*

8.7. Correct Answer: **b**

The interaction of epinephrine and tricyclic antidepressants like amitriptyline (Elavil) or phenelzine (Nardil), a monoamine oxidase inhibitor, can produce severe hypertension and tachycardia. These medications increase sympathetic storage of norepinephrine (NE). Giving sympathomimetic medications such as epinephrine can release stored NE and produce unpredictable and exaggerated adrenergic responses.

Skoog, RE: Monoamine Oxidase Inhibitors: Pharmacology and Implications in the Perioperative Period. J Post Anesth Nurs *4(4): 264-267, 1989; Edwards, MW: Premedication in* Dripps/Eckenhoff/Vandam Introduction to Anesthesia, *8th ed. (Longnecker, DE & Murphy, FL, Eds). Philadelphia, Saunders, pp. 38-39, 1992.*

8.8. Correct Answer: **a**

Some clinicians believe the size of the needle used to puncture the dura is the most important determinant of whether postdural puncture headache (PDPH) will occur. Very small gauge needles reduce potential for leakage of cerebrospinal fluid through the dural puncture. Specially designed needles split, not cut, fibers of the dura. PDPH typically occurs 1-5 days postoperatively, well after the ambulatory surgery (ASU) patient is discharged.

Kang, SB: Postanesthesia Nursing Care for Ambulatory Surgery Patients Post-Spinal Anesthesia. J Post Anesth Nurs *9(2): 101-106, 1994; Burden, N:* Ambulatory Surgical Nursing. *Philadelphia, Saunders, pp. 103-104 & 310-311, 1993.*

8.9. Correct Answer: **b**

Ability to control and empty the bladder and to stand without profound *hypo*tension indicates postspinal recovery of function of sacral nerves S-3 to S-5 and of sympathetic tone. Peripheral vasoconstriction and bladder control are the first functions to be blocked and the last to return. Return of movement and sensation (sympathetic block) after spinal anesthesia occurs in reverse from the order of loss. Requirements that a patient urinate before leaving Phase II vary among facilities; this expectation is recommended for specific situations, including spinal and epidural blocks.

Kang, SB: Postanesthesia Nursing Care for Ambulatory Surgery Patients Post-Spinal Anesthesia. J Post Anesth Nurs *9(2): 101-106, 1994; Burden, N:* Ambulatory Surgical Nursing. *Philadelphia, Saunders, p. 349, 1993.*

8.10. Correct Answer: **c**

Every patient has risk of nerve, soft tissue, and eye injury related to intraoperative position and anesthetic effects. Though he does have diabetes and perhaps some vascular compromise, this patient is relatively young and his surgery lasted less than 2 hours. He probably was in the supine position, which provides greatest safety. Long surgical procedures (more than 2 hours), obesity or extreme thinness, vascular impairment from diabetes or peripheral vascular disease, or movement-limiting problems like arthritis or artificial joints are most associated with damage to body tissue.

Litwack, K: Post Anesthesia Care Nursing, *2nd ed. St. Louis, Mosby, pp. 480-483, 1995; Walsh, J: Postop Effects of OR Positioning.* RN *56(2): 50-58, 1993.*

8.11. Correct Answer: **b**

Expect labile and exaggerated blood pressures after surgical manipulation of the carotid artery. Baroreceptors in a diseased carotid artery grew accustomed to adjusting blood pressure through a veil of plaque. Manipulation or removal of this plaque that coats the carotid artery's intima exposes pressure-sensitive baroreceptors to unfiltered pressure. Baroreceptors are primary feedback mechanisms that sense and alter blood pressure and blood flow. Theoretically true pressures can be temporarily "misinterpreted" and the neurological responses exaggerated.

Johnson, SM & Anderson, B: Carotid Endarterectomy: A Review. Crit Care Clin North Am *3(3): 499-505, 1991; Lowdon, JC & Isaacson, IJ: Postoperative Considerations After Major Vascular Surgery in* Post Anesthesia Care *(Vender, JS & Speiss, BD, Eds). Philadelphia, Saunders, pp. 120-124, 1993.*

8.12. Correct Answer: **d**

The trigeminal nerve (cranial nerve V) moves the jaw and provides sensation to the face, scalp, cornea and interior nose and mouth. Following cerebellar tumors or resection of acoustic neuroma, one postoperative assessment is determining proper motor function of jaw muscles.

Mitchell, PH: Neurological Data Acquisition in AACN's Clinical Reference for Critical-Care Nursing *(Kinney, MR, Packa, DR & Dunbar, SB, Eds). St. Louis, Mosby, pp. 781-792, 1993; Stupple, L: Brain Tumors in* The Clinical Practice of Neurological and Neurosurgical Nursing, *3rd ed (Hickey, JV, Ed). Philadelphia, Lippincott, p. 489, 1992.*

8.13. Correct Answer: **c**

Malignant hyperthermia (MH) appears more commonly in the 1-30 year age group, in all racial groups. Infants are seldom affected; boys and girls are equally susceptible until puberty, then men seem affected twice as often as adult women. MH rarely occurs in patients older than 50 years of age. Preexisting muscular diseases, history of anesthetic complications, intraoperative death of a relative or unexplained perioperative fever are "red flags" that alert health care providers to an MH susceptible patient.

Holtzclaw, B: Temperature Problems in the Post-Operative Period. Crit Care Nurs Clin North Am *2: 589-597, 1990; Murphy, FL: Hazards of Anesthesia in* Dripps/Eckenhoff/Vandam Introduction to Anesthesia, *8th ed (Longnecker, DE & Murphy, FL, Eds). Philadelphia, Saunders, pp. 420-422, 1992.*

8.14. Correct Answer: **b**

Prior to *any* medication for his restlessness, this patient must be assessed for contributing reasons. Hypoxia and pain are suspect causes and must be addressed before administering a sedative. Midazolam is a highly potent benzodiazepine that quickly causes respiratory depression and hemodynamic alterations. A 3 mg intravenous dose is too large and must be questioned. Elderly, frail, or debilitated patients or children or patients who have received narcotics receive one-half to two-thirds dose reductions. The nurse slowly titrates incremental 0.5-1 mg midazolam doses to clinical effect.

Product literature: Versed. Nutley, NJ, Hoffmann-La Roche, 1993; Burden, N: Ambulatory Surgical Nursing. *Philadelphia, Saunders, pp. 244-245, 1993.*

8.15. Correct Answer: **a**

Sympathetic block occurs when local anesthetic medication acts on spinal nerves to prevent vasoconstriction below the level of injection. The size of the vascular compartment expands for the duration of the block's effect, particularly above the T-10 dermatome. Filling this compartment with additional intravenous fluid minimizes or prevents significant hypotension.

Kang, SB: Postanesthesia Nursing Care for Ambulatory Surgery Patients Post-Spinal Anesthesia. J Post Anesth Nurs *9(2): 101-106, 1994; Burden, N:* Ambulatory Surgical Nursing. *Philadelphia, Saunders, pp. 103-104 & 310-311, 1993.*

8.16. Correct Answer: **c**

Gentamicin (and other "mycin" antibiotics) affect the neuromuscular junction. These medications can increase muscle weakness by reversing the cholinergic effects of the anticholinesterase (pyridostigmine) used to treat Ms N's myasthenia gravis. Neostigmine is sometimes used during acute illness to manage myasthenia symptoms. Narcotics and sedatives may have exaggerated effects, so doses should be reduced. Myasthenia gravis gradually destroys acetylcholine receptors.

Burden, N: Ambulatory Surgical Nursing. *Philadelphia, Saunders, pp. 281, 1993; Lazear, SE: Neuromuscular Disorders in* Critical Care Nursing, *2nd ed (Vazquez, M, Lazear, SE & Larson, EL, Eds). Philadelphia, Saunders, pp. 198-202, 1992.*

8.17. Correct Answer: **d**

Inadequate amounts of anticholinesterase medication in the system produce myasthenic crisis. Symptoms include progressive respiratory failure, ptosis, increased secretions and hypertension. Absence of nausea, diarrhea, miosis and bradycardia distinguish myasthenic crisis from its opposite, cholinergic crisis. In the PACU, a myasthenia gravis patient could develop increasing muscle weakness when anticholinesterases are withheld or as an effect of neuromuscular blocking medications. Both produce anticholinesterase deficiency.

Drain, C: Post Anesthesia Care Nursing: A Critical Care Approach to Post Anesthesia Nursing, *3rd ed. Philadelphia, Saunders, pp. 521-522, 1994; Lazear, SE: Neuromuscular Disorders in* Critical Care Nursing, *2nd ed (Vazquez, M, Lazear, SE & Larson, EL, Eds). Philadelphia, Saunders, pp. 198-202, 1992.*

8.18. Correct Answer: **b**

Hypertension, edema, distended neck veins or increased central venous pressure and a heart gallop indicated by an S_3 sound suggest fluid volume excess. Temporarily, Mr. Y's intravascular space increased due to moderate blood loss and vasodilation from spinal anesthetic. The space was filled intraoperatively with blood, colloid and crystalloid. As the spinal effect recedes and capacity of arterioles to vasoconstrict returns postoperatively, this increased total body volume circulates through a smaller space—and overloads the cardiovascular system.

Silinsky, J: The Hematologic System in ASPAN's Core Curriculum for Post Anesthesia Nursing Practice, *3rd ed (Litwack, K, Ed). Philadelphia, Saunders, p. 196, 1994; Tuman, KJ: Fluid and Electrolytes Abnormalities and Management in* Post Anesthesia Care *(Vender, JS & Speiss, BD, Eds). Philadelphia, Saunders, pp. 160 & 167-169, 1992.*

8.19. Correct Answer: **a**

Fever and chills, nausea and chest or flank pain occur early during a transfusion as the patient's antibodies destroy incompatible red blood cells in the transfused blood. An acute hemolytic reaction is due to ABO-type incompatibility between the blood donor's red blood cell antigens and the recipient's antibodies. Blood-fluid incompatibility or sepsis from blood contamination also causes hemolysis. ABO incompatibility produces severe symptoms of hypotension with tachycardia, renal failure and disseminated intravascular coagulation (DIC).

Coffland, FI & Shelton, DM: Blood Component Replacement Therapy. Nurs Clin North Am *5(3): 543-556, 1993; Morgan, GE & Mikhail, MS:* Clinical Anesthesiology. *Norwalk, CT, Appleton & Lange, pp. 484-486, 1992.*

8.20. Correct Answer: **d**

A postoperative spinal surgery patient must avoid twisting and malalignment. The technique of "log rolling" assures spinal alignment, decreases spinal muscle spasms, and limits twisting of back while repositioning.

Shpritz, DW: The Neurosurgical Patient in ASPAN's Core Curriculum for Post Anesthesia Nursing Practice, *3rd ed (Litwack, K, Ed). Philadelphia, Saunders, pp. 386-392, 1994; Partyka, MB: Practical Points in the Care of the Post-Lumbar Spine Surgery Patient.* J Post Anesth Nurs *6(3): 185-187, 1991.*

8.21. Correct Answer: **a**

Blood is highly irritating to neural tissue and produces severe pain. Hematoma formation in the spine compresses nerves and augments neurologic deficits, decreasing sensation and increasing motor weakness below the hematoma. Though most primary spinal tumors are benign, resecting an intramedullary tumor (one that develops within the spinal cord) is technically difficult and can damage nerve structures.

Shpritz, DW: The Neurosurgical Patient in ASPAN's Core Curriculum for Post Anesthesia Nursing Practice, *3rd ed (Litwack, K, Ed). Philadelphia, Saunders, pp. 387-392, 1994; Hawkins, J & Hawkins, VC: Post Anesthesia Care of the Neurosurgical Patient in* The Post Anesthesia Care Unit: A Critical Care Approach to Post Anesthesia Nursing, *3rd ed (Drain, C, Ed). Philadelphia, Saunders, p. 442, 1994.*

8.22. Correct Answer: **c**

Bupivacaine and tetracaine are long-acting local anesthetics, though bupivacaine's effect generally lasts about 2-4 hours and tetracaine's duration is about 1.5-3 hours. Chemical structure, dose and lipid solubility alter duration. Injected volume and concentration of the anesthetic solution determine the dose. Procaine 10% is a low-potency, short-acting medication with less than 60 minutes' effect. A lidocaine 5% solution has a moderate duration of action, approximately 60 minutes. Diluting a local anesthetic medication in dextrose increases its density relative to cerebrospinal fluid (CSF); adding dextrose helps extend the drug's spread across dermatomes but does not alter the block's duration. Adding a narcotic provides postoperative analgesia but does not lengthen motor and sensory block.

Covino, BG & Lambert, DH: Management of Anesthesia in Clinical Anesthesia, *2nd ed (Barash, PG, Cullen, BE, Stoelting, RK, Eds). Philadelphia, Lippincott, pp. 828-829, 1992; Drain, C:* The Post Anesthesia Care Unit: A Critical Care Approach to Post Anesthesia Nursing, *3rd ed. Philadelphia, Saunders, pp. 247-249 & 252-253, 1994; Brown, DL:* Atlas of Regional Anesthesia. *Philadelphia, Saunders, pp. 5-7, 1992.*

8.23. Correct Answer: **a**

Epinephrine or phenylephrine added to a local anesthetic solution prolongs the duration of effect. Anesthesia could continue up to 50% longer. Vasoconstriction and delayed elimination of medication mean neural tissue has contact with the local anesthetic medication for a longer time. Longer contact extends the effect.

Covino, BG & Lambert, DH: Management of Anesthesia in Clinical Anesthesia, *2nd ed (Barash, PG, Cullen, BE, Stoelting, RK, Eds). Philadelphia, Lippincott, pp. 828-829, 1992; Litwack, K:* Post Anesthesia Care Nursing, *2nd ed. St. Louis, Mosby, pp. 157-158, 1995.*

8.24. Correct Answer: **d**

Distribution of anesthetic block (spread) is influenced by the patient's position and the density (weight or baricity) of the solution. *Gravity* greatly affects movement of local anesthetic in spinal fluid. A patient who remains in a sitting position for 5-10 minutes after insertion of medication has a more localized block than the patient who is immediately placed in a supine position so the medication can spread to affect several dermatomes. Anesthetic *density* is influenced by the diluting solution. Hyperbaric solutions diluted in dextrose extend the block; isobaric solutions in saline affect only a small area.

Drain, C: The Post Anesthesia Care Unit: A Critical Care Approach to Post Anesthesia Nursing, *3rd ed. Philadelphia, Saunders, pp. 252-253, 1994; Riegler, FX: Spinal and Epidural Anesthesia in* Dripps/Eckenhoff/Vandam Introduction to Anesthesia, *8th ed (Longnecker, DE & Murphy, FL, Eds). Philadelphia, Saunders, pp. 216-220, 1992.*

8.25. Correct Answer: **b**

Hypotension is a likely consequence of spinal blockade due to the anesthetic's vasodilating effects and paralysis of neurovascular response. Vasodilation increases the vascular space; circulating blood volume is suddenly insufficient in this enlarged compartment. Blocked peripheral blood vessels cannot constrict in response to decreased blood pressure. Thus increasing fluid volume, assuring tissue oxygenation, and maintaining cerebral blood flow with a head-low position are appropriate.

Litwack, K: Post Anesthesia Care Nursing, *2nd ed. St. Louis, Mosby, pp. 172-175, 1995; Drain, C:* The Post Anesthesia Care Unit: A Critical Care Approach to Post Anesthesia Nursing, *3rd ed. Philadelphia, Saunders, pp. 253-255, 1994.*

8.26. Correct Answer: **b**

A patient who can lift a knee from the bed surface has regained motor function to approximately the L-2 or L-3 dermatome. Ability to plantar flex toes indicates the block has receded to the S-1 to S-2 dermatomes. Risk of hypotension is high when blockade is at the T-5 dermatome and significantly decreases with block resolution to the level of the umbilicus (T-10).

Riegler, FX: Spinal and Epidural Anesthesia in Dripps/Eckenhoff/Vandam Introduction to Anesthesia, *8th ed (Longnecker, DE & Murphy, FL, Eds). Philadelphia, Saunders, pp. 216-220, 1992; Burden, N:* Ambulatory Surgical Nursing. *Philadelphia, Saunders, pp. 101-106, 1993.*

8.27. Correct Answer: **c**

As spinal anesthetic blockade resolves, motor function generally returns before either sensory function or sympathetic tone. Usually neurofunction returns in the reverse order from blockade. Evidence of sympathetic blockade can continue after both motor and sensory functions return. Sympathetic block causes vasodilation; symptoms are related to hypotension and the relative fluid volume deficit vasodilation creates. The nurse tests Mr. J's sensory block by assessing the patient's perception of cold, pinprick, or touch.

Litwack, K: Post Anesthesia Care Nursing, *2nd ed. St. Louis, Mosby, pp. 172-177, 1995; Riegler, FX: Spinal and Epidural Anesthesia in* Dripps/Eckenhoff/Vandam Introduction to Anesthesia, *8th ed (Longnecker, DE & Murphy, FL, Eds). Philadelphia, Saunders, p. 220, 1992.*

8.28. Correct Answer: **a**

Cholinergic receptors in the midbrain affect alertness. Acetylcholine is the designated transmitter for the "cholinergic arousal system" at the midbrain portion of the brain stem. Anticholinergic medications like scopolamine and atropine therefore affect arousal.

Sloan, TB: Postoperative Central Nervous System Dysfunction in Post Anesthesia Care *(Vender, JE & Speiss, BD, Eds). Philadelphia, Saunders, pp. 179-181, 1992; Stalheim-Smith, A & Fitch, GK:* Understanding Human Anatomy and Physiology. *Minneapolis/St. Paul, West Publishing, p. 409, 1994.*

8.29. Correct Answer: **b**

Sudden and intense headache, neck pain or stiffness, and nausea with vomiting are classic indicators of subarachnoid bleeding. Seizures, visual impairment, confusion, disorientation or complete loss of consciousness may coincide. This patient has high risk for a subarachnoid hemorrhage; his already leaking aneurysm can spontaneously rupture at any time, filling the subarachnoid space with blood. The brain loses its autoregulatory ability and cerebral perfusion pressure plummets as intracranial pressure rapidly increases. Hemorrhage may spread through subarachnoid fluid and compress intracranial structures, producing other neurologic deficits.

Whitney-Rainbolt, CM: Patients with Cerebral Vascular Disorders in Critical Care Nursing *(Clochesy, JM, Breu, C, Cardin, S, et al, Eds). Philadelphia, Saunders, pp. 718-721, 1992.*

8.30. Correct Answer: **b**

Place the patch on a flat area of the upper torso after a *water* wash and *clipping* body hair. Heat and skin nicks increase absorption of any transdermal drug.

Do not scrub or shave hair. Patients often need premedication with intravenous medication before the fentanyl patch has effect; however, a 3 ml (150 mcg) single dose of IV fentanyl is excessive

and likely will alter consciousness and breathing.

Willens, JS: Giving Fentanyl for Pain Outside the OR. Am J Nurs *94(2): 24-28, 1994.*

SET II

Answer Key

8.31. c
8.32. b
8.33. a
8.34. d
8.35. b
8.36. c
8.37. a
8.38. c
8.39. a
8.40. b
8.41. b
8.42. c
8.43. b
8.44. a
8.45. a
8.46. d
8.47. b
8.48. c
8.49. d
8.50. c
8.51. d
8.52. a
8.53. c
8.54. d
8.55. c
8.56. a
8.57. c
8.58. d
8.59. b
8.60. d

SET II

Rationales and References

8.31. Correct Answer: **c**

A drowsy patient who rouses to follow simple commands when stimulated is *lethargic*. An *awake* patient becomes fully oriented and appropriate when stimulated, whereas a *stuporous* patient is very difficult to rouse and only with strong stimuli. Descriptions of nursing observations are best to describe a patient's level of consciousness, as any distinctions among these states are subjective.

Hawkins, JK & Hawkins, VC: Post Anesthesia Care of the Neurosurgical Patient in The Post Anesthesia Care Unit: A Critical Care Approach to Post Anesthesia Nursing, *3rd ed (Drain, C, Ed). Philadelphia, Saunders, p. 425, 1994; Provenzano, SM: Assessment: Nervous System in* Critical Care Nursing: A Holistic Approach, *6th ed (Hudak, CM & Gallo, BM, Eds). Philadelphia, Lippincott, pp. 651-652, 1994.*

8.32. Correct Answer: **b**

Hypocarbia is desirable to help reduce cerebral blood flow and intracranial volume, thereby minimizing intracranial pressure fluctuations. Mr. Q's postoperative drowsiness and suppressed level of consciousness can represent residual effects of anesthetic medications or physiologic imbalances like hypothermia, inadequate ventilation with hypoxemia and hypercarbia, or an acid base, chemical (hypoglycemia) or electrolyte imbalance. Especially in the immediate postanesthesia period, these factors must be considered while evaluating the possibility of increased intracranial pressure related to neurologic damage.

Hawkins, JK & Hawkins, VC: Post Anesthesia Care of the Neurosurgical Patient in The Post Anesthesia Care Unit: A Critical Care Approach to Post Anesthesia Nursing, *3rd ed (Drain, C, Ed). Philadelphia, Saunders, p. 425, 1994; Kenner, CV: Neurologic Assessment in* Critical Care Nursing; Body-Mind-Spirit *(Dossey, BM, Guzzetta, CE & Kenner, CV, Eds). Philadelphia, Lippincott, p. 541, 1992.*

8.33. Correct Answer: **a**

Reporting to the neurosurgeon Mr. G's decrease in sensorium from lethargic to stuporous is appropriate—and essential. Even a subtle alteration in level of consciousness, the "most sensitive indicator of neurologic function," is one early clue of intracranial changes. Neurologic changes occur quickly, within 15 minutes. Signs indicating intracranial pressure increases progress in a rostral (top) to caudal (down) direction within the brain, or from cerebrum to brain stem. Therefore brain stem signs like respiratory and pupillary changes suggest that either early changes were undetected or intracranial hypertension occurred quickly. Respiratory depression, perhaps from renarcotization, is another possible reason for Mr. Q's lethargy, though the suggested naloxone dose (0.8 mg) is excessive. Naloxone is more appropriately titrated in small increments to Mr. Q's level of response to avoid treatment-related intracranial pressure increases.

Shpritz, DW: The Neurosurgical Patient in ASPAN's Core Curriculum for Post Anesthesia Nursing Practice, *3rd ed (Litwack, K, Ed). Philadelphia, Saunders, pp. 347-348, 1994; Mitchell, PH: Neurological Disorders in* AACN's Clinical Reference for Critical-Care Nursing, *(Kinney, MR, Packa, DR & Dunbar, SB, Eds). St. Louis, Mosby, pp. 815-817, 1993.*

8.34. Correct Answer: **d**

Mr. Q has observable responses only to an unpleasant (noxious) stimulus. The Glasgow Coma Scale is a widely accepted and objective assessment tool used to document trends in several neurologic functions. Applying this scale, Mr. Q's best eye opening response occurs only *to pain;* his best verbal response is *no sound* (mute); and his best motor response is left arm *flexion.* These responses are each assessed when Mr. Q is considered maximally stimulated by voice, touch or painful stimulus. Both left- and right-sided responses are scored. His right-sided responses are scored in a similar manner and his pupil size and reactions to light are documented. His overall Glascow Coma Scale score is 6.

Kenner, CV: Neurologic Assessment in Critical Care Nursing: Body-Mind-Spirit *(Dossey, BM, Guzzetta, CE & Kenner, CV, Eds). Philadelphia, Lippincott, p. 541, 1992; Mitchell, PH: Neurological Disorders in* AACN's Clinical Reference for Critical-Care Nursing *(Kinney, MR, Packa, DR & Dunbar, SB, Eds). St. Louis, Mosby, pp. 815-817, 1993.*

8.35. Correct Answer: **b**

Pressure pain to the toe, fingernails, or knuckles is a legitimate assessment technique; strong pinches or tissue twisting, direct eyeball pressure, and breast or genital touch are not. A multiinstitution study of motor responses to painful stimuli yielded the most consistent responses when pressure was applied to the nailbed. A painful, noxious stimulus may elicit a physical response or increase awareness of a patient with decreased level of consciousness. Mr. Q's skin must be protected from bruises, abrasions or breaks in integrity. Pressure may be applied to the area *above* the eye (supraorbital ridge).

Provenzano, SM: Assessment: Nervous System in Critical Care Nursing: A Holistic Approach, *6th ed (Hudak, CM & Gallo, BM, Eds). Philadelphia, Lippincott, p. 652, 1994.*

8.36. Correct Answer: **c**

Mr. Q's response to pain is *decortication,* indicated interrupted corticospinal pathways with a "functional disconnection" of inhibiting impulses. A lesion or pressure affects neurofunction at the level of the cerebrum or thalamus. Greater deterioration to the midbrain or pons level produces decerebration with rigid extension of all extremities.

Litwack, K: Post Anesthesia Care Nursing, *2nd ed. St. Louis, Mosby, pp. 236-237, 1995; Shpritz, DW: The Neurosurgical Patient in* ASPAN's Core Curriculum for Post Anesthesia Nursing Practice, *3rd ed (Litwack, K, Ed). Philadelphia, Saunders, pp. 348-349, 1994.*

8.37. Correct Answer: **a**

Mr. Q's symptoms indicate a dire emergency to prevent herniation of brain tissue into linings of the cranial cavity. Compensatory adaptations that adjust CSF and blood flow (autoregulation) have been exhausted. The closed cranial cavity cannot expand to accommodate long-term increases in brain tissue, CSF volume or blood flow. Compression of intracranial structures occurs instead—until the pressure exceeds cranial capacity and contents push through the most available, least resistant opening.

Mitchell, PH: Neurological Disorders in AACN's Clinical Reference for Critical-Care Nursing, *(Kinney, MR, Packa, DR & Dunbar, SB, Eds). St. Louis, Mosby, pp. 805-820, 1993; Hawkins, JK & Hawkins, VC: Post Anesthesia Care of the Neurosurgical Patient in* The Post Anesthesia Care Unit: A Critical Care Approach to Post Anesthesia Nursing, *3rd ed (Drain, C, Ed). Philadelphia, Saunders, pp. 416-420, 1994.*

8.38. Correct Answer: **c**

A lesion or increased pressure predominately in the *left* cerebral hemisphere will produce same-sided, or *ipsilateral,* changes in the *left* pupil. Right-sided cranial lesions likely affect the right pupil. Cranial nerve III nuclei responsible for controlling pupil size are located in the brain stem. By the time pupillary changes occur, pressure from herniating brain structures has already compressed cranial nerve III and prevented constriction, so pupils become unequal (anisocoria). When observed in the less than alert patient, particularly one with documented trauma or intracranial lesion, one dilated, or "blown," pupil is a true neurologic emergency.

Provenzano, SM: Assessment: Nervous System in Critical Care Nursing: A Holistic Approach, *6th ed (Hudak, CM & Gallo, BM, Eds). Philadelphia, Lippincott, p. 656-661, 1994. Shpritz, DW: The Neurosurgical Patient in* ASPAN's Core Curriculum for Post Anesthesia Nursing Practice, *3rd ed (Litwack, K, Ed). Philadelphia, Saunders, pp. 341-343, 1994.*

8.39. Correct Answer: **a**

Decreasing pCO_2 to 21-25 mm Hg by manually hyperventilating Mr. Q after reintubation reduces blood flow and may prevent further rises in intracranial pressure (ICP). Immediate CT scanning may pinpoint intracranial bleeding for a likely surgical reexploration. Subdural veins bleed quickly and cause acute hematoma, compression of intracranial contents and potential for rapid herniation. Meanwhile, mannitol or urea may temporarily decrease ICP. Suctioning, stir-up activities and positions that increase cerebral blood flow (flat) or flex the neck further stress labile patients who have limited intracranial adaptive reserves.

Mitchell, PH: Neurological Disorders in AACN's Clinical Reference for Critical-Care Nursing *(Kinney, MR, Packa, DR & Dunbar, SB, Eds). St. Louis, Mosby, pp. 824 & 805-820, 1993; Morgan, GE & Mikhail, MS:* Clinical Anesthesiology. *Norwalk, CT, Appleton & Lange, pp. 431-434, 1992.*

8.40. Correct Answer: **b**

Dexamethasone (Decadron) may decrease edema in cerebral tissues, thereby reducing the intracranial volume. Tissue edema occurs with surgical manipulation. The adaptive capacity that compensates for shifting blood flow, cerebrospinal fluid volume and brain tissue mass may improve. This medication is a synthetic adrenocorticoid with a long duration of effect.

Broderson, JM: Surgical Options for Brain Tumor Treatment. Crit Care Nurs Clin North Am. *7(1): 95, 1995; Smith, RN: Management Modalities: Nervous System in* Critical Care Nursing: A Holistic Approach, *6th ed (Hudak, CM & Gallo, BM, Eds). Philadelphia, Lippincott, p. 675-676 & 685, 1994.*

8.41. Correct Answer: **b**

Respiratory depression often follows pain relief with fentanyl. Kappa receptor stimulation produces constricted, pinpoint-sized pupils. Fentanyl is a highly potent opioid agonist with mu receptor effects that are similar to morphine. Fentanyl is approximately 100 times more potent than morphine, acts quickly (within 5 minutes) and provides analgesia of moderate duration. Patients who receive high doses of fentanyl may develop a second, delayed effect when stored fentanyl is released back into the circulation. This "delayed-onset respiratory depression" occurs after initial depressant and analgesic effects have abated and the patient is awake.

Drain, C: The Post Anesthesia Care Unit: A Critical Care Approach to Post Anesthesia Nursing, *3rd ed. Philadelphia, Saunders, pp. 217-218, 1994; Shannon, MT, Wilson, BA & Stang, CL:* Govoni & Hayes Drugs and Nursing Implications, *8th ed. Norwalk, CT, Appleton & Lange, pp. 515-516, 1995.*

8.42. Correct Answer: **c**

This patient needs adequate arm support so that his fingers are elevated above his heart level to promote venous return. Ideally this position also promotes comfort. After replantation of an amputated body part, medical and nursing goals focus on promoting circulation and decreasing any factors that vasoconstrict. Frequent neurovascular assessment is critical to quickly detect any circulatory compromise. The surgeon may request temperature monitoring or pulse detection to monitor blood flow. Warmth and adequate hydration promote blood flow. Analgesics promote comfort and interrupt the physiologic stress response that also produces peripheral vasoconstriction.

Kull, L: The Orthopedic Surgical Patient in ASPAN's Core Curriculum for Post Anesthsia Nursing Practice, *3rd ed (Litwack, K, Ed). Philadelphia, Saunders, pp. 531-532, 1994.*

8.43. Correct Answer: **b**

The reticular activating system (RAS) originates at the midbrain in an organized group of functional neurons, the reticular formation. Axons extend upward through to the thalamus and cortex to bring cerebral awareness of sensory and chemical input from environmental stimuli to conscious attention. The RAS is sensitive to depression by medication, hypoxia- or hypoglycemia-induced metabolic alterations, and even small changes in brain stem pressure.

Mitchell, PH: Neurological Anatomy and Physiology in

AACN's Clinical Reference for Critical-Care Nursing *(Kinney, MR, Packa, DR & Dunbar, SB, Eds). St. Louis, Mosby, pp. 758-761, 1993.*

8.44. Correct Answer: **a**

The corpus callosum is a band of transverse nerve fibers that link symmetrical portions of the left and right cerebral cortex. The longitudinal fissure separates cortical hemispheres, and the central sulcus is the fissure separating the parietal and frontal lobes.

Shpritz, DW: The Neurosurgical Patient in ASPAN's Core Curriculum for Post Anesthesia Nursing Practice, *3rd ed (Litwack, K, Ed). Philadelphia, Saunders, pp. 339-340, 1994.*

8.45. Correct Answer: **a**

Hypoglycemia, a measured glucose of less than 50 mg/dl, can cause irreversible damage to the nervous system. Preoperative fasting, symptom-masking sedative and anesthetic medications, excessive insulin doses and renal failure (a likelihood for the over 30 year old insulin-dependent patient) can mask recognition and prevent treatment of low glucose levels.

Drain, C: The Post Anesthesia Care Unit: A Critical Care Approach to Post Anesthesia Nursing, *3rd ed. Philadelphia, Saunders, pp. 522-523, 1994; Kraft, SA, Mihm, FG & Feeley, TW: Postoperative Endocrine Problems in* Post Anesthesia Care *(Vender, JS & Speiss, BD, Eds). Philadelphia, Saunders, pp. 216-222, 1992.*

8.46. Correct Answer: **d**

Mannitol is an osmotic diuretic that increases the serum osmolarity. Solute or particle concentration is then greater in circulating blood than in tissue, creating a pressure disparity. Mannitol is a "staple" medication in neurosurgery; the osmotic pressure gradient pulls water from intracellular (brain) tissue into the vascular compartment for excretion through the kidneys. Reducing cerebral edema decreases intracranial pressure.

Shannon, MT, Wilson, BA & Stang, CL: Govoni & Hayes Drugs and Nursing Implications, *8th ed. Norwalk, CT, Appleton & Lange, pp. 708-709, 1995; Morgan, GE & Mikhail, MS:* Clinical Anesthesiology. *Norwalk, CT, Appleton & Lange, pp. 431-434, 1992.*

8.47. Correct Answer: **b**

A single dose of epidural morphine (Duramorph) can depress respirations early, within the first hour or two after injection, and again several hours later. Ms R's greatest hypoventilation risk continues for another 8-12 hours (up to 16 hours after injection). Morphine spreads slowly and gradually up (cephalad) through the cerebrospinal fluid, eventually reaching the brain's respiratory centers. This migration is termed *rostral spread.* Protocols for postepidural monitoring often recommend close consciousness and respiratory observation for up to 24 hours. Fentanyl is sometimes used as an epidural analgesic because its clearance from the body is more rapid, with less opportunity for spread through CSF to alter ventilation.

Drain, C: The Post Anesthesia Care Unit: A Critical Care Approach to Post Anesthesia Nursing, *3rd ed. Philadelphia, Saunders, pp. 255-256, 1994; Litwack,*

K: Post Anesthesia Care Nursing, *2nd ed. St. Louis, Mosby, pp. 167-172 & 509-517, 1995.*

8.48. Correct Answer: **c**

Alterations or pressure changes in the *left* side of the brain alter motor function *contralaterally,* or on the body's *right* side. Likewise, trauma or pressure changes in the right side of the brain alter left-sided movement. Anatomically, cortical fibers cross (decussate) below the brain stem to form the lateral corticospinal tract. These pyramidal tracts descend from the cerebral cortex to control voluntary movement of muscle groups on the opposite side. Ascending spinothalamic tracts relay sensory information through the spinal cord to the thalamus.

Provenzano, SM: Assessment: Nervous System in Critical Care Nursing: A Holistic Approach, *6th ed (Hudak, CM & Gallo, BM, Eds). Philadelphia, Lippincott, p. 661, 1994; Mitchell, PH: Neurological Anatomy and Physiology in* AACN's Clinical Reference for Critical-Care Nursing *(Kinney, MR, Packa, DR & Dunbar, SB, Eds). St. Louis, Mosby, pp. 757-762, 1993.*

8.49. Correct Answer: **d**

Observing single, dilated pupil in this young patient likely reflects brain edema or rebleeding at the surgical site that displaces brain tissue. First, though, the nurse should distinguish new anisocoria (unequal pupils) from a pupil that is dilated from a congenital condition, from medications or from prior eye surgery. Document pupil status, prior eye surgery, and use of mydriatic (dilating) ocular medications preoperatively to provide an important postoperative reference. Uncal displacement, the movement of part of the cerebrum's temporal lobe through the tentorium, is the most common herniation syndrome. Brain compression has occurred and contents press on nuclei of cranial nerve III in the brain stem.

Shpritz, DW: The Neurosurgical Patient in ASPAN's Core Curriculum for Post Anesthesia Nursing Practice, *3rd ed (Litwack, K, Ed). Philadelphia, Saunders, pp. 352-353, 1994. Mitchell, M: Common Neurological Disorders in* Critical Care Nursing: A Holistic Approach, *6th ed (Hudak, CM & Gallo, BM, Eds). Philadelphia, Lippincott, pp. 739-748, 1994.*

8.50. Correct Answer: **c**

Mr. P's procedure was most likely performed while he was in the prone position. Specific attention assured that bony prominences were adequately padded and body weight did not unduly compress soft tissues. Eye abrasions, especially during turning, and inadvertent ear bending can cause damage. Body weight might rest against the rib cage and iliac crests, causing skin redness or open breaks in skin integrity during the hours of surgery. The nurse should document and report apparent injury and improvement in skin condition during the PACU stay.

Litwack, K: Post Anesthesia Care Nursing, *2nd ed. St. Louis, Mosby, pp. 488-490, 1995.*

8.51. Correct Answer: **d**

Supplemental doses of intravenous narcotics provide analgesia until concentrations of epidurally infused narcotics reach therapeutic levels. In this situation, small (2-3 mg) doses of IV morphine sulfate provide pain relief—within 7 minutes—while the pharmacy and nursing staff promptly ready the fentanyl solution and epidural infusion pump. As a single postoperative dose in PACU intravenous fentanyl 150 mcg and intramuscular morphine sulfate 15 mg are excessive.

Burden, N: Ambulatory Surgical Nursing. *Philadelphia, Saunders, pp. 294-298, 1993; Litwack, K:* Post Anesthesia Care Nursing, *2nd ed. St. Louis, Mosby, pp. 509-517, 1995.*

8.52. Correct Answer: **a**

Before any infusion is initiated, the epidural catheter *must* be gently aspirated to determine catheter contents; the PACU nurse must also document that catheter tubing is securely taped. Aspirating bloody fluid may reflect entry into the dura during spinal surgery or may signal catheter migration into an epidural blood vessel; a bolus of fentanyl could be inadvertently injected into the circulation. Easy aspiration of clear fluid may indicate catheter movement across the dura into the subarachnoid space to obtain cerebrospinal fluid. When sanctioned by state law, facility policy, and unit protocols, the nurse's responsibility includes pain and epidural catheter management. Whenever catheter movement is suspected or unexpected fluid is aspirated, the anesthesia provider must be informed and the infusion deferred.

American Society of Post Anesthesia Nurses (ASPAN): Standards for Perianesthesia Nursing Practice, Resource 13. Thorofare, NJ, 1995; Wild, L & Coyne, C: The Basics and Beyond. Am J Nurs *92(4): 26-36, 1992.*

8.53. Correct Answer: **c**

A purely *narcotic* epidural solution that contains no local anesthetic seldom causes profound hypotension. Narcotics do not directly block sympathetic fibers that control vascular constriction and dilation. Over time, a moderate blood pressure decrease may reflect increased comfort. Potential for respiratory depression must be a primary concern during continuous narcotic infusion as fentanyl circulates and affects the brain's respiratory center. Nausea, itching and urinary retention are also common. Ms A should be able to move her legs; sensory or motor loss is unlikely with a purely narcotic infusion.

Litwack, K: Post Anesthesia Care Nursing, *2nd ed. St. Louis, Mosby, pp. 167-172, 1995; Wild, L & Coyne, C: The Basics and Beyond.* Am J Nurs *92(4): 26-36, 1992.*

8.54. Correct Answer: **d**

Transfer from PACU should be delayed pending further nursing observation and notification and evaluation by the physician. These symptoms are new and raise concern. Severe pain unrelated to the surgical site or incision is significant and requires further investigation. Backache and neurologic changes may result from epidural hematoma; thrombosis in an abdominal artery can produce weakness and buttock or leg pain.

Burden, N: Ambulatory Surgical Nursing. *Philadelphia, Saunders, pp. 104-105, 1993; Cohen, MS: Continuous Epidural Infusions of Acute Postoperative Pain: Part III.* Curr Rev PACN *11(12): 97-104, 1989.*

8.55. Correct Answer: **c**

In this young and healthy patient, prolonged muscle relaxation probably results from atypical pseudocholinesterase, a genetically determined inability to metabolize succinylcholine. Pseudocholines-terase may be deficient in either amount or effectiveness. The patient remains weak, and vigilant nursing observation and possibly respiratory support will be necessary until succinylcholine's effects naturally dissipate. Pseudocholinesterase deficiency can also be acquired. Normally the enzyme pseudocholinesterase rapidly destroys succinylcholine, the depolarizing muscle relaxant, in the plasma.

Litwack, K: Post Anesthesia Care Nursing, *2nd ed. St. Louis, Mosby, pp. 144-145, 1995; Fisher, DM: Muscle Relaxants in* Dripps/Eckenhoff/Vandam Introduction to Anesthesia, *8th ed (Longnecker, DE & Murphy, FL, Eds). Philadelphia, Saunders, pp. 113-114, 1992.*

8.56. Correct Answer: **a**

Wound drainage in PACU is generally minimal after shoulder reconstruction and less than 150 ml/8 hours. The patient's arm often is immobilized in a sling to maintain an adducted, internal rotation. Capillary refill should be within 2-3 seconds, indicating neither venous congestion or compromised blood flow. Finger movement indicates intact motor function, fine coordination and ability to discern position of other fingers. Extremity reassessment should occur hourly in PACU.

Kull, L: The Orthopedic Surgical Patient in ASPAN's Core Curriculum for Post Anesthesia Nursing Practice, *3rd ed (Litwack, K, Ed). Philadelphia, Saunders, pp. 513-514 & 528, 1994.*

8.57. Correct Answer: **c**

Rapid development of Ms D's symptoms strongly suggests local anesthetic toxicity, which quickly penetrates the blood-brain barrier to produce dizziness, tingling, and tinnitus. Toxic effects may soon result in muscle twitching, tremors and generalized seizure. Depending upon the amount of circulating local anesthetic, vasodilation, hypotension, and delayed intracardiac conduction could also occur with toxicity; providing adrenergic antagonism with labetalol is probably unnecessary. Significance of Ms D's symptoms is determined by the dose of local anesthetic absorbed. Oxygen, close nursing observation and physican notification are primary first interventions. The toxicity occurs when a local anesthetic rapidly enters the circulation, either by rapid or unanticipated injection.

Litwack, K: Post Anesthesia Care Nursing, *2nd ed. St. Louis, Mosby, pp. 158-161, 1995.*

8.58. Correct Answer: **d**

Adequate capillary refill (within 3 seconds) and skin color indicate the circulatory status in Ms D's casted extremity. Though after 6 hours, Ms D's brachial plexus block has most likely resolved, return of motor and sensory function is not usually a discharge requirement after a regional block. Ms D must know how to protect her arm until these functions do return. Her discharge instructions will include use of her analgesic prescription and how to regularly assess her hand circulation.

Litwack, K: Post Anesthesia Care Nursing, *2nd ed. St. Louis, Mosby, p. 164, 1995; Burden, N:* Ambulatory Surgical Nursing.

Philadelphia, Saunders, pp. 344-350, 1993.

8.59. Correct Answer: **b**

Ms D's plaster cast will not dry for up to 24 hours and so is at risk for damage and deformity from dents, pressure, and hard surfaces. A deformed cast can increase pressure against her arm, compressing blood flow and impairing nerve and muscle function. Ice may help reduce pain and arm edema. Though her skin may itch, nothing should be inserted between the cast and her skin to prevent skin breaks and possible infection.

Kull, L: The Orthopedic Surgical Patient in ASPAN's Core Curriculum for Post Anesthesia Nursing Practice, *3rd ed (Litwack, K, Ed). Philadelphia, Saunders, pp. 518-519, 1994.*

8.60. Correct Answer: **d**

Ms D's cast may still feel warm as it dries, although the normal, initial "burning" sensation probably has abated; the exterior surface may now feel cool. She should report fever, unrelenting pain, and cast odor to her surgeon as indicators of possible infection or compartment syndrome. The purplish hand color may be bruising but could also indicate venous congestion and impaired circulation from a too tight cast. Always compare the right and left fingers, hands and arms for similarity in color, degree of swelling, temperature, pulses (if discernible), sensation, and capillary refill.

Kull, L: The Orthopedic Surgical Patient in ASPAN's Core Curriculum for Post Anesthesia Nursing Practice, *3rd ed (Litwack, K, Ed). Philadelphia, Saunders, pp. 518-519, 1994.*

SET III

Answer Key

8.61. d
8.62. c
8.63. a
8.64. b
8.65. b
8.66. a
8.67. b
8.68. a
8.69. a
8.70. c
8.71. c
8.72. b
8.73. c
8.74. d
8.75. d
8.76. a
8.77. a
8.78. c
8.79. c
8.80. b
8.81. c
8.82. d
8.83. b
8.84. b
8.85. a
8.86. c
8.87. d
8.88. a
8.89. b
8.90. b
8.91. c
8.92. d

SET III

Rationales and References

8.61. Correct Answer: **d**

The primary purpose of the occipital lobes is to receive and understand visual images. Specialized neurotissue in areas of the cerebral cortex have specific functions.

Shpritz, DW: The Neurosurgical Patient in ASPAN's Core Curriculum for Post Anesthesia Nursing Practice, *3rd ed (Litwack, K, Ed). Philadelphia, Saunders, p. 340, 1994.*

8.62. Correct Answer: **c**

Maintaining hip alignment is essential for Ms O. After repair of a fracture to the femoral neck, adduction, hip flexion, and often positioning on the operative side are specifically avoided. Ms O also still has spinal anesthetic effects and no motor control of her legs; the legs will naturally externally rotate and adduct. Limiting leg movement, securing an abduction pillow between her thighs, perhaps placing a trochanter roll next to the left thigh and maintaining a flat position without hip flexion promote hip safety. Ice may reduce swelling and pain. Avoid placing pillows behind Ms O's knees that could impair circulation and compress nerves; do observe for hip drainage that could seep from the dressing and pool beneath the patient.

Litwack, K: Post Anesthesia Care Nursing, *2nd ed. St. Louis, Mosby, pp. 251-253, 1995; Kull, L: The Orthopedic Surgical Patient in* ASPAN's Core Curriculum for Post Anesthesia Nursing Practice, *3rd ed (Litwack, K, Ed). Philadelphia, Saunders, pp. 518-519, 1994.*

8.63. Correct Answer: **a**

Ms S's ability to form the words to state her name indicate that she can speak. An intact left cortical hemisphere is essential to both spoken language and comprehension. The dominant frontal lobe area at the inferior portion of the third gyrus controls motor speech. Damage to this area renders the patient able to understand written and oral language but unable to produce words.

Mitchell, PH: Neurological Anatomy and Physiology in AACN's Clinical Reference for Critical-Care Nursing, *3rd ed (Kinney, MR, Packa, DR & Dunbar, SB, Eds). St. Louis, Mosby, pp. 760-761, 1993; Willis, WD: The Nervous System and Its Components in* Physiology, *3rd ed (Berne, RM & Levy, MN, Eds). St. Louis, Mosby, pp. 260-261, 1993.*

8.64. Correct Answer: **b**

A lesion at *Broca's area,* at the third convolution of the person's dominant frontal lobe (usually the left), impairs the ability to speak and causes motor (expressive) aphasia. Producing words is difficult even though muscles controlling the mouth move adequately and ability to understand remains intact. Understanding spoken words, assuming auditory capability is intact, is governed by Wernicke's area. Damage here produces sensory aphasia.

Mitchell, M: Anatomy and Physiology of the Nervous System in Critical Care Nursing: A Holistic Approach, *6th ed (Hudak, CM & Gallo, BM, Eds). Philadelphia,*

Lippincott, pp. 633-634, 1994; Stalheim-Smith, A & Fitch, GK: Understanding Human Anatomy and Physiology. *Minneapolis/St. Paul, West Publishing, p. 406, 1994.*

8.65. Correct Answer: **b**

Coordinated (conjugate) eye movements with no jerking (nystagmus) and with pupils that constrict briskly to light and simultaneously (consensually) indicate proper oculomotor function. Cranial nerves III (oculomotor), IV (trochlear), and VI (abducens) team to control optic function. Pupil size inequity, nonsymmetric pupillary response to light or extraocular movements can indicate extreme pressure on brain stem structures (midbrain and pons) that contain the nuclei of these cranial nerves. In the postcraniotomy patient, such unilateral changes are critical events.

Stalheim-Smith, A & Fitch, GK: Understanding Human Anatomy and Physiology. *Minneapolis/St. Paul, West Publishing, p. 431-436, 1994; Mitchell, PH: Neurological Anatomy and Physiology in* AACN's Clinical Reference for Critical-Care Nursing, *3rd ed (Kinney, MR, Packa, DR & Dunbar, SB, Eds). St. Louis, Mosby, pp. 782-787, 1993.*

8.66. Correct Answer: **a**

Upper arm muscle strength and tone is assessed when both arms are extended with palms facing up. Ms S's eyes are closed during assessment. Loss of strength causes a weak arm to rotate and begin to fall (termed "pronator drift"). Increasing intracranial pressure likely produces noticeable upper extremity weakness before the lower arm is affected. Therefore a traditional "squeeze my hand" command does not provide reliable information to detect small, early changes in the relationships among cerebral function and muscle control, strength and tone that occur long before consciousness changes. Even decerebrate patients can seem to squeeze a hand, though not to command.

Mitchell, PH: Neurological Anatomy and Physiology in AACN's Clinical Reference for Critical-Care Nursing, *3rd ed, (Kinney, MR, Packa, DR & Dunbar, SB, Eds). St. Louis, Mosby, pp. 816-821, 1993; Shpritz, DW: The Neurosurgical Patient in* ASPAN's Core Curriculum for Post Anesthesia Nursing Practice, *3rd ed (Litwack, K, Ed). Philadelphia, Saunders, pp. 347-350, 1994.*

8.67. Correct Answer: **b**

Capillaries in the choroid plexus of the lateral and third ventricles produce 500-600 ml of CSF each day. Osmotic pressure and active transport systems contribute to production. Subarachnoid spaces contain most (about 100 ml) of the approximately 140 ml of CSF continuously circulating through the brain's ventricular system and subarachnoid space.

Willis, WD: The Nervous System and Its Components in Physiology, *3rd ed (Berne, RM & Levy, MN, Eds). St. Louis, Mosby, pp. 96-97, 1993; Mitchell, M: Anatomy and Physiology of the Nervous System in* Critical Care Nursing: A Holistic Approach, *6th ed (Hudak, CM & Gallo, BM, Eds). Philadelphia, Lippincott, pp. 632-633, 1994.*

8.68. Correct Answer: **a**

Systolic blood pressure increases, diastolic blood pressure decreases, and profound bradycardia develops as the brain's adaptive capacity succumbs to continuous increases in intracranial pressure. A patient presenting these three signs of Cushing's triad faces imminent death. Clinicians *must act* earlier to reverse more subtle signs of increasing intracranial pressure and potential herniation long before continued ischemia and medullary pressure produce this triad of signs and herald irreversible neurodamage.

Shpritz, DW: The Neurosurgical Patient in ASPAN's Core Curriculum for Post Anesthesia Nursing Practice, *3rd ed (Litwack, K, Ed). Philadelphia, Saunders, p. 350, 1994; Mitchell, PH: Neurological Anatomy and Physiology in* AACN's Clinical Reference for Critical-Care Nursing, *3rd ed (Kinney, MR, Packa, DR & Dunbar, SB, Eds). St. Louis, Mosby, pp. 822-823, 1993.*

8.69. Correct Answer: **a**

Most connections between the higher and lower brain structures (tracts) emerge from the medulla (brain stem) after the pyramids decussate, or cross, to the opposite side. Voluntary muscle activity is controlled by the pyramidal system, which arises in the frontal lobes and descends through the brain stem. The right lateral pyramidal tract, therefore, carries impulses to control left contralateral functions.

Shpritz, DW: The Neurosurgical Patient in ASPAN's Core Curriculum for Post Anesthesia Nursing Practice, *3rd ed (Litwack, K, Ed). Philadelphia, Saunders, pp. 341-344, 1994.*

8.70. Correct Answer: **c**

Hemoglobin is generally measured early in the postoperative period and regularly thereafter. Surgical intervention for scoliosis is associated with potential for major blood loss, and replacing lost blood cells may be necessary to assure adequate tissue oxygenation. Patients with significant scoliosis may have altered lung capacity; deep breathing is essential to help maintain lung tissue expansion. To prevent instrument displacement, Angela should *not* use her arms to reposition herself or be lifted under her arms by others. Facial edema *is* likely from gravity-induced migration fluid to lips, eyes, nose and cheeks during several intraoperative hours in a prone position; these fluids gradually reshift over days. Gastric distention and potential for ileus are best relieved by nasogastric tube, not position.

Kull, L: The Orthopedic Surgical Patient in ASPAN's Core Curriculum for Post Anesthesia Nursing Practice, *3rd ed (Litwack, K, Ed). Philadelphia, Saunders, pp. 529-530, 1994; Salem, MR & Klowden, AJ: Anesthesia for Orthopedic Surgery in* Pediatric Anesthesia, *3rd ed (Gregory, GA, ed). New York, Churchill-Livingstone, pp. 607-634, 1994.*

8.71. Correct Answer: **c**

"Salvage" of intraoperative blood loss, washing away many contaminants then reinfusing, provides the patient with immediately available blood. Viability, function and numbers of platelets, and specific clotting factors remain near normal for up to 24 hours; these factors diminish as blood is banked and stored. Processing of shed blood washes away most, but not all, of the citrate that can alter function of coagulation factors. Blood must be reinfused within 6 hours through tubing with microaggregate filters.

Hudak, CM & Gallo, BM: Critical Care Nursing: A Holistic Approach, *6th ed. Philadelphia, Lippincott, pp. 284-292, 1994.*

8.72. Correct Answer: **b**

No medications, including patient controlled analgesia (PCA) narcotics, should infuse with blood. Evidence of hemolysis (hematuria) transfusion reaction (fever, chills, nausea, flank pain, oliguria), particulate microembolism, and sepsis *can* occur with autotransfusion. Procedures for reinfusing processed, shed intraoperative blood resemble procedures for transfusion of banked blood: infuse within 4 hours, follow established facility protocols for tubing requirements and patient identification, and closely monitor temperature, vital signs, and the patient response. Cramping, tingling, or new cardiac arrhythmias may indicate altered calcium balance or acidosis; increased wound drainage can indicate developing coagulopathy.

Hudak, CM & Gallo, BM: Critical Care Nursing: A Holistic Approach, *6th ed. Philadelphia, Lippincott, pp. 284-292, 1994.*

8.73. Correct Answer: **c**

Nitroprusside can actually increase intracranial pressure (ICP) even when the effect on blood pressure is small. Normal ICP is 0-15 mm Hg. To maintain ICP within normal parameters, attention to specific details of patient management is necessary. Hyperventilation maintains pCO_2 in the hypocapnic range of 30-35 mm Hg; a head-elevated position of 15-30 degrees with *no* knee flexion and straightly aligned neck encourages venous drainage from the head; a 20% mannitol solution initiated within the first hour effectively decreases ICP by 15-20 mm Hg.

Shpritz, DW: The Neurosurgical Patient in ASPAN's Core Curriculum for Post Anesthesia Nursing Practice, *3rd ed (Litwack, K, Ed). Philadelphia, Saunders, pp. 354-356, 1994; Mitchell, PH: Neurological Disorders in* AACN's Clinical Reference for Critical-Care Nursing, *3rd ed (Kinney, MR, Packa, DR & Dunbar, SB, Eds). St. Louis, Mosby, pp. 808-813, 1993.*

8.74. Correct Answer: **d**

Plateau waves, or "A" waves, indicate a trend toward above-normal intracranial pressures (ICP) and correlate with cerebral ischemia. Patient management includes interventions to reduce pressure. Patients with invasive ICP catheters or bolts have significantly increased risk of infection; use of steroids suppresses immunity and further increases infection potential. Aseptic technique and reporting any drainage are essential. *Never* "flush" the monitoring system! Though nursing actions certainly are planned according to changes and trends in intracranial pressure, calculating intracranial compliance is the physician's responsibility.

Guanci, MM: Increased Intracranial Pressure in The Clinical Practice of Neurological and Neurosurgical Nursing, *3rd ed (Hickey, JV, Ed). Philadelphia, Lippincott, pp. 272-276, 1992; Hawkins, JK & Hawkins, VC:*

Post Anesthesia Care of the Neurosurgical Patient in The Post Anesthesia Care Unit: A Critical Care Approach to Post Anesthesia Nursing, *3rd ed (Drain, C, Ed). Philadelphia, Saunders, pp. 420-426, 1994.*

8.75. Correct Answer: **d**

The Monro-Kellie hypothesis reflects the principles of intracranial volume. This volume is a dynamic relationship equal to the volume of the brain plus volume of cerebral blood plus cerebrospinal fluid volume. Altering any one of these factors affects the others. Usually, when brain volume increases, autoregulatory processes decrease cerebral blood flow to maintain a constant intracranial volume. Volume translates to pressure. As autoregulatory mechanisms fail, the volume of intracranial contents increases; as the skull cannot expand to accommodate the increased volume, pressure increases.

Smith, RN: Management Modalities: Nervous System in Critical Care Nursing: A Holistic Approach, *6th ed (Hudak, CM & Gallo, BM, Eds). Philadelphia, Lippincott, pp. 674-677, 1994; Guanci, MM: Increased Intracranial Pressure in* The Clinical Practice of Neurological and Neurosurgical Nursing, *3rd ed (Hickey, JV, Ed). Philadelphia, Lippincott, pp. 249-253, 1992.*

8.76. Correct Answer: **a**

A cerebral perfusion pressure (CPP) of only 43 mm Hg in a nonanesthetized patient indicates inadequate blood flow and ischemia. To adequately perfuse the brain, CPP must be at least 60 mm Hg; normal CPP is 80-90 mm Hg. CPP is the calculated difference between mean arterial pressure (MAP)—blood entering the brain—and intracranial pressure (ICP)—resistance to this flow. Therefore, CPP = MAP – ICP.

Guanci, MM: Increased Intracranial Pressure in The Clinical Practice of Neurological and Neurosurgical Nursing, *3rd ed (Hickey, JV, Ed). Philadelphia, Lippincott, pp. 249-253, 1992; Shpritz, DW: The Neurosurgical Patient in* ASPAN's Core Curriculum for Post Anesthesia Nursing Practice, *3rd ed (Litwack, K, Ed). Philadelphia, Saunders, pp. 351-352, 1994.*

8.77. Correct Answer: **a**

The vascularity of meningiomas makes bleeding a high-potential intraoperative complication; blood is usually cross-matched for possible use. Meningiomas are typically slow-growing, usually benign, and often vascular tumors and represent up to 20% of all intracranial tumors. Incidence is age-related and highest among adult men. Location in the brain determines symptoms. As the tumor size increases, surrounding brain structures are *compressed* rather than invaded. Though well-encapsulated, size and tumor location complicate resection.

Stewart-Amidei, C: Meningioma: Nursing Care Considerations. J Post Anesth Nurs *6(4): 269-278, 1991; Stupple, L: Brain Tumors in* The Clinical Practice of Neurological and Neurosurgical Nursing, *3rd ed (Hickey, JV, Ed). Philadelphia, Lippincott, pp. 487-488, 1992.*

8.78. Correct Answer: **c**

CSF contains glucose. Yellowish drainage from surgical site, ear, eye, or nose could be CSF, indicating dural tear. Potential for infection rises. Do not suction drainage! Do not "pack" dressings into any site when CSF leak is suspected! Confirm glucose presence and report to the physician.

Kane, DM: Practical Points in the Postoperative Management of a Craniotomy Patient. J Post Anesth Nurs *6(2): 121-124, 1992; Lazear, SE: Postoperative Care of the Neurosurgical Patient in* Critical Care Nursing, *2nd ed (Vazquez, M, Lazear, SE & Larson, EL, Eds). Philadelphia, Saunders, pp. 166-171, 1992.*

8.79. Correct Answer: **c**

Particularly following an infratentorial approach, difficulty in maintaining airway patency or abnormal breathing pattern heralds a complication requiring that the PACU nurse notify the surgeon. Edema or postoperative bleeding in the posterior fossa, the area below the tentorium, compresses brain stem structures. Altered respiratory status, cardiovascular stability and function of cranial nerves with nuclei in the medulla result. The cerebellum, located in the infratentorium, coordinates, not initiates, movement; fine motor incoordination more likely indicates postoperative cerebellar dysfunction than does paralysis.

Chisari, R: Care of the Patient Undergoing Intracranial Surgery in The Clinical Practice of Neurological and Neurosurgical Nursing, *3rd ed (Hickey, JV, Ed). Philadelphia, Lippincott, pp. 304 & 310-313, 1992; Mitchell, PH: Neurological Disorders in* AACN's Clinical Reference for Critical-Care Nursing, *3rd ed (Kinney, MR, Packa, DR & Dunbar, SB, Eds). St. Louis, Mosby, p. 845, 1993.*

8.80. Correct Answer: **b**

Interventions that move the patient's body as a unit (without bends or twists) minimize neck flexion, extension, or malalignment. "Log roll" turns avoid brain stem pressure or circulatory impairment that potentially compromise respiratory function. Coughing and suction are avoided when possible. PEEP increases intrathoracic pressure, reduces venous return and therefore increases intracranial pressure.

Mitchell, PH: Neurological Disorders in AACN's Clinical Reference for Critical-Care Nursing, *3rd ed (Kinney, MR, Packa, DR & Dunbar, SB, Eds). St. Louis, Mosby, p. 845, 1993; Hawkins, JK & Hawkins, VC: Post Anesthesia Care of the Neurosurgical Patient in* The Post Anesthesia Care Unit: A Critical Care Approach to Post Anesthesia Nursing, *3rd ed (Drain, C, Ed). Philadelphia, Saunders, pp. 427-428, 1994.*

8.81. Correct Answer: **c**

Right-sided deficits below the brain stem must raise nursing concern for this patient's neurologic health. For this patient, dilation of the right pupil probably has less ominous significance than motor dysfunction on the left side. Corticospinal tracts connecting this patient's left cerebral cortex with spinal cord cells in the anterior horn decussate, or cross, to control function on his right side. Control of pupillary constriction occurs at the midbrain, above the area where pyramidal tracts cross.

Shpritz, DW: The Neurosurgical Patient in ASPAN's Core Curriculum for Post Anesthesia Nursing Practice, *3rd ed (Litwack, K, Ed). Philadelphia, Saunders, pp. 347-*

351, 1994; Mitchell, PH: Neurological Anatomy and Physiology in AACN's Clinical Reference for Critical-Care Nursing, *3rd ed (Kinney, MR, Packa, DR & Dunbar, SB, Eds). St. Louis, Mosby, pp. 762-766, 1993.*

8.82. Correct Answer: **d**

For each patient, the physician determines the rate and volume of cerebrospinal fluid to be removed through the ventriculostomy. A ventriculostomy system is inserted to manage hydrocephalus (impaired cerebrospinal fluid circulation) that significantly dilates cerebral ventricles and increases intracranial pressure. Infection from this invasive system and ventricular collapse from excessive drainage are the greatest associated risks. The system must remain sterile, is generally "leveled" with the zero-point near the patient's ear (approximately the foramen of Monro) and often is positioned by the neurosurgeon. Negative pressure is *never* applied to the system.

Guanci, MM: Increased Intracrainial Pressure in The Clinical Practice of Neurological and Neurosurgical Nursing, *3rd ed (Hickey, JV, Ed). Philadelphia, Lippincott, p. 270, 1992; Smith, RN: Management Modalities: Nervous System in* Critical Care Nursing: A Holistic Approach, *6th ed (Hudak, CM & Gallo, BM, Eds). Philadelphia, Lippincott, pp. 684-685, 1994.*

8.83. Correct Answer: **b**

This patient easily moves her right leg and can raise her knee, indicating the strength to overcome gravity. She cannot, however, maintain her own muscle strength against resistance applied by the nurse-examiner. Physician expectations are important to determine. Wynona's weakness may be similar to her preoperative weakness and of little current concern. Inform the surgeon of new or increasing weakness. Strength of Wynona's arms and left leg muscles is normal. Observations of muscle activity are often rated on a scale (typically with grades 0-5) to objectively communicate muscle strength. Whether a rating scale is used or not, extremity muscle strength must be frequently documented—as clinically indicated in PACU or as physician-ordered.

Hickey, JV: The Clinical Practice of Neurological and Neurosurgical Nursing, *3rd ed. Philadelphia, Lippincott, pp. 75-79, 1992; Provenzano, SM: Assessment: Nervous System in* Critical Care Nursing: A Holistic Approach, *6th ed (Hudak, CM & Gallo, BM, Eds). Philadelphia, Lippincott, pp. 652-654, 1994.*

8.84. Correct Answer: **b**

To decrease edema after spinal trauma, "megadoses" of steroids have improved neurologic function. Though some consider this a controversial practice, some practitioners rapidly infuse methylprednisolone 30 mg/kg, followed by a smaller dose each hour for 23 hours. When initiated promptly after injury (surgical trauma with decreased neurologic function, in Wynona's situation), motor and sensory function has significantly improved for some patients.

Poyner, M: Vertebral and Spinal Cord Trauma in The Clinical Practice of Neurological and Neurosurgical Nursing, *3rd ed (Hickey, JV, Ed). Philadelphia, Lippincott, p. 414, 1992; Shan-*

non, MT, Wilson, BA & Stang, CL: Govoni & Hayes Drugs & Nursing Implications, *8th ed. Norwalk, CT, Appleton & Lange, pp. 763-764, 1995.*

8.85. Correct Answer: **a**

Symptoms of gastrointestinal irritability (nausea, vomiting, and peptic ulcers) are likely consequences of steroid administration. Often, concurrent doses of medications to reduce gastric acidity are also provided. When caring for Wynona, the PACU nurse must be mindful of Wynona's increasing infection risk due to the acute antiinflammatory influence of high-dose steroids. Eventually, a schedule of tapered steroid dose reduction will be needed to prevent adrenal crisis associated with abrupt withdrawal.

Poyner, M: Vertebral and Spinal Cord Trauma in The Clinical Practice of Neurological and Neurosurgical Nursing, *3rd ed (Hickey, JV, Ed). Philadelphia, Lippincott, p. 414, 1992; Shannon, MT, Wilson, BA & Stang, CL:* Govoni & Hayes Drugs & Nursing Implications, *8th ed. Norwalk, CT, Appleton & Lange, pp. 763-764, 1995.*

8.86. Correct Answer: **c**

Recurrent respiratory depression and resedation are likely; the effects of sufentanil likely will "outlive" any reversal provided by naloxone. Sufentanil (Sufenta) is often delivered by continuous infusion, particularly for long surgical procedures. Sufenta is similar to fentanyl in action but 5-7 times more potent. Inhaled anesthetics and sedatives further potentiate the effects.

Drain, C: The Post Anesthesia Care Unit: A Critical Care Approach to Post Anesthesia Nursing, *3rd ed. Philadelphia, Saunders, p. 218, 1994.*

8.87. Correct Answer: **d**

Nystagmus is disconjugate, jerking or oscillating movement of the eyes and an abnormal ocular response. The eyes of a normally alert person do not show involuntary movements.

Hawkins, JK & Hawkins, VC: Post Anesthesia Care of the Neurosurgical Patient in The Post Anesthesia Care Unit: A Critical Care Approach to Post Anesthesia Nursing, *3rd ed (Drain, C, Ed). Philadelphia, Saunders, p. 426, 1994.*

8.88. Correct Answer: **a**

Mr. R has normal reflex responses. Assessment of reflexes compares left and right responses for symmetry and reaction strength. Deep tendon (or muscle stretch) reflexes are commonly graded on a 0-4 scale; "2" is the normal response, "0" indicates no response to a reflex hammer tap. Brisk, hyperactive reflexes suggest disease or chemical imbalance and are scored as "4." Presence of a downward toe sign to plantar stroking (Babinski's sign), is not numerically graded and always indicates positive results—and pathology.

Provenzano, SM: Assessment: Nervous System in Critical Care Nursing: A Holistic Approach, *6th ed (Hudak, CM & Gallo, BM, Eds). Philadelphia, Lippincott, p. 655, 1994.*

8.89. Correct Answer: **b**

An autologous bone graft moves healthy bone pieces from one site in the patient's body to stabilize bone at another, usually for fusion of vertebrae or after fractures. Often bone from the iliac crest is used; pain from the donor site may be intense and require ice and narcotic analgesia.

Mussler, CA: Post Anesthesia Care of the Plastic Surgical Patient in The Post Anesthesia Care Unit: A Critical Care Approach to Post Anesthesia Nursing, *3rd ed (Drain, C, Ed). Philadelphia, Saunders, pp. 493-494, 1994.*

8.90. Correct Answer: **b**

Blood may drain unnoticed beneath Mr. C's leg; the accumulated drainage can be a significant volume. In addition, drainage collected in the wound drain can easily be more than 100 ml, particularly if a tourniquet was applied to the leg intraoperatively. Mr. C has increased potential for venous thrombosis; leg movement is encouraged. In addition, range of motion activities increase circulation while promoting joint mobility. Pillow pressure behind the knee (popliteal area) is avoided; a pillow inhibits knee movement and compromises limb circulation.

Kull, L: The Orthopedic Surgical Patient in ASPAN's Core Curriculum for Post Anesthesia Nursing Practice, *3rd ed (Litwack, K, Ed). Philadelphia, Saunders, p. 527, 1994.*

8.91. Correct Answer: **c**

Alternating compression and decompression pressures and soft, loose leg wraps of the 65 year old man's sequential compression devices are least likely to restrict circulation. Patients with soft tissue or crush injuries, bleeding with hematoma into the skin, casted fractures, and prolonged compression by casts, weight, or pressure have high risk for compartment syndrome. When in lithotomy position for 3 hours, circulation in the anesthetized woman's posterior lower legs can be restricted; she is unable to feel the pain and alter her position to relieve pressure. Compartment syndrome occurs when extremity circulation and nerve function are compromised by greatly elevated pressures within the extremity. Greatest risk is within 6 hours after the precipitating event.

Kull, L: The Orthopedic Surgical Patient in ASPAN's Core Curriculum for Post Anesthesia Nursing Practice, *3rd ed (Litwack, K, Ed). Philadelphia, Saunders, pp. 514-515, 1994; Walsh, J: Postop Effects of OR Positioning.* RN *56(2): 50-58, 1993.*

8.92. Correct Answer: **d**

Pain, paresthesia, pallor, paralysis, and decreased pulse ("the five Ps") are the hallmark signs of compartment syndrome. Circulatory impairment and nerve compression in an increasingly tight, high-pressure extremity segment (compartment) produces these symptoms. Burning indicates sensory damage (paresthesia); decreasing motor strength and decreasing pulse quality are relatively early signs of increasing compartment pressure. Pulse absence and true cyanosis (not pallor) develop much later, after significant tissue damage has occurred.

Litwack, K: Post Anesthesia Care Nursing, *2nd ed. St. Louis, Mosby, p. 25, 1995; Kull, L: The Orthopedic Surgical Patient in* ASPAN's Core Curriculum for Post Anesthesia Nursing Practice, *3rd ed (Litwack, K, Ed). Philadelphia, Saunders, pp. 512-523, 1994.*

Section 9

Intraabdominal and Retroperitoneal Observations

Scenarios and items in this section focus *on the renal, genitourinary, gynecologic, hepatic, and gastrointestinal* systems. Though specific function of these systems varies, these concepts are considered together because:

- anatomically, the primary organs for these systems are located within the abdomen or retroperitoneum.
- nursing assessments related to potential postsurgical complications are similar.
- the nursing process focuses include detection of hidden bleeding; restoring thermal, fluid, and electrolyte balance; promoting oxygenation and pulmonary function; and assuring integrity of surgical drains, stomas, or anastomoses.

ESSENTIAL CORE CONCEPTS	AFFILIATED CORE CURRICULUM CHAPTERS
Nursing Process	
Assessment	
Planning and Intervention	Chapters 2, 21, 22 & 23
Evaluation	
Renal and Genitourinary Systems	
Nursing Process	
Anatomy, Structure, and Function	
Adrenals and Lymphatics	
Nephron, Cortex, and Medulla	
Sex-Related Variations	
Ureters, Bladder, Urethra, and Sphincters	
Physiologic Concerns	
Hormonal	
Prostaglandins and Erythropoietin	
Renin-Angiotensin	
Vitamin D	
Metabolic	Chapter 21
Fluid and Chemical	
Aldosterone and ADH	
Filtration and Clearance	

Pathology
- Acute Tubular Necrosis
- Acute vs. Chronic Renal Failure: Cause and Effect
- Azotemia and Oliguria
- Blood Flow, Pressure, and Ischemia
- End-Stage Renal Disease (ESRD)
- Prerenal-Intrarenal-Postrenal Alterations
- Stones, Toxicity, Trauma, and Chemical Changes

Perianesthesia Priorities
- Hemorrhage, Fluid Shifts, Chemical Changes
- Stomas, Stents, and Catheters
- Strain (Urine), Drain (Wound), and Pain

Surgical Interventions
- Lasers, Shocks, and Scopes
- Position-Related Outcomes
- Resections, Suspensions, and Organ Removal

Gastrointestinal and Hepatic Systems

Nursing Process

Anatomy, Structure, and Organ Function
- Esophagus, Stomach, Intestine, and Colon
- Gallbladder, Liver, Pancreas, and Spleen

Pathology
- Polyps, Tumors, and Stones
- Strictures, Obstructions, Trauma, and Adhesions
- Ulcers, Infarcts, and -itises

Physiologic Balance
- Nutrition, Fluid, and Electrolytes
- Temperature, Hemostasis, and Sepsis

Perianesthesia Priorities
- Drains, Tubes, and Stomas
- Hydration, Clots, and Electrolytes
- Lungs, Circulation, and Distention
- Position, Pain, and Thrombus

Surgical Interventions
- Anastomoses and Pouches
- Biopsies, Scopes, and Scans
- -ectomies, Bypasses, -plasties and -otomies
- Position-Related Outcomes

Gynecologic System

Nursing Process

Anatomy, Structure, and Organ Function

Pathologic Conditions
- -celes, Hormones, Tumors, and Infections
- Ectopic Pregnancies and Abortions

Perianesthesia Priorities
- Catheters, Drains, and Tubes
- Embolus, Electrolytes, and Hydration
- Sepsis, Position, and Hemostasis

Surgical Interventions
Aspirations, Dilations, and Ligations
Hysterectomy, Oophorectomy, and Salpingectomy
Lasers, -scopes, and Suspensions
Position-Related Outcomes

SET I

Items 9.1-9.30

9.1. Oliguria refers to:
a. retention of nitrogenous waste products
b. approximately 400 ml daily urine production
c. unrecognized obstruction of urinary catheter
d. a syndrome of uremia, alkalosis and absent urine

9.2. Insufficient circulating cortisone would most likely cause the physiologic outcome of:
a. hypotension
b. hyperglycemia
c. hypernatremia
d. hypothermia

NOTE: Consider scenario and items 9.3-9.6 together.

Following abdominoperineal resection, Mr. V arrives in PACU in supine, head-flat position. He is drowsily responsive, moans and indicates abdominal cramping and nausea. Pneumatic sequential compression leg wraps are functioning, and his nasogastric tube drains scant amounts of dark red fluid. One abdominal wound drain is in compressed position and a perineal sump drain is attached to low suction.

9.3. Mr. V's *most* immediate postoperative risk is potential for:
a. deep vein thrombosis
b. dumping syndrome
c. inhalation of aspirated particles
d. malnutrition from impaired absorption syndrome

9.4. During assessment of Mr. V's surgical condition, the PACU nurse is *most* concerned to observe:
a. 75 ml serosanguineous perineal drainage in 1 hour
b. absent bowel sounds and a soft abdomen
c. 45 ml tan nasogastric fluid and potassium = 4.7 mEq/L
d. clear yellow urine and a light grey stoma

NOTE: The scenario continues.

Mr. V received an inhalation anesthetic with intravenous narcotic. The anesthesiologist placed an epidural catheter for postoperative pain management but did not instill any medication. The PACU nurse observes that Mr. V is "splinting" his respirations and chooses to begin the infusion promptly. The protocol for epidural bupivacaine and morphine includes a bolus dose and parameters for titration.

9.5. Prior to initiating the epidural infusion, the nurse assures that the anesthesiologist administers the test dose and that:
a. Mr. V rates his pain as ">7" on a pain scale of 0-10
b. an opioid agonist/antagonist accompanies Mr. V
c. the intravenous catheter is patent and nonreddened
d. Mr. V moves his feet, indicating the catheter rests in the intrathecal space

9.6. After 1 hour of epidural medication, Mr. V rates his pain at a "7" on the 0-10 pain scale. With support of hospital protocols and physician collaboration, the PACU nurse should:
a. administer meperidine 100 mg intramuscularly while awaiting effect of epidural medication
b. reinject the epidural catheter with a small supplemental bolus
c. double the infusion's opioid concentration, then expand dosing parameters
d. reposition the catheter, then adjust the infusion rate

9.7. Decreased blood and renal perfusion pressures prompt:
a. renin release with renovascular constriction
b. decreased urine excretion due to ADH suppression
c. aldosterone-induced sodium excretion
d. renal vasodilation from angiotensin II effect

NOTE: Consider scenario and item 9.8 together.

A 32 year old woman with chronic renal insufficiency fell at home 24 hours ago and hit her head. She is hypertensive in PACU after today's trephination and hematoma evacuation. Her intracranial pressure is 15 cm H_2O.

9.8. Administering hydralazine to this patient is *least likely* to:
a. impair renal clearance
b. increase cerebral blood flow
c. enhance adaptive cerebral autoregulation
d. decrease cardiac afterload

9.9. The type of hepatitis transmitted through nonparenteral routes is:
a. hepatitis D
b. hepatitis C
c. hepatitis B
d. hepatitis A

NOTE: Consider scenario and item 9.10 together.

Following open cholecystectomy, a patient remains in PACU for 4 hours due to an unanticipated high census on the nursing unit. During this period, the PACU nurse measures T-tube drainage of 60 ml each hour. Dressings are dry, and the abdomen is soft and round with moderate incisional tenderness.

9.10. The PACU nurse intervenes by:
a. documenting this normal hourly drainage volume
b. power-stripping the tubing for patency
c. informing the surgeon of the abdominal status
d. attaching the T-tube to suction

NOTE: Consider items 9.11-9.13 together.

9.11. Following pancreaticoduodenectomy, the patient will *most likely* require regular:
a. serum glucose assessment
b. glucocorticoid doses
c. potassium supplementation
d. cryoprecipitate infusions

9.12. With regard to this patient's gastrointestinal assessment, the *most appropriate* nursing plan of care includes:
a. irrigating the nasogastric tube with 30 ml normal saline each hour
b. asking the surgeon to identify tube locations and expected drainage
c. swiftly reinserting the nasogastric tube removed by a rambunctious patient
d. anticipating absent bowel sounds and a firm, tympanic abdomen

9.13. This patient's surgery involves:
a. pancreatic reconstruction and removal of a liver lobe, duodenum, and gallbladder
b. removing the spleen, biliary decompression with bile duct dilation, and creating an ileostomy
c. cholecystectomy and diverting ascitic and pancreatic fluid into the superior vena cava
d. resecting the pancreas, duodenum, lower stomach, and bile duct and constructing a gastrojejunostomy

NOTE: Consider scenario and items 9.14-9.17 together.

Fifty-five year old Ms E has a long history of postoperative nausea and vomiting (PONV). Today's anesthetic plan during her vaginal hysterectomy includes preoperative placement of a scopolamine patch behind the left ear.

9.14. Scopolamine is classified as a/an:

a. class I antiemetic
b. anticholinergic
c. class II neuroleptic
d. acetylcholinesterase

9.15. The PACU nurse anticipates the scopolamine may affect Ms E's PACU care by contributing to:

a. emergence delirium
b. malignant hyperthermia
c. delayed awakening
d. prolonged muscle relaxation

9.16. These potential scopolamine-related symptoms could be effectively managed with:

a. glycopyrrolate
b. nalbuphine
c. physostigmine
d. dantrolene

9.17. Two hours postoperatively, the PACU nurse prepares Ms E for transfer from PACU. With regard to Ms E's surgical outcomes, the nurse is *most* concerned when nursing assessment reveals:

a. lumbar pain and occipital headache
b. soft abdomen and menstrual-like cramps
c. leg pain during foot dorsiflexion
d. no sanguineous fluid in wound drain or perineal pad

9.18. Intervention for oliguria from prerenal causes may include:

a. ureteral stent placement for clot-free patency
b. aminoglycoside antibiotics to prevent infection
c. furosemide to promote sodium excretion
d. dopamine infusion at 3.5 mg/kg to augment perfusion

NOTE: Consider scenario and item 9.19 together.

A patient is scheduled for a vasectomy, using a local anesthetic and IV conscious sedation with fentanyl and midazolam. A Phase I PACU nurse with extensive operating room experience monitors the patient's status during the procedure and has no other responsibilities. Cardiac and noninvasive blood pressure monitors and a pulse oximeter are attached to the patient. The surgeon arrives and demands the nurse remove the equipment as he believes such monitoring is unnecessary.

9.19. The nurse's *most* effective response is to:

a. refuse to remain in the room during the procedure
b. inform the surgeon of IV conscious sedation policy
c. discontinue the monitors and auscultate respirations
d. tactfully request the surgeon cancel the procedure

NOTE: Consider scenario and item 9.20 together.

Mr. U's surgeon resected 15 g of prostate tissue during today's transurethral resection of the prostate (TURP) and placed a suprapubic catheter. After 30 minutes in PACU, Mr. U has epigastric, suprapubic and left shoulder pain and a firm abdomen. His blood pressure is 94/50 and heart rate is 126 beats per minute. He is diaphoretic and nauseated.

9.20. The nurse pages the physician and further assesses the patient for possible:

a. evolving myocardial infarction
b. septic bacteremia
c. perforated bladder
d. bladder spasm with prostatic bleeding

9.21. Deficits related to intraoperative positioning are *least* affected by a patient's:

a. duration of surgery
b. anesthetic technique
c. geriatric age
d. physical condition

9.22. Patient education priorities following extracorporeal shock wave lithotripsy focus primarily on:

a. hematuria prevention
b. forced hydration
c. scheduled analgesia
d. antibiotic effects

NOTE: Consider scenario and items 9.23-9.25 together.

Ms A is a spry 73 year old woman who arrives in PACU after pelvic exenteration and lymphadenectomy. She is settled in PACU and is currently stable. Her health history includes rheumatoid arthritis and a recently resolved pneumonia. Medications include ibuprofen prn and prednisone 60 mg daily.

9.23. The PACU nurse scans Ms A's record to determine the preoperative baseline oxygen saturation and verify Ms A has:

a. no chemical addictions
b. estrogen replacement therapy
c. hydrocortisone coverage
d. no risk factors for thromboembolism

9.24. When aware of her surroundings, Ms A is *best* positioned:

a. with her head elevated 30 degrees
b. however she wishes
c. flat and on her left side
d. in Fowler's position with her feet elevated

9.25. With regard to her chronic steroid use, Ms A has increased postoperative risk for:

a. pulmonary edema
b. wound infection
c. diabetes insipidus
d. fluid deficit

9.26. Renal failure from prerenal origins differs from acute tubular necrosis (ATN) by the amount of:

a. urine production
b. concentrating ability
c. nephron damage
d. renin release

NOTE: Consider scenario and items 9.27-9.29 together.

Following a 4 hour exploratory laparotomy, transverse colon and tumor resection and creation of colostomy, Mr. L has persistent hypotension in PACU with blood pressure 80/42. Cardiac rhythm is sinus with heart rate 102 beats/minute. Mr. L has a preoperative history of seasonal allergy, migraine headaches and osteoarthritis. No hemodynamic monitoring catheters were inserted. Urine volume remains 40 ml/h and 5% dextrose in 0.45% normal saline with 20 mEq of potassium chloride infuse at 150 ml/h. His temperature is 37° C, and he is easily responsive, with moderate pain managed with morphine delivered with patient-controlled analgesia (PCA) technique. Hemoglobin is 12.5 g/dl, and potassium 3.8 mEq/L.

9.27. The *most likely* potential explanation for Mr. L's hypotension is:

a. ECF deficit from hypertonic intravenous infusions
b. perioperative myocardial infarction with shock
c. unrecognized preoperative gastrointestinal fluid loss
d. fluid relocation with altered capillary permeability

9.28. Perianesthesia nursing and medical goals for Mr. L focus on:

a. instituting renal replacement therapy
b. supporting cardiac output and renal perfusion
c. recirculating intraintestinal fluid
d. increasing osmotic pressure with whole blood

NOTE: The scenario continues.

Mr. L ultimately receives 3000 ml of lactated Ringer's solution during a 3 hour stay in PACU. When approved for discharge from Phase I PACU, he is alert, has moderate pain, no audible rales, and denies dyspnea. Urine output remains 35 ml/h; blood pressure is consistently 100/52, heart rate is 98 beats per minute with normal sinus rhythm, and oxygen saturation is 98%.

9.29. The PACU nurse communicates Mr. L's fluid status to his nurse on the medical nursing unit and anticipates that:

a. fluid reabsorption will occur when capillaries heal
b. spontaneous diuresis will begin within 6 hours
c. low rate hypotonic fluids will prevent tissue edema
d. pain will increase cardiac tone and decrease afterload

NOTE: Consider scenario and item 9.30 together.

A 38 year old dental assistant and hygienist is scheduled for a cystoscopy, ureteral stent placement and extracorporeal shock wave lithotripsy (ESWL). His preoperative history and physical assessment document allergies to fish, milk, and eggs and recent episodes of conjunctivitis, eye swelling and itchy, red hands at work.

9.30. The preanesthesia nurse consults the anesthesia provider to express her concern about this patient's increased risk to develop:

a. bronchospasm during endotracheal intubation
b. anaphylaxis after propofol sedation
c. corneal abrasion from lateral position
d. upper quadrant pain with IV morphine sulfate

SET II

Items 9.31-9.60

9.31. The capacity of a normally functioning bladder is approximately:
a. 250 ml
b. 500 ml
c. 1 L
d. 1500 ml

9.32. Renal effects from this antidiuretic hormone deficiency include:
a. sodium and water retention
b. renin-angiotensin activation
c. hypoconcentrated urine excretion
d. glucocorticoid depletion

9.33. Risk of nephrotoxicity from aminoglycoside antibiotics may be reduced by providing concurrent:
a. nonsteroidal antiinflammatory medications
b. adequate intravascular volume
c. high-dose thiazide diuretics
d. slight metabolic acidosis

NOTE: Consider scenario and items 9.34-9.35 together.

Ms H was scheduled for pelviscopy to evaluate recurrent abdominal pain. The surgeon anticipated a left salpingectomy and oophorectomy. Ms H received succinylcholine for intubation, midazolam, and fentanyl. The surgeon's plan changed intraoperatively and Ms H's surgery ended quickly after lysis of adhesions and laser treatment of endometriosis. Ms H arrives in PACU apneic and not moving. Respiratory support is provided with a mechanical ventilator, a rash scatters across her chest and upper arm, and she shows no muscle response to nerve stimulator impulses.

9.34. The nurse considers Ms H's response to intraoperative muscle relaxants and anticipates:
a. a tragic permanent paralysis from atypical response
b. any arm movements will precede intercostal action
c. abdominal muscle function will precede eye opening
d. brief sensory deficit from allergic reaction

NOTE: The scenario continues.

Within 90 minutes, Ms H is alert, demonstrates adequate muscle strength, and is extubated. By late afternoon, she is fully awake, sipping fluids and slowly preparing for discharge home. Ms H mentions pain when smiling, turning her head, and moving about.

9.35. This discomfort is *most likely* related to:
a. nerve compression during lithotomy position
b. intraabdominal tissue burn
c. muscle strain from postanesthetic vomiting
d. intraoperative muscle fasciculation

9.36. Parasympathetic nervous system effects on the urinary bladder are *most* altered by:
a. droperidol and fentanyl
b. atropine and glycopyrrolate
c. neostigmine and edrophonium
d. morphine and midazolam

NOTE: Consider scenario and items 9.37-9.38 together.

During a 90 minute bilateral orchiectomy, 73 year old Mr. X, who was anxious preoperatively, received nitrous oxide, fentanyl 200 mcg, vecuronium 10 mg, and midazolam 7 mg. This minimally responsive patient now has an oral airway, a temperature of 36.4° C, and a respiratory rate of 10 breaths per minute. During consultation in

PACU, the anesthesiologist recommends that Mr. X receive flumazenil 0.8 mg IV push, to be repeated in 5 minutes if needed.

9.37. Before giving the flumazenil, the PACU nurse consults the anesthesiologist to discuss the ordered dose and Mr. X's:

a. allergy to tricyclic antidepressants
b. need for dose adjustment related to age
c. history of panic attacks
d. analgesic needs after fentanyl reversal

9.38. Thirty minutes after receiving 0.4 mg flumazenil, Mr. X is conversant, oriented, and breathing adequately and has stable vital signs. The PACU nurse is relieved for lunch and advises her nurse colleague to observe Mr. X in PACU for another half hour, *primarily* because:

a. respiratory failure is a concern for up to 60 minutes after a flumazenil dose
b. flumazenil reverses amnesia; Mr. X will probably recall frightening intraoperative events
c. muscle weakness might return when flumazenil's effect on residual vecuronium abates
d. flumazenil is less effective than physostigmine when reversing midazolam sedation

NOTE: Consider scenario and items 9.39-9.41 together.

Following a motor vehicle accident, a comatose motorcyclist was admitted to the hospital with multiple injuries. Six hours later, a depressed skull fracture was surgically repaired. Now, 24 hours after injury, his abdomen has been explored, his spleen excised, and a fractured hip opened, reduced, and internally fixed.

9.39. During initial assessment, the PACU nurse would be *most* concerned about:

a. platelets of 98,000/mm3
b. temperature of 39.8° C
c. urine output of 29 ml/h
d. hemoglobin of 9.8 mg/dl

NOTE: The scenario continues.

During PACU admission procedures, this patient actively shivers, blood pressure is 100/50, and respiratory rate is 28 breaths per minute. EKG indicates sinus tachycardia; shivering artifact makes initial SpO_2 measurement difficult.

9.40. The PACU nurse:

a. automatically initiates analgesia protocol
b. applies active rewarming air blanket
c. administers butorphanol to suppress shivering
d. documents skin warmth, dryness and redness

9.41. Classic indicators of *early* respiratory distress in an adult with septic shock are:

a. hyperventilation with respiratory alkalosis and elevated lactate
b. hypoventilation with decreased pulse pressure and excess circulating corticosteroids
c. hyperventilation with peripheral cyanosis and acidosis
d. hypoventilation with elevated lactate and low serum glucose

NOTE: Consider scenario and items 9.42-9.44 together.

A 60 year old woman is admitted to PACU after revision of an arteriovenous access in her left arm under regional anesthesia and sedation. The patient has a VVI pacemaker and underlying first degree heart block. The pacemaker is unipolar, and the pulse generator is implanted in the left subclavian area.

9.42. The PACU nurse interprets the cardiac rhythm on the following page as failure to:

a. sense
b. capture
c. stimulate
d. pace

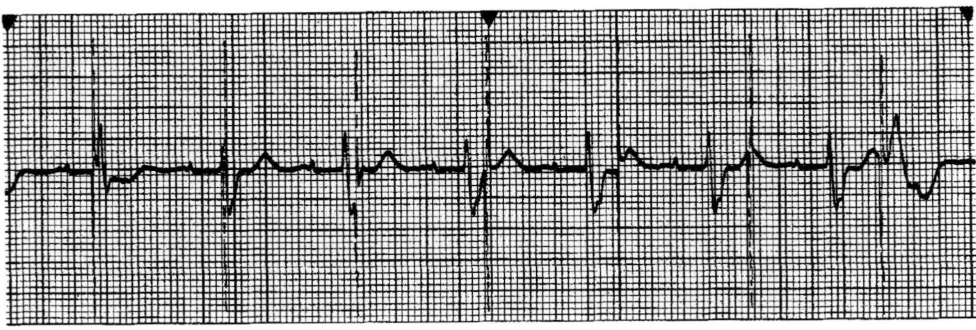

Figure 9.1. From Wiederhold, R, *Electrocardiography: The Monitoring Lead.* Philadelphia, Saunders, p. 312, 1988

9.43. If this pacemaker rhythm continues, the nurse anticipates this patient's *most likely* potential outcome is:

a. ventricular asystole
b. atrioventricular delay
c. ventricular tachycardia
d. atrial fibrillation

9.44. With regard to this pacemaker rhythm and potential outcomes, the PACU nurse anticipates need to:

a. initiate lidocaine infusion at 6 mg/kg
b. deliver electrical cardioversion energy
c. manually decrease the pacemaker's milliamperage
d. administer intravenous labetalol 5 mg

NOTE: Consider scenario and items 9.45-9.47 together.

Ms B is a healthy middle-aged woman whose uneventful abdominal hysterectomy ended 2 hours ago; intraoperative blood loss was 100 ml. She is drowsy and states moderate abdominal pain. Blood pressure is low-normal, though generally only 10% less than her preoperative measures; in PACU her blood pressure dipped to 88/48 twice. Ms B's cardiac rhythm is sinus at a consistent rate of 128 beats per minute.

9.45. The PACU nurse's ongoing assessment of this patient considers this situation's *most likely* explanation is:

a. fever-induced tachycardia related to hyperdynamic sepsis
b. neurogenic vasodilation related to untreated hypothermia
c. decreased venous return related to evolving silent myocardial infarction
d. reflex tachycardia related to intravascular volume deficit

9.46. The *most appropriate* collaborative nurse-physician interventions for Ms B's immediate care are:

a. restrict fluids, oxygen and neosynephrine 0.3 mg prn
b. rapid crystalloid infusion and measure hemoglobin
c. acetaminophen suppository and titrate esmolol infusion
d. active rewarming, labetalol 5 mg, and measure prothrombin time

9.47. A patient with a blood urea nitrogen (BUN) of 55 mg/dl and serum creatinine of 5.2 mg/dl is considered:

a. anuric
b. cachectic
c. oliguric
d. azotemic

NOTE: Consider scenario and items 9.48-9.53 together.

At 0200, an "on-call" PACU nurse is phoned to care for 25 year old Ms M after an emergency laparoscopy and salpingectomy to remove an ectopic pregnancy.

9.48. According to ASPAN's *Standards of Perianesthesia Nursing Practice,* recommended postanesthesia care for Ms M includes:

a. observation in the ICU by a PACU nurse and an ICU nurse in the adjacent isolation room
b. care by a registered nurse and visitation in PACU by two family members
c. presence of two licensed nurses for duration of PACU period
d. one registered nurse at the bedside and anesthesiologist available by pager in obstetric suite

9.49. Prior to transfer to an inpatient hospital bed, the PACU nurse administers Rho(D) immune globulin (RhoGAM) to Ms M, who is Rh negative, to prevent:

a. hemolysis of maternal erythrocytes
b. maternal Rh sensitivity and antibody formation
c. antibody stimulation in a future Rh negative fetus
d. maternal conversion to Rh positivity

9.50. A preoperative intervention intended to reduce potential adverse outcomes related to Ms M's position during laparoscopy may include:

a. H_2 antagonists
b. bladder distention
c. antiembolic stockings
d. beta blockers

9.51. At 0420, 30 minutes after admission to PACU, the nurse is most concerned when Ms M's assessment reveals:

a. bradycardia and moderate vaginal bleeding
b. severe right shoulder pain and nausea
c. tachycardia and a flat, silent abdomen
d. painful, firm abdomen and bloody bandages

9.52. The PACU nurse discovers that Ms M is unable to dorsiflex the great toe on her right foot. This deficit may indicate intraoperative:

a. sciatic nerve injury
b. posterior tibial nerve compression
c. femoral nerve pressure
d. peroneal nerve dysfunction

9.53. During laparoscopy, peripheral nerve injury is *most* related to:

a. lithotomy position
b. intramuscular injection
c. retractor pressure
d. prolonged hip extension

NOTE: Consider scenario and items 9.54-9.56 together.

A 43 year old woman with diabetes mellitus and end-stage renal disease is in PACU after bilateral nephrectomy to control severe hypertension. A mature arteriovenous fistula in her right arm provides hemodialysis access. Her most recent dialysis was 12 hours ago.

9.54. When planning this patient's postoperative analgesia and sedation, the PACU nurse considers that:

a. hydrophilic medications bind strongly to protein
b. morphine's active metabolites may stimulate seizures
c. midazolam's rapid elimination leaves few active metabolites
d. lipophilic medications are ineffective and require renal excretion

9.55. The perianesthesia nurse's plan of care for this patient emphasizes blood pressure, glucose, and pain and fluid management and considers the increased potential for:

a. hyperkalemia and orthopedic fracture
b. infection and oliguria
c. impaired ventilation and hypercoagulation
d. anemia and dilutional hypokalemia

9.56. While caring for this patient, the greatest potential infection risk to the PACU nurse is:

a. CMV from a vomitus spill onto a fresh skin abrasion
b. HBV from spilled wound drainage onto the nurse's finger papercut
c. HIV from a mucous splash to upper lip during a cough
d. HAV from a blood splash to the cornea during sampling for laboratory tests

NOTE: Consider items 9.57-9.59 together.

9.57. During his hemorrhoidectomy, sphincterotomy, and repair of a large rectal fistula, Mr. T received mivacurium. This medication is notable as a/an:

a. intermediate-acting, depolarizing muscle relaxant
b. drug with the same onset time as succinylcholine
c. depolarizing relaxant reversible with flumazenil
d. nondepolarizing muscle relaxant of short duration

9.58. Potentiation of mivacurium's effects is *least likely* with:

a. postoperative neostigmine 2.5 mg
b. isoflurane at 1.25 MAC to maintain anesthesia
c. intraoperative tobramycin 60 mg
d. concurrent administration of hydrocortisone 100 mg

9.59. With regard to Mr. T's surgical procedure, the Phase I PACU nurse has *greatest* concern when:

a. sanguineous drainage saturates dressings twice in 1 hour
b. postoperative urination is difficult
c. Mr. T states significant perineal pressure and severe rectal pain
d. no drainage and absent perineal sensation occur

NOTE: Consider scenario and item 9.60 together.

Today Ms K's Crohn's disease was surgically treated with a 3.5 hour total proctocolectomy and creation of a continent ileostomy. Now in Phase I PACU, she mentions right heel pain and an aching back.

9.60. At this time, the *most appropriate* nursing intervention is to:

a. request an anticoagulation protocol to monitor risk of deep vein thrombus
b. reposition Ms K's feet to limit contact with the stretcher
c. further assess Ms K for right leg compartment syndrome
d. provide sedation and frequent analgesia so Ms K will relax and doze

SET III

Items 9.61-9.87

NOTE: Consider items 9.61-9.62 together.

9.61. Upon admission to PACU, Mr. J cannot hold his head up and has shallow respiratory effort with hiccoughs and jerky arm movements after his vecuronium, fentanyl, nitrous oxide and midazolam anesthetic. These signs *most likely* indicate:

a. anticipated outcomes after a "balanced" anesthetic
b. incomplete muscle relaxant reversal
c. narcotic effect masking postanesthesia shaking
d. weak vomiting effort with upper airway obstruction

9.62. The anesthesiologist requests that Mr. J receive intravenous edrophonium. The PACU nurse anticipates that edrophonium will:

a. antagonize blockade more slowly than neostigmine
b. potentiate the effect of reversal medications when given with atropine
c. shorten vecuronium's half-life by speeding Hofmann elimination
d. continue blockade if hypothermia is not treated

9.63. Ms V's surgeon orders that she receive 500 mg vancomycin prior to her choledochoduodenostomy. The preanesthesia nurse administers the vancomycin over at least 30 minutes to reduce the potential for:

a. postoperative ototoxicity
b. painful bile duct spasm
c. hypotensive response
d. delayed muscle relaxant metabolism

NOTE: Consider items 9.64-9.68 together.

9.64. Mr. O's temperature is 34.9° C when he is admitted to PACU following general anesthesia for exploratory laparotomy and insertion of a peritoneovenous shunt. Physiologic consequences related to this temperature include:

a. rapid return to alertness and lower oxygen demand
b. respiratory alkalosis with metabolic acidosis
c. increased hepatic circulation and drug clearance
d. peripheral vasoconstriction with dysrhythmia risk

9.65. Initial nursing interventions to address Mr. O's hypothermia include all of the following goals *except:*

a. reversing metabolic acidosis
b. improving tissue perfusion
c. preventing radiant heat loss
d. suppressing muscle activity

9.66. As Mr. O's core temperature approaches 35.5° C, he begins to shiver. Physiologic concerns during rewarming include:

a. fibrinogenesis and rewarming hypervolemia
b. hypotension and carbon dioxide production
c. bradycardia and preventing evaporative heat loss
d. diuresis and metabolic alkalosis

9.67. The purpose of Mr. O's surgical procedure is to:

a. reinfuse accumulated peritoneal fluid to vena cava
b. divert bile flow obstructed by hepatic tumor
c. drain the omentum and a jejunal abscess to a skin pouch
d. decompress liver cirrhosis by aspirating ascites

9.68. The PACU nurse visits Mr. O on his first postoperative day. To determine any adverse hypothermia-related outcomes, she assesses Mr. O for:

a. epinephrine depletion
b. overcompensated hypothermia
c. generalized myalgia
d. renewed curarization

9.69. Renal autoregulation is *least* affected by:

a. isoflurane
b. systolic blood pressure of 200 mm Hg
c. dobutamine
d. stimulation of alpha adrenergic receptors

9.70. Oliguria from prerenal causes often improves after:

a. irrigation and traction to urinary catheter
b. 300 ml crystalloid bolus
c. gentamicin 60 mg for a patient with myoglobinuria
d. a flat and supine position

9.71. The most sensitive indicator of renal function is serum:

a. urea nitrogen
b. osmolality
c. potassium
d. creatinine

NOTE: Consider scenario and items 9.72-9.73 together.

A patient with acute renal failure (ARF) is admitted to PACU for observation after a double lumen subclavian catheter was surgically inserted for hemodialysis access. The patient received midazolam with intraoperative monitoring by the anesthesia provider.

9.72. This patient is particularly at risk to develop:

a. respiratory alkalosis
b. intravascular sepsis
c. nosocomial peritonitis
d. serum potassium deficit

9.73. The PACU nurse observes tall, peaked T waves on this patient's cardiac monitor. The QRS complex extended from 0.10 seconds to 0.14 seconds. The most likely source of this observation is:

a. ventricular hypertrophy
b. hyperkalemia
c. hypocalcemia
d. myocardial ischemia

9.74. During a preadmission interview the patient discloses a history of "yeast infections" that are resistant to antifungal antibiotics. The interviewing nurse explores this patient's risk for:

a. HIV positivity
b. cervical cancer
c. acute hepatitis A
d. unconfirmed pregnancy

NOTE: Consider items 9.75-9.77 together.

9.75. After a bupivacaine spinal anesthetic and resection of 52 g of prostate tissue by transurethral approach, Mr. P's bladder should be irrigated with titrated:

a. sterile distilled water
b. hypertonic colloid solution
c. sterile normal saline
d. hypotonic electrolyte solution

9.76. Mr. P states sensation to his iliac crests and cannot move his legs. Urinary returns are currently bright red and clot free. During his visit with Mr. P in PACU, the urologist applies traction to Mr. P's triple lumen urinary catheter. The nurse now expects to observe:

a. strong abdominal pain, large urinary clots and tissue shreds
b. tachycardia and urge incontinence around the catheter
c. pink tinged urine and suprapubic pain as spinal effect ends
d. referred flank pain and cherry red, clotless irrigation returns

NOTE: The scenario continues.

As Mr. P's spinal anesthetic metabolizes, the nurse notes that Mr. P's blood pressure is consistently 180/92. He is oriented, conversant, breathes comfortably, and denies pain or urge to void. The nurse consults with the anesthesiologist, who orders 2 doses of intravenous esmolol 10 mg to achieve a systolic blood pressure of less than 160 mm Hg.

9.77. While evaluating Mr. P's blood pressure response to esmolol, the PACU nurse anticipates the *most likely* change in cardiac rhythm on EKG will be:

a. sinus bradycardia
b. right bundle branch block
c. multifocal premature ventricular contractions
d. reflexive supraventricular tachycardia

9.78. A middle-aged man is scheduled for left knee arthroplasty at 1500 today. He uses a nonsteroidal anti-inflammatory drug (NSAID) to manage pain in his arthritic left knee, and so he has increased risk to develop:

a. delayed joint healing
b. gastric ulceration
c. hypercoagulability
d. hydronephrosis

NOTE: Consider scenario and items 9.79-9.81 together.

For the past 9 months, Ms A has dialyzed herself at home even though she still produces about 500 ml of urine each day. She was admitted to the hospital 18 days ago for peritonitis treatment. One week ago, a small colon lesion was discovered, and today Ms A had an intraoperative colonoscopy and transverse colon resection.

9.79. Ms A's renal disease affects the pharmacokinetics of anesthetic medications in a way that increases:

a. circulating unbound medication
b. protein-bound anesthetic
c. blood-brain barrier permeability
d. Hofmann elimination

9.80. When assessing Ms A's postoperative condition in PACU, the nurse is *most* concerned when the:

a. abdominal dressing is colored by a small circle of sanguineous drainage
b. intermittent nasogastric suction is set at –80 mm Hg
c. peritoneal dialysis catheter has a pale pink and nontender skin exit site
d. antibiotic tubing connects by "piggyback" into the total parenteral nutrition (TPN) solution

NOTE: The scenario continues.

Prior to dialyzing herself at home with continuous peritoneal dialysis (CAPD), Ms A received hemodialysis twice each week. A synthetic graft was inserted into her left arm and used as her hemodialysis access. Hemodialysis is now planned postoperatively, again using this access.

9.81. The nursing plan of care related to this dialysis access considers all of the following *except* that the:

a. blood sampling occurs in the right arm
b. bruit is audible during left blood pressure cuff inflation
c. nurse's fingertips palpate a venous thrill
d. neurovascular status of left arm is unaltered

9.82. The *greatest priority* in the Phase I PACU nurse's plan of care for Ms G after her Billroth I procedure is:

a. stimulating frequent deep breaths and position shifts
b. monitoring reoccurrence of peritoneal ascites
c. reporting 25 ml bright red nasogastric returns
d. assuring patency and traction on double balloon gastric tube

9.83. The nurse caring for Ms H after her vaginal hysterectomy is *most concerned* when:

a. Ms H mentions low back pain and tingling toes
b. no tension is applied to the suprapubic catheter
c. Ms H states abdominal pressure and cramping
d. one perineal pad saturates with blood in an hour

NOTE: Consider scenario and item 9.84 together.

The PACU nurse observes blue discoloration along 25 year old Ms Y's right flank after her lysis of adhesions and resection of a perforated appendix. Ms Y's respirations are shallow, she states pain and nausea, and she curls her knees to her chest. There are no audible bowel sounds.

9.84. The nurse's *most appropriate* nursing intervention related to these observations is to promptly:

a. measure abdominal girth and blood pressure
b. assess gastric hemoglobin and provide analgesia
c. reposition Ms Y and administer her antibiotic
d. obtain arterial blood gasses and insist Ms Y breathe more deeply

9.85. The obese patient is *most likely* to develop postoperative:

a. hyperventilation syndrome
b. hypermetabolism of narcotics
c. hyperglycemia
d. hypercarbia while asleep

NOTE: Consider scenario and item 9.86 together.

Upon arrival in PACU after a general anesthetic with enflurane and narcotic, a middle-aged man repeatedly attempts to sit up, states he wants to get out of bed, removes his oxygen face tent and picks at his abdominal dressing.

9.86. The PACU nurse attempts to reassure and reorient this man and assesses him for the most likely causes of his restlessness, including hypoxia, pain and:

a. recurrent angina
b. halogenated-gas toxicity
c. distended bladder
d. renarcotization

9.87. *Early* hemorrhagic hypovolemia in a child is usually indicated by:

a. restlessness
b. tachycardia
c. hypotension
d. somnolence

SET I

Answer Key

9.1.	b
9.2.	a
9.3.	c
9.4.	d
9.5.	c
9.6.	b
9.7.	a
9.8.	a
9.9.	d
9.10.	c
9.11.	a
9.12.	b
9.13.	d
9.14.	b
9.15.	a
9.16.	c
9.17.	c
9.18.	c
9.19.	b
9.20.	c
9.21.	b
9.22.	b
9.23.	c
9.24.	a
9.25.	b
9.26.	c
9.27.	d
9.28.	b
9.29.	a
9.30.	a

SET I

Rationales and References

9.1. Correct Answer: **b**

Oliguria is defined as "diminished urine secretion in relation to fluid intake" and clinically indicates urine production of less than 400 ml/day. This may (or may not) result in retention of nitrogenous wastes and acidosis. Urinary catheter obstruction may be one cause of postrenal failure; patency must be determined prior to any intervention for suspected acute renal failure.

Miller, BF & Keane, CB: Encyclopedia and Dictionary of Medicine, Nursing and Allied Health, *4th ed. Philadelphia, Saunders, p. 883, 1987; Clement, JM: Assessment: Renal System in* Critical Care Nursing: A Holistic Approach, *6th ed (Hudak, CM & Gallo, BM, Eds). Philadelphia, Lippincott, pp. 576-594, 1994.*

9.2. Correct Answer: **a**

An insufficient amount of circulating adrenocorticosteroids is called Addison's disease. The cause may be either adrenal disease or the unrecognized chronic use or insufficient replacement of exogenous steroids. Without adequate cortisol replacement, severe hypotension with low cardiac output and vasodilation can develop. This response indicates the body's inability to respond to surgical stress. Hypoglycemia, fever, lethargy, and electrolyte shifts are also associated with corticosteroid suppression.

Genuth, SM: The Endocrine System in Physiology, *3rd ed (Berne, RM & Levy, MN, Eds). St. Louis, Mosby, pp. 955-966 & 977, 1993; Gervasio, BA: The Endocrine Surgical Patient in* ASPAN's Core Curriculum for Post Anesthesia Nursing Practice, *3rd ed (Litwack, K, Ed). Philadelphia, Saunders, pp. 549-550, 1994.*

9.3. Correct Answer: **c**

Aspiration is a concern for any sedated patient with a nasogastric tube. Assuring tube patency and elevating Mr. V's head to semi-Fowler's position help decrease risk. A nasogastric tube snaked into the stomach enhances the likelihood of gastroesophageal reflux by passing through (opening) the lower esophageal sphincter. Acidic stomach contents can creep up the outside of the tube, particularly if obstructed. Like fluid traveling on a wick, gastric contents then move down the trachea to the lungs. Gastric peristalsis slowly returns 1-4 days postoperatively. Thrombophlebitis *is* a potential complication, though less immediate than the risk of aspiration in a sedated patient with a gastric tube in place.

Ahrens, T: Respiratory Disorders in AACN's Clinical Reference for Critical-Care Nursing, *3rd ed (Kinney, MR, Packa, DR & Dunbar, SB, Eds). St. Louis, Mosby, p. 710, 1993; Pelligrini, C: Postoperative Complications in* Current Surgical Diagnoses and Treatment *(Way, LW, Ed). Appleton & Lange, Norwalk, CT, pp. 25-41, 1992.*

9.4. Correct Answer: **d**

A newly created stoma should be pink or red, not bluish or light grey. The nurse must inform the surgeon of this observation, as interrupted blood flow to the stoma is possible. The nurse can expect no bowel sounds, a soft abdomen when palpated, and small amounts of nasogastric returns.

O'Brien, DD: The Gastrointestinal Surgical Patient in ASPAN's Core Curriculum for Post Anesthesia Nursing Practice, *3rd ed (Litwack, K, Ed). Philadelphia, Saunders, pp. 452-454, 1994; O'Brien, D: Post Anesthesia Care of the Gastrointestinal, Abdominal, and Anorectal Surgical Patient in* The Post Anesthesia Care Unit: A Critical Care Approach to Post Anesthesia Nursing, *3rd ed (Drain, C, Ed). Philadelphia, Saunders, p. 455-456, 1994.*

9.5. Correct Answer: **c**

Mr. B requires a patent intravenous line. Significant cardiopulmonary compromise could immediately occur during the test dose. Malposition or migration of the epidural catheter after insertion could result in an unplanned intravascular or intraspinal injection. Emergency treatment of the resulting hypotension and respiratory suppression may include rapid intravenous fluid volume and infusion of vasopressors and a pure opioid agonist (naloxone). The registered nurse's responsibility when delivering intraspinal medications is clear: administering a test or initial dose to determine catheter placement is the responsibility only of "licensed professionals who are educated in the specialty of anesthesia."

Litwack, K: Post Anesthesia Care Nursing, *2nd ed. St. Louis, Mosby, pp. 167-172, 1995; American Society of Post Anesthesia Nurses (ASPAN): Standards of Perianesthesia Nursing Practice, Resource 13. Thorofare, NJ, ASPAN, pp. 52-53, 1995.*

9.6. Correct Answer: **b**

The PACU nurse's scope of practice may permit the nurse to *reinject* and *alter* the infusion *rate* when managing the analgesia of a nonobstetric patient *with physician direction.* State law, practice codes and facility policies must state this. Establishing dosage parameters and catheter placement are specific physician responsibilities. Up to 2 hours may be needed to achieve an effective dose of an epidural narcotic. Therefore an alternative approach could be to administer supplemental doses of intravenous narcotic in addition to reconsidering the dose of epidural narcotic.

Litwack, K: Post Anesthesia Care Nursing, *2nd ed. St. Louis, Mosby, pp. 167-172, 1995; American Society of Post Anesthesia Nurses (ASPAN):* Standards of Perianesthesia Nursing Practice, *Resource 13. Thorofare, NJ, ASPAN, pp. 52-53, 1995.*

9.7. Correct Answer: **a**

The kidney "interprets" altered blood flow from any cause as reason to increase blood pressure and retain fluid. Renin released from the kidney activates angiotensin, which constricts renal vessels and tries to increase blood pressure. Unfortunately this further decreases renal blood flow. Aldosterone's effect on the nephron's distal tubule promotes sodium reabsorption. Antidiuretic hormone secretion, not suppression, prompts fluid retention, and decreases urine volume.

Nagle, GM: The Urologic Surgical Patient in ASPAN's Core Curriculum for Post Anesthesia Nursing Practice, *3rd ed (Litwack, K, Ed). Philadelphia, Saunders, pp. 404-407, 1994; Morgan, GE & Mikhail, MS:* Clinical Anesthesiology. *Norwalk, CT, Appleton & Lange, pp. 463-464 & 514-517, 1992.*

9.8. Correct Answer: **a**

Hydralazine has little overall effect on renal blood flow and is often selected for the hypertensive patient with renal failure. However, a patient with limited intracranial adaptive capacity (compliance) risks an ever higher intracranial pressure if given hydralazine. Hydralazine vasodilates arterioles and decreases systemic vascular resistance (afterload). Intracranial pressure increases when cerebral blood flow increases. As a "potent cerebral vasodilator," hydralazine inhibits the physiologic response of autoregulation that maintains consistent cerebral blood flow.

Morgan, GE & Mikhail, MS: Clinical Anesthesiology. *Norwalk, CT, Appleton & Lange, pp. 169-172, 1992; Drain, C:* The Post Anesthesia Care Unit: A Critical Care Approach to Post Anesthesia Nursing, *3rd ed. Philadelphia, Saunders, p. 102, 1994.*

9.9. Correct Answer: **d**

Hepatitis A, eliminated through the feces, is transmitted when an infected source is orally ingested by an uninfected person. Sources include fecally contaminated water or food. Hepatitis B is more virulent and spreads through contact between the carrier's infected blood or blood-containing secretions and the mucous membrane or broken skin barrier of a noninfected person. Hepatitis C and D are also spread parenterally.

Krumberger, JM: Gastrointestinal Disorders in AACN's Clinical Reference for Critical-Care Nursing, *3rd ed (Kinney, MF, Packa, DR & Dunbar, SB, Eds). St. Louis, Mosby, pp. 1171-1177, 1993.*

9.10. Correct Answer: **c**

This patient's bile drainage should be reported. Postoperative drainage of bile after cholecystectomy is typically less than 30 ml/hour. Obstruction, fistula or severed common bile duct are conditions that increase volume of bile drainage. Bleeding with the bile drainage can indicate cystic artery hemorrhage, a serious consequence.

O'Brien, DD: Post Anesthesia Care of the Gastrointestinal, Abdominal and Anorectal Surgical Patient in The Post Anesthesia Care Unit: A Critical Care Approach to Post Anesthesia Nursing, *3rd ed (Drain, C, Ed). Philadelphia, Saunders, p. 460, 1994.*

9.11. Correct Answer: **a**

Glucose-insulin imbalance is expected after a pancreaticoduodenectomy (Whipple procedure) to resect a pancreatic tumor. The pancreas' insulin-producing function is disrupted by both the tumor and the surgery. Frequent measures of serum glucose determine the required insulin dose to maintain a glucose level between 200-300 mg/dl. These often poorly nourished patients also frequently receive hyperalimentation, a high-glucose fluid that contributes to serum glucose elevations.

O'Brien, DD: Post Anesthesia Care of the Gastrointestinal, Abdominal and Anorectal Surgical Patient in The Post Anesthesia Care Unit: A Critical Care Approach to

Post Anesthesia Nursing, *3rd ed (Drain, C, Ed). Philadelphia, Saunders, p. 460, 1994; Krumberger, JM: Gastrointestinal Disorders in* AACN's Clinical Reference for Critical-Care Nursing, *3rd ed (Kinney, MF, Packa, DR & Dunbar, SB, Eds). St. Louis, Mosby, pp. 1181-1183, 1993.*

9.12. Correct Answer: **b**

Particularly after a major resection and "reconnection" of gastrointestinal structures, the surgeon should inform the nurse of type and purpose of any abdominal tubes and of expected drainage volumes. To avoid disrupting a fragile anastomosis after gastric surgery, a nasogastric tube should *never* be irrigated, manipulated at whim, or reinserted by the nurse until approved by the surgeon. Often the nasogastric tube is precisely positioned by direct visualization during surgery. Abdominal distention after this surgery could herald a leaking anastomosis with intraabdominal hemorrhage or leaking gastric contents.

O'Brien, DD: Post Anesthesia Care of the Gastrointestinal, Abdominal and Anorectal Surgical Patient in The Post Anesthesia Care Unit: A Critical Care Approach to Post Anesthesia Nursing, *3rd ed (Drain, C, Ed). Philadelphia, Saunders, p. 460, 1994; Krumberger, JM: Gastrointestinal Disorders in* AACN's Clinical Reference for Critical-Care Nursing, *3rd ed (Kinney, MF, Packa, DR & Dunbar, SB, Eds). St. Louis, Mosby, pp. 1181-1183, 1993.*

9.13. Correct Answer: **d**

A pancreaticojejunostomy involves resection of major gastrointestinal organs and creating new connections, usually to treat pancreatic cancer. The distal (lower) stomach, part of the common bile duct, ampulla (head) of the pancreas and adjoining duodenum are removed. Appropriate biliary, hepatic, gastric and intestinal reconnections (anastomoses) are made to restore some integrity and function to the gastrointestinal tract.

O'Brien, DD: Post Anesthesia Care of the Gastrointestinal, Abdominal and Anorectal Surgical Patient in The Post Anesthesia Care Unit: A Critical Care Approach to Post Anesthesia Nursing, *3rd ed (Drain, C, Ed). Philadelphia, Saunders, p. 450, 1994.*

9.14. Correct Answer: **b**

Scopolamine, like atropine, is an anticholinergic medication that blocks the action of the neurotransmitter acetylcholine on the brain's vomiting center. As such, it can be a potent antiemetic. In addition, disorientation or drowsiness may develop. Some gynecologic surgical procedures have been associated with higher likelihood for postoperative nausea.

Belatti, RG: Common Post Anesthetic Problems in Post Anesthesia Care *(Vender, JE & Speiss, BD, Eds). Philadelphia, Saunders, pp. 13-18, 1992; Harbut, RE: Anesthetic Agents and Adjuncts in* ASPAN's Core Curriculum for Post Anesthesia Nursing Practice, *3rd ed (Litwack, K, Ed). Philadelphia, Saunders, pp. 124-125, 1994.*

9.15. Correct Answer: **a**

Central nervous system (CNS) effects of anticholinergic medications include delirium with disorientation, combativeness and agitation. Hypoxia and acid-base imbalances *must* be excluded as causes of any delirium before attributing delirium solely to the scopolamine. The likelihood of emergence delirium increases when narcotics are not used with the anticholinergic. Preoperative anxiety and fear, pain, and hypoxia also contribute to emergence delirium.

Belatti, RG: Common Post Anesthetic Problems in Post Anesthesia Care *(Vender, JE & Speiss, BD, Eds). Philadelphia, Saunders, pp. 11, 14-16 & 196, 1992; Burden, N:* Ambulatory Surgical Nursing. *Philadelphia, Saunders, p. 291, 1993.*

9.16. Correct Answer: **c**

Physostigmine (Antilirium) in 1 mg doses successfully reverses the CNS effects and toxicity (confusion and agitation) of anticholinergic medications like scopolamine. The effect of the reversal agent may be shorter than the anticholinergic's influence on the CNS, though. If agitation recurs, repeat the physostigmine—to a maximum total dose of 3 mg. This minimizes bradycardic symptoms from large doses or overzealous administration.

Burden, N: Ambulatory Surgical Nursing. *Philadelphia, Saunders, p. 291, 1993; Herbert, DW: Manual of Drugs in* Anesthesia and Critical Care. *Philadelphia, Saunders, pp. 58-59, 1993.*

9.17. Correct Answer: **c**

The nurse must consider Ms E's potential for deep vein thrombosis (DVT) in her legs, suggested by calf or posterior knee tenderness, redness or heat. Both her surgery (gynecologic) and her intraoperative position (lithotomy) can alter circulation and damage nerves. Gynecologic procedures reportedly reduce blood flow from the legs by more than 50%, though the actual incidence of DVT is less than 10%. The nurse should assess and document that Ms E's peripheral pulses are present. Back, hip and leg pain likely are of muscular origin and, therefore, self-limiting. Though abdominal cramping is expected, true distention and unrelieved pain may indicate uterine perforation. Most patients have minimal postoperative drainage in PACU.

Miller, KM: Post Anesthesia Care of the Obstetric and Gynecologic Surgical Patient in ASPAN's Core Curriculum for Post Anesthesia Nursing Practice, *3rd ed (Litwack, K, Ed). Philadelphia, Saunders, pp. 481-483, 1994; Burden, N:* Ambulatory Surgical Nursing. *Philadelphia, Saunders, pp. 505-507, 1993.*

9.18. Correct Answer: **c**

Renal function arising from prerenal failure may be improved by increasing cardiac output and sodium excretion. Furosemide (Lasix) is a potent diuretic that increases sodium excretion (followed by fluid) at the loop of Henle and distal renal tubules. Sodium (and fluid) are retained in prerenal failure when the kidneys "sense" low fluid volume and low cardiac output. Correcting a fluid volume deficit and supporting cardiac output also may sufficiently increase renal blood flow to improve the renal failure. Dopamine promotes renal perfusion, though the "renal dose" of dopamine is small, approximately 0.5 mg/kg; aminoglycosides are strongly nephrotoxic and should not be used in azotemic patients. Patency of any ureteral stent is essential to renal function but addresses a *post*renal cause of oliguria.

Nagle, GM: The Urologic Surgical Patient in ASPAN's Core Curriculum for Post Anesthesia Nursing Practice, *3rd ed (Litwack, K, Ed). Philadelphia, Saunders, pp. 409-410, 1994; Clement, JM: Assessment: Renal System in* Critical Care Nursing: A Holistic Approach, *6th ed (Hudak, CM & Gallo, BM, Eds). Philadelphia, Lippincott, pp. 576-594, 1994.*

9.19. Correct Answer: **b**

Hospital protocols and state laws govern criteria for administering medications for intravenous conscious sedation. Nursing responsibility includes continuous monitoring and assessment of airway, respiratory rate, oxygen saturation, blood pressure and cardiac rate and rhythm. The nurse observing the patient must have no other responsibilities and must be able to both intervene in emergency situations and contact additional personnel for support.

American Society of Post Anesthesia Nurses (ASPAN): Standards of Post Anesthesia Nursing Practice, *Resource 14. Thorofare, NJ, ASPAN, pp. 54-55, 1995; Burden, N:* Ambulatory Surgical Nursing. *Philadelphia, Saunders, pp. 95-96, 1993.*

9.20. Correct Answer: **c**

Mr. U's symptoms after a transurethral resection of the prostate (TURP) are consistent with bladder perforation. Fluid pouring into the abdomen contribute to the referred pain into the shoulder. Mr. U's urologist must be contacted; best outcomes require cystectomy, preferably within 1-2 hours after perforation. Bladder spasm is a frequent event after TURP and can cause pain (usually over the bladder area) and a strong urge to urinate. Increased bleeding and perhaps clots in the returns of the bladder irrigation system may be noted with spasms; bladder relaxation, increased rate of irrigation and observation are interventions for bladder spasms.

Miller, KM: Post Anesthesia Care of the Genitourinary Surgical Patient in The Post Anesthesia Care Unit: A Critical Care Approach to Post Anesthesia Nursing, *3rd ed (Drain, C Ed). Philadelphia, Saunders, p. 472, 1994; Jacobsen, WK:* Manual of Post Anesthesia Care. *Philadelphia, Saunders, pp. 119-120, 1992.*

9.21. Correct Answer: **b**

Both regional and general anesthetic techniques expose the patient to changes in muscle and vascular tone, ability to move and feel pain and altered circulation to surface areas, particularly the pressure-susceptible bony sites. More than 2 hours in a surgical position, elderly age, preexisting (and often age-related) arthritis, diabetes, cardiovascular diseases, and nutritional status greatly affect the potential for position-related injury.

Walsh, J: Postop Effects of OR Positioning. RN *56(2): 50-58, 1993; Litwack, K:* Post Anesthesia Care Nursing, *2nd ed. St. Louis, Mosby, pp. 480-492, 1995.*

9.22. Correct Answer: **b**

Following extracorporeal shock wave lithotripsy (ESWL), patients often are discharged to home and so must understand that high-volume fluid intake and straining urine are essential. ESWL directs multiple high-frequency shocks through the skin to pulverize renal calculi. The patient must excrete the stone fragments through the urine. Copious fluid intake is expected to promote strong urine volumes to flush the stones through the renal system. Pain is usually minimal after ESWL, though flank tenderness and slight skin redness occur.

Burden, N: Ambulatory Surgical Nursing. *Philadelphia, Saunders, p. 504, 1993; Nagle, GM: The Urologic Surgical Patient in* ASPAN's Core Curriculum for Post Anesthesia Nursing Practice, *3rd ed (Litwack, K, Ed). Philadelphia, Saunders, p. 423, 1994.*

9.23. Correct Answer: **c**

Ms A regularly takes prednisone; her steroid-induced adrenal atrophy requires timely postoperative hydrocortisone supplementation to support her stress responses. If an intraoperative dose of hydrocortisone was not administered and no postoperative doses are ordered, the PACU nurse contacts the physician. Steroids cannot be abruptly interrupted without physiologic consequences; dexamethasone does not provide sufficient replacement. Cortisol is not stored in the body, yet is essential to systemic function, particularly to sustain adequate serum glucose and for stress adaptation. Ms A's surgical procedure and intraoperative position increase her potential for thromboembolism; she needs antiembolic stockings or pneumatic leg compression devices.

Steelman, VM: Surgical Client in Basic Nursing: Theory and Practice, *3rd ed (Potter, PA & Perry, AG, Eds). St. Louis, Mosby, p. 1082, 1994; Litwack, K:* Post Anesthesia Care Nursing, *2nd ed. St. Louis, Mosby, p. 279, 1995.*

9.24. Correct Answer: **a**

This elderly woman has risk for hypoxia and hypercarbia from age-related alterations in respiratory volumes. A moderate head-elevated position and encouraged deep breathing allow the greatest chest expansion. Surgically, this patient can assume a position of comfort. A high-Fowler's position is avoided to better promote blood flow to and from the legs and prevent stasis.

Miller, KM: Post Anesthesia Care of the Obstetric and Gynecologic Surgical Patient in The Post Anesthesia Care Unit: A Critical Care Approach to Post Anesthesia Nursing, *3rd ed (Drain, C, Ed). Philadelphia, Saunders, pp. 481-483, 1994.*

9.25. Correct Answer: **b**

Unrecognized infection, impaired wound healing, thinner, more fragile skin tissue, osteoporosis, fluid retention and hyperglycemia are among physiologic changes produced by chronic use of synthetic corticosteroids. Any symptoms of infection can be masked by suppressed inflammatory responses. Therefore, Ms A requires particular attention to her nutritional status and asepsis during wound observation and dressing changes.

Burden, N: Ambulatory Surgical Nursing. *Philadelphia, Saunders, pp. 405-406; Goldfien, A: Adrenocorticosteroids and Adrenocortical Antagonists in* Basic and Clinical Pharmacology, *6th ed (Katzung, BG, Ed). Norwalk, CT, Appleton & Lange, pp. 595-601, 1995.*

9.26. Correct Answer: **c**

In prerenal failure, the nephron remains undamaged even though the volume of blood filtered at the glomerulus, and therefore the amount of urine produced, decreases. Hypovolemia from overdiuresis, shock, cardiac failure or dehydration—outcomes produced by events unrelated to kidney anatomy—cause prerenal failure. Acute tubular necrosis results from actual damage to kidney tissue, thereby affecting the kidney's ability to concentrate fluid and excrete wastes.

Weems, J: Quick Reference to Renal Critical Care Nursing. *Gaithersburg, MD, Aspen, pp. 39-42, 1991; Clement, JM: Assessment: Renal System in* Critical Care Nursing: A Holistic Approach, *6th ed (Hudak, CM & Gallo, BM, Eds). Philadelphia, Lippincott, pp. 576-594, 1994.*

9.27. Correct Answer: **d**

Despite adequate overall fluid volume replacement, Mr. L's hypotension likely results when fluid translocates from his vascular compartment into abdominal tissues and spaces that normally contain little fluid. This sequestered volume is unavailable to support cardiac output. Extensive bowel manipulation, tissue trauma or infection, decreased serum protein and altered capillary permeability are among forces that could allow fluids to exit the vascular compartment after a major abdominal surgical procedure.

Tuman, KJ: Fluid and Electrolyte Abnormalities and Management in Post Anesthesia Care *(Vender, JS & Speiss, BD, Eds). Philadelphia, Saunders, pp. 163-169, 1992; DeFranco, M: Fluid and Electrolyte Balance in* ASPAN's Core Curriculum for Post Anesthesia Nursing Practice, *3rd ed (Litwack, K, Ed). Philadelphia, Saunders, pp. 161-163, 1994.*

9.28. Correct Answer: **b**

To improve cardiac output and assure sufficient renal blood flow are appropriate responses to treat Mr. L's decreased circulating blood volume and fluid shifts. Supporting circulation may initially require several liters of crystalloid or, alternatively and controversially, colloid support, and then judicious monitoring to detect evidence of cardiac overload.

Tuman, KJ: Fluid and Electrolyte Abnormalities and Management in Post Anesthesia Care *(Vender, JS & Speiss, BD, Eds). Philadelphia, Saunders, pp. 163-169, 1992; DeFranco, M: Fluid and Electrolyte Balance in* ASPAN's Core Curriculum for Post Anesthesia Nursing Practice, *3rd ed (Litwack, K, Ed). Philadelphia, Saunders, pp. 161-163, 1994.*

9.29. Correct Answer: **a**

The fluid volume given in PACU to fill Mr. L's vascular compartment and support his cardiac output eventually is reabsorbed and renally excreted. Intestinal tissue injuries must first heal and capillary permeability must return to normal; fluid translocation can continue for up to 72 hours. Until then, Mr. L still has risk of circulatory overload and requires close observation of vital signs, renal output and urine concentrating ability, and pulmonary infiltration. He still requires fluids as prescribed by the physician, as much as 200 ml/hour of hypertonic fluid. Pain can increase both preload and afterload, possibly overtaxing cardiac muscle.

Tuman, KJ: Fluid and Electrolyte Abnormalities and Management in Post Anesthesia Care *(Vender, JS & Speiss, BD, Eds). Philadelphia, Saunders, pp. 163-169, 1992; DeFranco, M: Fluid and Electrolyte Balance in* ASPAN's Core Curriculum for Post Anesthesia Nursing Practice, *3rd ed (Litwack, K, Ed). Philadelphia, Saunders, pp. 161-163, 1994.*

9.30. Correct Answer: **a**

This patient may be sensitive to latex. Eye swelling and hand dermatitis at work are important bits of preoperative information. Exposing him to the array of latex products in the anesthesia environment can result in systemic responses like bronchospasm, severe hypotension or cardiac arrest (anaphylaxis). Health care workers like dentists, hygienists, physicians and nurses regularly wear latex gloves. Over time, multiple exposures to latex antigen sensitizes the health care worker either by direct contact with a latex product or by inhaling airborne particles. Latex reactions range from a localized rash with redness and itching to a systemic hypersensitivity reaction with anaphylaxis.

Benner, SD: Latex Allergy. CPANewsletter *pp. 3-4, 8 Nov, 1994; Weiss, ME & Levy, JH: Allergic and Transfusion Reactions in* Post Anesthesia Care *(Vender, JS & Speiss, BD, Eds). Philadelphia, Saunders, pp. 233-239, 1992.*

SET II

Answer Key

9.31. b
9.32. c
9.33. b
9.34. c
9.35. d
9.36. b
9.37. c
9.38. a
9.39. b
9.40. d
9.41. a
9.42. a
9.43. c
9.44. b
9.45. d
9.46. b
9.47. d
9.48. c
9.49. b
9.50. a
9.51. d
9.52. d
9.53. a
9.54. c
9.55. a
9.56. b
9.57. d
9.58. a
9.59. a
9.60. b

SET II

Rationales and References

9.31. Correct Answer: **b**

Normal bladder volume ranges from about 300-800 ml. Urge to void generally occurs when the bladder fills with 300-400 ml. Deferring micturation stretches bladder walls and over time could alter muscle contraction and emptying. Regional anesthesia, surgical procedures, lack of privacy, and "unnatural" positions can affect bladder emptying during the immediate postanesthetic period.

Nagle, GM: The Urologic Surgical Patient in ASPAN's Core Curriculum for Post Anesthesia Nursing Practice, *3rd ed (Litwack, K, Ed). Philadelphia, Saunders, p. 401, 1994; Stalheim-Smith, A & Fitch, GK:* Understanding Human Anatomy and Physiology. *Minneapolis/St. Paul, West Publishing, p. 888, 1994.*

9.32. Correct Answer: **c**

Diabetes insipidus occurs when the hypothalamus fails to respond to sensed need for antidiuretic secretion (ADH, vasopressin). Great quantities of dilute, poorly concentrated and "sugar-free" urine are excreted by the kidneys. Dehydration results from this deficiency.

Provenzano, SM: Head Injury in Critical Care Nursing: A Holistic Approach, *6th ed. Philadelphia, Lippincott, pp. 710-711, 1994.*

9.33. Correct Answer: **b**

Reversing fluid volume deficits and acidemia are among interventions that can reduce renal damage (nephrotoxicity) from aminoglycoside antibiotics. Elderly age, nonsteroidal antiinflammatories, and large doses of potent diuretics are other risk factors that can increase the incidence of renal damage during treatment with this class of antibiotics. Up to 20% of patients develop renal dysfunction after receiving aminoglycoside antibiotics.

Bauman, LA & Prough, DS: Acute Perioperative Renal Dysfunction in Post Anesthesia Care *(Vender, JS & Speiss, BD, Eds). Philadelphia, Saunders, pp. 143-144, 1992.*

9.34. Correct Answer: **c**

After succinylcholine-induced relaxation, muscle function returns first to the respiratory (intercostal) muscles and then to shoulders and abdomen, followed by neck and extremities. Eye, finger and toe muscles recover last. Ms H is presumed to have an atypical (congenital) pseudocholinesterase response that delayed her metabolism of succinylcholine; succinylcholine is usually hydrolyzed quickly. Recovery of muscle function depends upon the amount of active circulating pseudocholinesterase. Her rash may result from a normal release of histamine.

Schweinefus, R & Schick, L: Succinylcholine: "Good Guy, Bad Guy." J Post Anesth Nurs *6(6): 410-419, 1991; Harbut, RE: Anesthetic Agents and Adjuncts in* ASPAN's Core Curriculum for Post Anesthesia Nursing Practice,

3rd ed (Litwack, K, Ed). Philadelphia, Saunders, pp. 97-101, 1994.

9.35. Correct Answer: **d**

Especially following brief surgical procedures and single intubating doses of succinylcholine, nearly one-half of patients state muscle aching when moving their face, neck, shoulder, rib, or abdomen. Postoperative bedrest seems to lessen the pain. Muscle tremors (fasciculations) occur during cellular depolarization; the contractions produce pain, which is noticed as the postoperative patient becomes mobile. Though nerve compression is possible from any intraoperative position, Ms H's lithotomy position more likely would produce back pain. Vomiting occurs after laparoscopic and endometrial surgery, though Ms H apparently tolerates fluids without emesis.

Schweinefus, R & Schick, L: Succinylcholine: "Good Guy, Bad Guy." J Post Anesth Nurs *6(6): 410-419, 1991; Harbut, RE: Anesthetic Agents and Adjuncts in* ASPAN's Core Curriculum for Post Anesthesia Nursing Practice, *3rd ed (Litwack, K, Ed). Philadelphia, Saunders, pp. 97-101, 1994.*

9.36. Correct Answer: **b**

Atropine and glycopyrrolate relax bladder smooth muscle and increase sphincter tone, therefore inhibiting urination. Atropine, a belladonna alkaloid, and glycopyrrolate, a belladonna alkaloid derivative, block the parasympathetic response to acetylcholine at the neuromuscular junction. Parasympathetic nerves control the urinary bladder and urge to void; a full bladder stimulates the parasympathetic nerves, relaxes the outlet sphincter, and contracts bladder muscle. By competing with acetylcholine at muscarinic receptors, anticholinergic (parasympatholytic) medications block bladder emptying. Neostigmine and edrophonium (Tensilon) stimulate muscarinic receptors and so oppose atropine's action.

Herbert, DW: Manual of Drugs in Anesthesia and Critical Care. *Philadelphia, Saunders, pp. 64-65, 1993; Kemp, B & Tabaka, N: Post Operative Urinary Retention in the PACU.* Curr Rev Post Anesth Nurs *13(12), 1992.*

9.37. Correct Answer: **c**

Flumazenil reportedly can provoke panic attacks in patients with prior history; agitation and labile emotions are among expected psychologic responses after flumazenil reverses midazolam's effects. In addition, the PACU nurse is correct in questioning this 0.6 mg dose of flumazenil. Usually flumazenil is titrated to effect (reawakening), typically in 0.2 mg doses each minute. Elderly patients like Mr. X do not require flumazenil dose reductions. Tricyclic antidepressant *use,* not allergy, is a reason to avoid flumazenil. Flumazenil does not alter narcotic-related (fentanyl) effects.

Herbert, DW: Manual of Drugs in Anesthesia and Critical Care. *Philadelphia, Saunders, pp. 128-129, 1993; Burden, N:* Ambulatory Surgical Nursing. *Philadelphia, Saunders, pp. 68-69, 1993.*

9.38. Correct Answer: **a**

Flumazenil's half-life is approximately 60 minutes; Mr. X should be closely observed for hypoventilation for at least 1 hour. Flumazenil is specifically designed to reverse the *central nervous system* effects of benzodiazepines. It has less effect on any respiratory hypoventilation caused by large midazolam doses. Flumazenil has no effect on muscle relaxant or narcotic-produced symptoms. Flumazenil's effect on amnesia produced by midazolam is unpredictable.

Herbert, DW: Manual of Drugs in Anesthesia and Critical Care. *Philadelphia, Saunders, pp. 128-129, 1993; Burden, N:* Ambulatory Surgical Nursing. *Philadelphia, Saunders, pp. 68-69, 1993.*

9.39. Correct Answer: **b**

Among the myriad of potential complications of multisystem organ failure, sepsis is a contributing cause of death in "as many as 42% of patients (Dossey)." Infection results from many possible sources and can initiate a progression of events that contributes to shock, disseminated intravascular coagulation, renal failure, gastrointestinal bleeding, and pulmonary failure. Vigilant effort is directed toward finding and eradicating the infectious source. The nurse will monitor the patient's currently acceptable platelets and urine output; the patient's hemoglobin level, though less than the accepted normal of 12-15, may reflect hemodilution, not necessarily new bleeding after abdominal exploration.

Dossey, BM, Guzzetta, CE & Kenner, CV: Critical Care Nursing: Body-Mind-Spirit, *3rd ed. Philadelphia, Lippincott, pp. 849-875, 1992; Mamaril, ME: Post Anesthesia Care of the Shock Trauma Patient in* The Post Anesthesia Care Unit: A Critical Care Approach to Post Anesthesia Nursing, *3rd ed (Drain, C, Ed). Philadelphia, Saunders, pp. 580-582, 1994.*

9.40. Correct Answer: **d**

A patient with early hyperdynamic septic shock has warm, dry extremities and flushed skin. This hyperdynamic phase of septic shock is characterized by peripheral vasodilation and markedly increased cardiac output, up to 2-3 times normal. Sepsis must be a primary concern for any patient with potential for multisystem organ failure, even though pain or hypothermia also occurs. This patient's shivering is not hypothermia induced; intravenous butorphanol (Stadol) might further increase intracardiac pressures, cardiac work, and vascular resistance; other medication options are preferable after determining respiratory adequacy. Providing analgesia should not be an "automatic" response.

Dossey, BM, Guzzetta, CE & Kenner, CV: Critical Care Nursing: Body-Mind-Spirit, *3rd ed. Philadelphia, Lippincott, pp. 840-875, 1992; Mamaril, ME: Post Anesthesia Care of the Shock Trauma Patient and Drain C: Opioid Intravenous Anesthetics in* The Post Anesthesia Care Unit: A Critical Care Approach to Post Anesthesia Nursing, *3rd ed (Drain, C, Ed). Philadelphia, Saunders, pp. 580-582 & 219-220, 1994.*

9.41. Correct Answer: **a**

Hyperventilation and $paCO_2$ of <25 mm Hg (respiratory alkalosis) are hallmarks of septic shock. The alkalosis is the body's initial attempt to compensate for metabolic acidosis, indicated by a still-elevated serum lactate. Hypoxemia heralds development of adult respiratory distress syndrome (ARDS). Sepsis stresses all body organ systems.

Dossey, BM, Guzzetta, CE & Kenner, CV: Critical Care Nursing: Body-Mind-Spirit, *3rd ed. Philadelphia, Lippincott, pp. 858-859, 1992; Hanson, CW: Managing the Desperately Ill Patient in* Dripps/Eckenhoff/Vandam Introduction to Anesthesia, *8th ed (Longnecker, DE & Murphy, FL, Eds). Philadelphia, Saunders, pp. 376-381, 1992.*

9.42. Correct Answer: **a**

This EKG indicates the pacemaker's failure to detect or recognize (sense) the patient's native cardiac activity (undersensing). Prompt intervention is required!! Pacemaker artifacts occur regularly and so competes with the patient's own cardiac rhythm. A VVI pacemaker paces the ventricle *(V* in the code's first position) when it senses no ventricular cardiac activity after a specific preset time interval (second *V* in the code). The pacemaker is either inhibited (*I*) or triggered, depending upon the electrical activity the pacemaker senses.

Witherell, CL: Cardiac Rhythm Control Devices. Crit Care Nurs Clin North Am *6(1): 85-95, 1994; Fetzer-Fowler, SJ: Caring for the Ambulatory Surgical Patient Who Has A Pacemaker: Part II.* J Post Anesth Nurs *8(4): 174-181, 1993.*

9.43. Correct Answer: **c**

Randomly delivered pacemaker energy can coincide with the T wave of the patient's intrinsic cardiac cycle and produce ventricular tachycardia. The T wave represents the vulnerable or relatively refractory period of the ventricle's cardiac cycle when less than the usual amount of electrical stimulation can produce an action potential.

Witherell, CL: Cardiac Rhythm Control Devices. Nurs Clin North Am *6(1): 85-95, 1994; Fetzer-Fowler, S: Caring for the Ambulatory Surgical Patient Who Has A Pacemaker: Part II.* J Post Anesth Nurs *8(4): 174-181, 1993.*

9.44. Correct Answer: **b**

Should ventricular tachycardia occur when a pacemaker fails to sense the patient's native cardiac rhythm, the patient's cardiac output must be preserved. The nurse applies electrical energy to the heart to cardiovert or defibrillate. Ideally, before any lethal rhythm develops, the implanted pacemaker would be reprogrammed at the bedside to increase the pacemaker's sensitivity to the patient's intrinsic rhythm. An implanted pacemaker cannot be manually adjusted.

Witherell, CL: Cardiac Rhythm Control Devices. Nurs Clin North Am *6(1): 85-95, 1994; Fetzer-Fowler, S: Caring for the Ambulatory Surgical Patient Who Has A Pacemaker: Part II.* J Post Anesth Nurs *8(4): 174-181, 1993.*

9.45. Correct Answer: **d**

Ms B's tachycardia and relatively low blood pressures may reflect absolute hypovolemia, either from hemoperitoneum and low hemoglobin or insufficient fluid volume replacement. To preserve adequate cardiac output, heart rate often reflexively increases to the tachycardic range (>100 beats per minute) to compensate for decreased venous blood return. The caregiver must recognize that only 2 hours after abdominal hysterectomy, Ms B may be actively bleeding into her abdomen, a not-so-rare complication in the first several postoperative hours. The nurse actually may consider sepsis, hypothermia, and myocardial infarction, as well as hypovolemia as causing Ms B's hypotension but must discern the correct underlying pathophysiologic process.

Mamaril, ME: Post Anesthesia Care of the Shock Trauma Patient in The Post Anesthesia Care Unit: A Critical Care Approach to Post Anesthesia Nursing, *3rd ed (Drain, C, Ed). Philadelphia, Saunders, pp. 577-578, 1994; Marymont, JH & O'Conner, BS: Postoperative Cardiovascular Complications in* Post Anesthesia Care *(Vender, JS & Speiss, BD, Eds). Philadelphia, Saunders, pp. 29-32, 1992.*

9.46. Correct Answer: **b**

Ms B's current hemoglobin should be verified and her abdomen examined for increased distention (girth), rigidity, and pain. The nurse increases the infusion rate of intravenous crystalloids and perhaps adds colloids or blood cell transfusions as ordered. Persistent tachycardia should not be treated with vasodilating or beta blocking medications until fluid volume deficits are corrected. Once adequate circulating volume is restored, tachycardia often self resolves.

Mamaril, ME: Post Anesthesia Care of the Shock Trauma Patient in The Post Anesthesia Care Unit: A Critical Care Approach to Post Anesthesia Nursing, *3rd ed (Drain, C, Ed). Philadelphia, Saunders, pp. 577-578, 1994.*

9.47. Correct Answer: **d**

Azotemia refers to retention of metabolic wastes in the blood due to lack of renal clearance. These by-products are nitrogen based. Urea, peptides, creatine, and creatinine result from protein or amino acid metabolism. Normal creatinine is 0.5-1.5 mg/dl, and BUN is less than 10 mg/dl. The azotemic patient who retains metabolic by-products may indeed have oliguria, with urine less than 400 ml/day.

Clement, JM: Assessment: Renal System in Critical Care Nursing: A Holistic Approach, *6th ed (Hudak, CM & Gallo, BM, Eds). Philadelphia, Lippincott, pp. 576-594, 1994; Drain, C:* The Post Anesthesia Care Unit: A Critical Care Approach to Post Anesthesia Nursing, *3rd ed. Philadelphia, Saunders, p. 138, 1994.*

9.48. Correct Answer: **c**

ASPAN's Standards of Perianesthesia Nursing Practice recommends that "two licensed nurses one of whom is an RN are present whenever a patient is recovering in Phase I."

American Society of Post Anesthesia Nurses (ASPAN): Standards of Perianesthesia Nursing Practice, *Resource 9. Thorofare, NJ, ASPAN, p. 47, 1995.*

9.49. Correct Answer: **b**

Ms M's fetus may have been Rh positive, having inherited this red blood cell antibody from the father. Ms M has no antibodies to the Rh-positive antigen. An Rh-positive fetus can stimulate antibody formation in the Rh-negative Ms M. Her future Rh-positive fetuses face erythrocyte destruction when these new Rh-positive maternal antibodies cross the placenta. Sensitivity to the Rh antigen can be reduced or eliminated by injecting immune globulin (RhoGAM) to Rh-negative women.

Stalheim-Smith, A & Fitch, GK: Understanding Human Anatomy and Physiology. *Minneapolis/St. Paul, West Publishing, pp. 690-692, 1994; Burden, N:* Ambulatory Surgical Nursing. *Philadelphia, Saunders, p. 511, 1993.*

9.50. Correct Answer: **a**

During laparoscopy, patients are placed in Trendelenburg's and lithotomy positions, increasing the potential for aspiration. Efforts to reduce gastric volume and acidity are necessary preoperatively. An empty bladder is desired for laparoscopy.

Burden, N: Ambulatory Surgical Nursing. *Philadelphia, Saunders, pp. 511-514, 1993.*

9.51. Correct Answer: **d**

Occurrence of hypotension, tachycardia, and significant abdominal distention, perhaps with severe pain and blood oozing through bandages that cover the laparoscope puncture sites, strongly suggests intraabdominal hemorrhage. Large amounts of blood can pour into the abdomen before severe pain, an initial symptom, occurs. Hemorrhage, viscous perforation, atelectasis, air (gas) embolism, and infection are among the serious, and rare, postlaparoscopic complications. Shoulder pain, typically right sided, some residual abdominal distention, and mild vaginal bleeding are expected events. Bradycardia may occur during the procedure due to peritoneal stretching.

Burden, N: Ambulatory Surgical Nursing. *Philadelphia, Saunders, pp. 510-514, 1993; Schell, RM & Applegate, RL: Obstetric and Gynecologic Recovery in* Manual of Post Anesthesia Care *(Jacobsen, WK, Ed). Philadelphia, Saunders, pp. 177-178, 1992.*

9.52. Correct Answer: **d**

One assessment of peroneal nerve function is determining the ability to dorsiflex the great toe and sensation atop the foot. Ischemia, compression or stretch from surgical position quite commonly affects the peroneal nerve during surgery and anesthesia. Recovery of function varies with extent of nerve damage and amount of regrowth necessary.

Sloan, TB: Postoperative Central Nervous System Dysfunction in Post Anesthesia Care *(Vender, JS & Speiss, BD, Eds). Philadelphia, Saunders, pp. 191-193, 1992.*

9.53. Correct Answer: **a**

During laparoscopy, lithotomy and Trendelenburg's positions are used. If improperly positioned or inadequately padded, the patient's leg could rest against leg supports. This lateral pressure against the leg can damage the peroneal nerve.

Sloan, TB: Postoperative Central Nervous System Dysfunction in Post Anesthesia Care *(Vender, JS & Speiss, BD, Eds). Philadelphia, Saunders, pp. 191-193, 1992; Burden, N:* Ambulatory Surgical Nursing. *Philadelphia, Saunders, pp. 510-514, 1993.*

9.54. Correct Answer: **c**

Elimination of midazolam from the body is quick and clean—the half-life is short, and few metabolites remain active. After bilateral nephrectomy to treat severe hypertension from end-stage renal disease, the pharmacokinetics of some medications are altered. Meperidine's primary metabolite, normeperidine, remains active for hours; over time, metabolites stimulate the central nervous system and can cause seizures. Morphine accumulates in the plasma and brain, potentially suppressing respirations. Renal failure reduces total protein; more unbound medication circulates freely and with prolonged effect.

Tobias, MD: Hepatic and Renal Disease in Dripps/Eckenhoff/Vandam Introduction to Anesthesia *(Longnecker, DE & Murphy, FL, Eds). Philadelphia, Saunders, pp. 299-300, 1992; Kay, J: Renal Disorders in* Manual of Anesthesia and the Medically Compromised Patient *(Cheng, EY & Kay, J, Eds). Philadelphia, Lippincott, pp. 254-264, 1990.*

9.55. Correct Answer: **a**

Tissue lysis and surgical stress can rapidly release intracellular potassium into the circulation, a potentially lethal occurrence for the patient with renal failure. Tall, peaked (tented) T waves and progressively widened QRS complexes develop on EKG as serum potassium increases. The nurse closely observes symptoms, monitors serum potassium often, and arranges prompt additional hemodialysis to treat severe hyperkalemia. A patient with chronic renal disease who is receiving dialysis often has osteodystrophy, anemia and clotting delays. Arranging position can promote fractures. A side-lying flank position during nephrectomy limits inflation of the dependent lung, promoting atelectasis. This anephric patient has no urine output, so oliguria is not a factor in her care.

Robins, K: Renal Transplantation in Critical Care Nursing: A Holistic Approach, *6th ed (Hudak, CM & Gallo, BM, Eds). Philadelphia, Saunders, pp. 596-601, 1994; Alexander, CM: Positioning the Surgical Patient in* Dripps/Eckenhoff/Vandam Introduction to Anesthesia, *8th ed (Longnecker, DE & Murphy, FL, Eds). Philadelphia, Saunders, pp. 186-187, 1992.*

9.56. Correct Answer: **b**

Frequent contact with blood or blood products increases risk of exposure to hepatitis B virus (HBV). Both HBV and human immunodeficiency virus (HIV) are transmitted through blood contact. However, the disease risk is 6-30% after needlestick with an HBV-contaminated needle; the risk after needlestick with an HIV-infected needle is less than 1%. Hepatitis A (HAV) exposure occurs through fecal, not blood, contamination to the mouth.

Sommargren, CE: Environmental Hazards in AACN's Clinical Reference for Critical-Care Nursing *(Kinney, MR, Packa, DR & Dunbar, SB, Eds). St. Louis, Mosby, pp. 99-100, 1993.*

9.57. Correct Answer: **d**

Mivacurium (Mivacron) has the shortest duration of action of the nondepolarizing muscle relaxants. Onset of effect lies about midway between succinylcholine's onset, the only depolarizing muscle relaxant, and onset times of intermediate-acting nondepolarizing muscle relaxants like atracurium or vecuronium. Spontaneous recovery is expected within 20 minutes and even more rapidly when reversal medications are used.

Drain, C: The Post Anesthesia Care Unit: A Critical Care Approach to Post Anesthesia Nursing, *3rd ed. Philadelphia, Saunders, p. 233, 1994; Miller, RD: Skeletal Muscle Relaxants in* Basic and Clinical Pharmacology *(Katzung, BG, Ed). Norwalk, CT, Appleton & Lange, p. 408, 1995.*

9.58. Correct Answer: **a**

Neostigmine is an anticholinesterase that *reverses* muscle relaxant effects to allow acetylcholine to remain active. Medications that potentiate the effects of other muscle relaxants, like "-mycin" antibiotics, glucocorticoids, and isoflurane anesthesia, may extend mivacurium's effect.

Product Information: Mivacron. Chicago, Burroughs Wellcome Co, 1994; Fisher, DM: Muscle Relaxants in Dripps/Eckenhoff/Vandam Introduction to Anesthesia, *8th ed (Longnecker, DE & Murphy, FL, Eds). Philadelphia, Saunders, pp. 115-121, 1992.*

9.59. Correct Answer: **a**

Drainage and bleeding are minimal after hemorrhoidectomy and repair of rectal fistulae. The nurse informs the surgeon when large volumes of sanguineous drainage are observed. Urinary retention is common after rectal surgery; some surgeons restrict fluids to prevent bladder distention until voiding occurs. Sharp or burning pain and rectal tenderness are likely; rectal packing often produces perineal pressure. Some surgeons infiltrate the rectal area with local anesthetic medications though, so absence of perineal pain and sensation immediately after surgery is also possible.

O'Brien, DD: Post Anesthesia Care of the Gastrointestinal, Abdominal and Anorectal Surgical Patient in The Post Anesthesia Care Unit: A Critical Care Approach to Post Anesthesia Nursing, *3rd ed (Drain, C, Ed). Philadelphia, Saunders, p. 457, 1994.*

9.60. Correct Answer: **b**

The nurse slightly supports Ms K's legs so her heels do not touch the mattress. Ms K's back pain and heel tenderness are probably results of her 3 1/2 hour anesthetized, supine position. Skin circulation over bony prominences like the heels, scapulae, elbows, and sacrum is easily compromised. Ischemia with blanching, edema, or even skin breakdown develop. Muscle aches respond to analgesia, reposition and heat. The nurse should also anticipate postural hypotension and assess for nerve injuries, particularly to upper extremities.

Litwack, K: Post Anesthesia Care Nursing, *2nd ed. St. Louis, Mosby, p. 482-485, 1995.*

SET III

Answer Key

9.61. b
9.62. d
9.63. c
9.64. d
9.65. a
9.66. b
9.67. a
9.68. c
9.69. a
9.70. b
9.71. d
9.72. b
9.73. b
9.74. a
9.75. c
9.76. c
9.77. a
9.78. b
9.79. a
9.80. d
9.81. b
9.82. a
9.83. d
9.84. a
9.85. d
9.86. c
9.87. b

SET III

Rationales and References

9.61. Correct Answer: **b**

Incomplete reversal of a nondepolarizing muscle relaxant medication accounts for partial paralysis and inability to hold his head up. Residual effects of Mr. J's intermediate-acting vecuronium produce weak, jerky muscle motion, "rocking," shallow respirations and a sensation of not "getting enough air." Even the elimination and reversal of a short-acting muscle relaxant like mivacurium can be altered in specific clinical and physiologic conditions. Volatile anesthetics can increase effect by up to 40%; aminoglycoside and "-mycin" antibiotics are well-known enhancers of neuromuscular block. Chronic glucocorticoid replacement can reduce plasma cholinesterase activity and possibly extend a block's effect.

Fisher, DM: Muscle Relaxants in Dripps/Eckenhoff/Vandam Introduction to Anesthesia, *8th ed (Longnecker, DE & Murphy, FL, Eds). Philadelphia, Saunders, pp. 115-121, 1992; Drain, C:* The Post Anesthesia Care Unit: A Critical Care Approach to Post Anesthesia Nursing, *3rd ed. Philadelphia, Saunders, pp. 233-234 & 237-244, 1994.*

9.62. Correct Answer: **d**

Hypothermia is one of several factors that can delay elimination of vecuronium. A dose of muscle relaxant reversal medication that is appropriate at normal temperature may not exert its full effect on a hypothermic patient. Edrophonium acts more quickly than neostigmine but can produce profound bradycardia. Edrophonium may reverse mivacurium's effects more effectively than neostigmine does. Though rapid spontaneous elimination (without reversal) of short-acting relaxants like mivacurium is expected, recovery of muscle function varies greatly among individuals and reversal may be used.

Kopman, AF: Reversal of Nondepolarizing Neuromuscular Blocking Agents. Semin Anesth *14(1): 1-15, 1995; Fisher, DM: Muscle Relaxants in* Dripps/Eckenhoff/Vandam Introduction to Anesthesia, *8th ed (Longnecker, DE & Murphy, FL, Eds). Philadelphia, Saunders, pp. 115-121, 1992; Litwack, K:* Post Anesthesia Care Nursing, *2nd ed. St. Louis, Mosby, pp. 148-149, 1995.*

9.63. Correct Answer: **c**

Blood pressure can plummet during vancomycin dosing if the drug is infused rapidly. The low blood pressure response resolves, but resolution occurs over hours. Recommended rate is 0.5-1 g delivered over 1/2-1 hour. While hearing loss (ototoxicity) is serious and common, rate of infusion does not affect its development.

Ma, MY: Antibacterial Agents in Clinical Pharmacology and Nursing, *2nd ed (Baer, CL & Williams, BR, Eds). Springhouse, PA, Springhouse Corp, pp. 1038-1040, 1992.*

9.64. Correct Answer: **d**

Hypothermia is signaled by core temperature measures of less than 36° C. Peripheral vasoconstriction, slowing blood flow and decreasing tissue perfusion occur. Cardiac work and the potential for both dysrhythmias and hypertension increase. Shivering increases oxygen consumption, decreases ventilation and promotes metabolic and respiratory acidosis. Hypothermia also decreases hepatic blood flow and alters rate of medication clearance, so Mr. O's return to alertness may be slowed.

Litwack, K: Post Anesthesia Care Nursing, *2nd ed. St. Louis, Mosby, pp. 462-470, 1995; Barash, PG, Cullen, BE & Stoelting, RK:* Handbook of Clinical Anesthesia. *Philadelphia, Lippincott, pp. 72-73, 1991.*

9.65. Correct Answer: **a**

The physiologic alterations associated with hypothermia increase oxygen consumption, alter oxygenation, and produce metabolic acidosis. Acidosis usually resolves as temperature increases; therefore sodium bicarbonate is not usually an *initial* therapy. Maintaining head and body skin coverage is important; nearly 50% of heat loss reportedly occurs by radiation from the head. Shivering reduction with rewarming techniques and/or medication minimizes physiologic damage and increases patient comfort.

Litwack, K: Post Anesthesia Care Nursing, *2nd ed. St. Louis, Mosby, pp. 462-470, 1995; Mecca, RS: Postoperative Recovery in* Clinical Anesthesia, *2nd ed (Barash, PG, Cullen, BF & Stoelting, RK, Eds). Philadelphia, Lippincott, pp. 1538-1539, 1992.*

9.66. Correct Answer: **b**

Peripheral vascular tone relaxes as the patient warms; the resulting vasodilation can produce major *hypo*tension. Shivering consumes energy, producing carbon dioxide and consuming oxygen. Rewarming after hypothermia should be gradual. As the hypothalamus regains temperature regulating control after general anesthesia, further significant heat loss is unlikely. The mildly hypothermic patient may have "cold-induced" diuresis and altered coagulation, including fibrinolysis and clot destruction.

Litwack, K: Post Anesthesia Care Nursing, *2nd ed. St. Louis, Mosby, pp. 462-470, 1995; Rosenberg, H & Horrow, JC: Causes and Consequences of Hypothermia and Hyperthermia in* Anesthesia and Perioperative Complications *(Benumof, JL & Saidman, LJ, Eds). St. Louis, Mosby, pp. 345-353, 1992.*

9.67. Correct Answer: **a**

Mr. O's surgical procedure is intended to manage his ascites. Fluid accumulating in the peritoneal cavity alters breathing by limiting movement of the diaphragm and lung expansion. Inserting a peritoneovenous shunt "recirculates" accumulated peritoneal fluid (ascites) into the general circulation. The LeVeen or Denver system includes a catheter with a one-way valve that is surgically placed in the peritoneum. Peritoneal fluid is diverted (shunted) through the catheter directly up to the right heart.

Busby, HC: Hepatic Disorders in Critical Care Nursing: A Holistic Approach, *6th ed (Hudak, CM & Gallo, BM, Eds). Philadelphia, Lippincott, p. 853, 1994.*

9.68. Correct Answer: **c**

Muscle movement involved in active shivering may produce muscle aching (myalgia) the next day. Both hypothermic and normothermic patients may shiver postoperatively. The hypothalamus begins to function when anesthesia suppression stops; "rebound" hyperthermia is unlikely the next day. Muscle relaxant effects, or recurarization, may recur while the patient rewarms in PACU, but residual effects are most certainly unlikely the next day.

Burden, N: Ambulatory Surgical Nursing. *Philadelphia, Saunders, pp. 288-290, 1993; Mecca, RS: Postoperative Recovery in* Clinical Anesthesia, *2nd ed (Barash, PG, Cullen, BF & Stoelting, RK, Eds). Philadelphia, Lippincott, pp. 1538-1539, 1992.*

9.69. Correct Answer: **a**

Anesthetic medications have little direct effect on renal autoregulation, though hypertension and vasoactive medications like dobutamine or alpha adrenergic stimulators do. Approximately one-fourth of cardiac output contributes to renal blood flow. Autoregulation assures a constant renal blood flow despite wide variations in mean arterial pressure (MAP). Cardiac output is minimally altered by isoflurane inhalation, so blood pressure can be expected to remain within normal limits, and altered renal blood flow is unlikely.

Drain, C: The Post Anesthesia Care Unit: A Critical Care Approach to Post Anesthesia Nursing, *3rd ed. Philadelphia, Saunders, pp. 140 & 200, 1994; Peschman, P: Renal Physiology in* Critical Care Nursing *(Clochesky, JM, Breu, C Cardin, S, et al, Eds). Philadelphia, Saunders, p. 835, 1992.*

9.70. Correct Answer: **b**

A fluid challenge with moderate volume of fluid can increase urine volume. Decreased urine output from prerenal causes arise from nonkidney origins. Examples include hypovolemia from hemorrhage, surgical blood losses, ascites removal, decreased myocardial performance, and "third space" fluid shifts or gastrointestinal losses. Diuretics do increase renal perfusion, but consider that a diuretic might further accentuate volume depletion. Catheter function addresses a postrenal cause. Myoglobin and aminoglycoside antibiotics like gentamicin are associated with acute renal failure and nephron damage, which are not prerenal conditions.

Whittaker, AA: Patients With Acute Renal Failure in Critical Care Nursing *(Clochesky, JM, Breu, C Cardin, S, et al, Eds). Philadelphia, Saunders, pp. 886-894, 1992; Jacobsen, WK:* Manual of Post Anesthesia Care. *Philadelphia, Saunders, p. 106, 1992.*

9.71. Correct Answer: **d**

Creatinine, a product of muscle metabolism, is filtered by the renal glomerulus and not reabsorbed. Blood urea nitrogen (BUN) varies with the rate of protein metabolism; osmolality and potassium also vary with nonrenal influences. Normal fasting serum creatinine (0.8-1.3 mg/dl) measures most often indicate adequate glomerular filtration, as the rate of muscle metabolism is constant.

Morgan, GE & Mikhail, MS: Clinical Anesthesiology. *Norwalk, CT, Appleton & Lange, p. 523, 1992.*

9.72. Correct Answer: **b**

Septicemia is a likely event for over 50% of patients with acute renal failure. Primary origins are pulmonary, urinary tract and wound infections. Renal failure promotes immunosuppression, which is associated with increased infection risk. Awareness of the patient's heightened risk and attention to aseptic technique are crucial to positive outcomes for this patient.

Giordano, B: Acute Renal Failure in Critical Care Nursing: Body-Mind-Spirit *(Dossey, BM, Guzzetta, CE & Kennter, CV, Eds). Philadelphia, Lippincott, pp. 636-637, 1992.*

9.73. Correct Answer: **b**

Stress, surgical lysis of tissues, and acidosis promote release of intracellular potassium to extracellular fluid. The failing kidney, whether due to acute or chronic disease, cannot adjust electrolyte imbalances; serum potassium increases to cardiotoxic, life-threatening levels. In all EKG leads, tall, peaked, narrow T waves appear when potassium reaches 5.5-6.5 mEq/L. Further serum potassium increases delay electrical conduction through the heart. The QRS gradually widens until ultimately either ventricular fibrillation or cardiac standstill occur. This patient requires immediate intervention to remove (dialyze) or shift potassium from the circulation.

Purcell, JA: Cardiac Electrical Activity in AACN's Clinical Reference for Critical-Care Nursing, *3rd ed (Kinney, MR, Packa, DR & Dunbar, SB, Eds). St. Louis, Mosby, pp. 293-294, 1993; Morgan, GE & Mikhail, MS:* Clinical Anesthesiology. *Norwalk, CT, Appleton & Lange, pp. 468-470, 1992.*

9.74. Correct Answer: **a**

Among women, early signs of positive HIV status include vaginal candidiasis, unresolved pelvic inflammatory disease (PID), menstrual changes or abnormal PAP smear. Many women do not know their own HIV status and are poorly aware of HIV risk factors. Yet behaviors and conditions that arise among women who develop HIV positivity may be different than high risk HIV-related indicators for men.

Kelly, PJ & Holman, S: The New Face of AIDS. Am J Nurs *93(3): 26-36, 1993.*

9.75. Correct Answer: **c**

Postoperatively, isotonic solutions (physiologic fluids that are neither hypertonic nor hypotonic) should be used to irrigate the bladder. Movement of solutions into the circulation by osmosis or vascular absorption can cause significant dilutional hyponatremia and produce symptoms of water intoxication. Water can hemolyze red blood cells after absorption into the bloodstream through highly vascular prostate tissue. Isotonic and nonhemolytic solutions are used during surgery to avoid electrical conduction through ionic solutions.

Miller, KM: Post Anesthesia Care of the Genitourinary Surgical Patient in The Post Anesthesia Care Unit: A Critical Care Approach to Post Anesthesia Nursing, *3rd ed (Drain, C, Ed). Philadelphia, Saunders, pp. 471-473, 1994; Fairchild, SS:* Perioperative Nursing: Principles and Practice. *Boston, Jones & Bartlett Publishers, pp. 486-487, 1993.*

9.76. Correct Answer: **c**

Traction on a urethral bladder catheter after transurethral resection of the prostate (TURP) applies pressure to the bladder outlet and is intended to decrease bleeding. Mr. P's urine should clear to a light red or pale pink color. The nurse observes the urinary returns while the sensory and smooth muscle effects of Mr. P's spinal anesthetic abate. Irrigation returns that again become either intermittently or continuously bright red suggest a bladder spasm. Clots may obstruct the catheter. Mr. P may feel strong bladder pain over his pubis. The nurse increases the irrigation's titrated rate to clear blood and clots from the bladder and administers a belladonna and opium suppository to relax irritable bladder muscle.

Miller, KM: Post Anesthesia Care of the Genitourinary Surgical Patient in The Post Anesthesia Care Unit: A Critical Care Approach to Post Anesthesia Nursing, *3rd ed (Drain, C, Ed). Philadelphia, Saunders, pp. 471-473, 1994.*

9.77. Correct Answer: **a**

Esmolol is a beta adrenergic blocking medication with a *very* brief duration of effect. While FDA-approved to decrease heart rate, esmolol is used perioperatively to decrease blood pressure. The nurse can expect heart rate and blood pressure reduction within 5 minutes; if response is inadequate, the nurse repeats the dose with anesthesiologist approval. The patient with congestive heart failure or AV conduction delays should not receive esmolol or any beta blocker. Because blood pressure reduction is both a desired outcome *and* a complication, the nurse assures reasonable hydration and fluid balance before beginning heart rate and blood pressure reduction.

Drain, C: The Post Anesthesia Care Unit: A Critical Care Approach to Post Anesthesia Nursing, *3rd ed. Philadelphia, Saunders, pp. 102-103, 1994; Vallerand, AH & Deglin, JH:* Davis's Guide to IV Medications, *2nd ed. Philadelphia, FA Davis, pp. 368-373, 1993.*

9.78. Correct Answer: **b**

Nonsteroidal antiinflammatory medications are associated with gastrointestinal irritation and ulceration, nephrotic syndrome and renal failure, and bleeding from antiplatelet effects. Stress related to today's surgical procedure may add to the patient's ulcer risk. Preanesthesia assessment might include questions to determine any unstated symptoms of gastrointestinal bleeding or renal disease.

Payan, DG & Katzung, BG: Nonsteroidal Anti-inflammatory Drugs; Nonopioid Analgesics; Drugs Used in Gout in Basic and Clinical Pharmacology *(Katzung, BG, Ed). Norwalk, CT, Appleton & Lange, pp. 546-547, 1995.*

9.79. Correct Answer: **a**

Ms A, like most patients receiving peritoneal dialysis, probably has a low serum albumin. Her recent peritonitis further decreased her protein supplies by causing protein losses of up to 40 g each day. When total protein decreases, the ability of proteins to bind medications decreases. Unbound drug circulates freely in the blood and has prolonged effect in a patient whose failing kidneys cannot eliminate the drug.

Holford, NHG & Benet, LZ: Pharmacokinetics and Pharmacodynamics: Rational Dose Selection and the Course of Drug Action in

Basic and Clinical Pharmacology *(Katzung, BG, Ed). Norwalk, CT, Appleton & Lange, pp. 44-47, 1995; Tobias, MD: Hepatic and Renal Disease and Kennedy, SK: Pharmacologic Principles of Anesthetics in* Dripps/Eckenhoff/Vandam Introduction to Anesthesia *(Longnecker, DE & Murphy, FL, Eds). Philadelphia, Saunders, pp. 67-73 & 297-301, 1992.*

9.80. Correct Answer: **d**

To assure that the hyperglycemic total parenteral nutrition (TPN) solution remains sterile, *no* other fluid or medication may be infused into the same tubing. To infuse antibiotics or other solutions, a separate IV site must be started. Ms A's nasogastric suction is appropriately set at around –80 mm Hg, and a small amount of bloody drainage may occur, especially if a Penrose-type wound drain was inserted. Saturated dressings should be reported to the surgeon. Infection of the peritoneal catheter site is a concern. Any local skin redness, tenderness and drainage around the catheter exit site in the abdomen suggest infection and are reported to the physician; the wound should be cultured.

Sieffert, WA: Management Modalities: Gastrointestinal System in Critical Care Nursing: A Holistic Approach, *6th ed (Hudak, CM & Gallo, BM, Eds). Philadelphia, Lippincott, pp. 568-573 & 830-836, 1994.*

9.81. Correct Answer: **b**

This vascular access has no external components. The graft is made from a synthetic, Teflon-like material. One end is grafted to Ms A's artery, then tunneled under her skin. The other end is anastomosed to a large vein. Nursing care includes avoiding situations that could compress blood flow through this graft or promote thrombosis obstruction. Therefore *no* blood pressure inflation or venipuncture tourniquets can be placed on Ms A's left arm. Hypotension can also compromise vascular flow. Patency of the access is detected by palpating above the venous anastomosis to feel a rush of blood flowing through the tubing. This bruit can also be audibly detected by stethoscope.

Zorzanello, M: Management Modalities: Renal System in Critical Care Nursing: A Holistic Approach, *6th ed (Hudak, CM & Gallo, BM, Eds). Philadelphia, Lippincott, pp. 558-560, 1994.*

9.82. Correct Answer: **a**

Poor ventilation, atelectasis and pneumonia are likely outcomes if Ms G does not move, breathe deeply and often, and have adequate pain management to participate in her pulmonary care. After the high upper abdominal incision used for gastrectomy, Ms G is likely to "splint" her incision and restrict her breathing to limit her pain. A Billroth I procedure involves significant partial gastrectomy, vagotomy and a stomach-duodenum anastomosis. Her nasogastric tube is likely to drain *small* amounts of bright residual gastric blood; more than 75 ml/h should be reported. After resection, a gastric tube for balloon tamponade should not be needed.

O'Brien, DD: Post Anesthesia Care of the Gastrointestinal, Abdominal and Anorectal Surgical Patient in The Post Anesthesia Care Unit: A Critical Care Approach to Post Anesthesia Nursing, *3rd ed*

(Drain, C, Ed). Philadelphia, Saunders, pp. 450-455, 1994; Busby, HC: Acute Gastrointestinal Bleeding in Critical Care Nursing: A Holistic Approach, *6th ed (Hudak, GM & Gallo, CM, Eds). Philadelphia, Lippincott, pp. 843-846, 1994.*

9.83. Correct Answer: **d**

Saturating through vaginal packing *and* a perineal pad is significant bleeding. The nurse notifies the surgeon and monitors Ms H closely for hypotension, fluid deficit and shock. Hypotension without overt bleeding may relate to surgical manipulation and pressure when vaginally removing the uterus. Abdominal cramping and pressure are expected and usually are adequately treated with narcotics in moderate doses. A suprapubic catheter should *not* have tension. Intraoperative lithotomy position commonly results in low back pain. Tingling likely indicates a position-related transient nerve ischemia from peroneal nerve compression; the nurse evaluates neurovascular status, checks for edema, then reassesses for improvement within 30 minutes.

Miller, KM: Post Anesthesia Care of the Obstetric and Gynecologic Surgical Patient in The Post Anesthesia Care Unit: A Critical Care Approach to Post Anesthesia Nursing, *3rd ed (Drain, C, Ed). Philadelphia, Saunders, p. 482, 1994; Alexander, CM: Positioning the Surgical Patient in* Dripps/Eckenhoff/Vandam Introduction to Anesthesia, *8th ed (Longnecker, DE & Murphy, FL, Eds). Philadelphia, Saunders, pp. 187-191, 1992.*

9.84. Correct Answer: **a**

The nurse assesses, then regularly monitors abdominal girth, vital signs, and possibly serum hemoglobin to detect hypotension and hypovolemia. Bluish discoloration around the umbilicus (Cullen's sign) or along the flanks (Turner's sign) suggests Ms Y may be bleeding either into her abdomen (hemoperitoneum) or retroperitoneally. Acute intraabdominal bleeding occurs rapidly and with evidence of shock, indicates organ rupture or trauma or release of ligature or anastomosis, and is life threatening. More gradual distention or increase in size *may* relate to slower intraabdominal bleeding or translocation of fluid into the peritoneum or intestine.

Beachley, M & Ferrar, J: Abdominal Trauma: Putting the Pieces Together. Am J Nurs *93(1): 26-35, 1993; Krumberger, JM: Acute Pancreatitis in* Critical Care Nursing: A Holistic Approach, *6th ed (Hudak, GM & Gallo, CM, Eds). Philadelphia, Lippincott, p. 861, 1994.*

9.85. Correct Answer: **d**

Obese patients are prone to sleep apnea and easy airway obstruction—and are very sensitive to airway depression. Decreased functional reserve capacity and greater oxygen consumption increase the obese patient's work of breathing. Supine position aggravates these factors, which all contribute to hypoventilation, hypoxia, and hypercarbia.

Mickler, TA: Patients with Metabolic and Endocrine Disorders in Dripps/Eckenhoff/Vandam Introduction to Anesthesia, *8th ed (Longnecker, DE & Murphy, FL, Eds). Philadelphia, Saunders, pp. 141 & 313-314, 1992.*

9.86. Correct Answer: **c**

Bladder distention can contribute to postoperative hypertension, tachycardia, and restlessness. These same symptoms also indicate hypoxia, which must be presumed as the primary cause of restlessness and disorientation until ruled out. Emergence delirium may be an additional cause of restlessness.

Kemp, B & Tabaka, M: Post Operative Urinary Retention in the PACU. Curr Rev Post Anesth Nurs *13(12), 1992; Burden, N:* Ambulatory Surgical Nursing. *Philadelphia, Saunders, p. 309, 1993.*

9.87. Correct Answer: **b**

Increased heart rate, a nonspecific indicator related to many situations, occurs first in the hypovolemic child. Hypovolemic tachycardia most likely is accompanied by weaker palpated peripheral pulses, oliguria, and slower capillary refill. A child can lose up to 25% of total blood volume before hypotension develops. Some clinicians use pulse quality and skin temperature to estimate volume depletion. For example, an arm that is cool from elbow to fingers suggests a 5% volume deficit; weak groin and axillary pulses suggest a 15% volume deficit.

Beachley, M & Ferrar, J: Abdominal Trauma: Putting the Pieces Together. Am J Nurs *93(1): 26-35, 1993; Cauldwell, CB: Induction, Maintenance and Emergence and Gregory, GA: Monitoring During Surgery in* Pediatric Anesthesia, *3rd ed (Gregory, GA, Ed). New York, Churchill-Livingstone, pp. 255-256 & 267-268, 1994.*

Section 10

Maxillofacial, Nasopharyngeal, Ophthalmic, Otologic, and Reconstructive Concepts

Scenarios and items in this section focus on perianesthesia considerations related to *ophthalmic* (eye), *otologic* (ear), *rhinologic* (nasal), *maxillofacial* (oral), *laryngologic* (neck or throat), and *reconstructive* (plastic) surgical procedures. These issues are considered together because:

- surgery on the eye, ear, mouth, nose, or throat involves facial and neck structures that often also require surgical reconstruction.
- to promote positive outcomes, eye, facial, and many reconstructive procedures share common postanesthesia priorities: assure hemostasis to promote healing, concern with airway and position, and limit pressure-increasing activities like coughing, stretching, straining, or vomiting.

ESSENTIAL CORE CONCEPTS	AFFILIATED CORE CURRICULUM CHAPTERS
Nursing Process	
Assessment	
Planning and Implementation	Chapters 2, 27
Evaluation	28 & 29
Ophthalmic Concerns	
Nursing Process	
Optic Structures and Physiology	
Pathology	
Abrasions, Ptosis, and Detachments	
Cataracts and Glaucoma	Chapter 28
Pharmacology	
Miotics and Mydriatics	
Cycloplegics and Osmotics	
Perianesthesia Priorities	
Nausea-Free, Coughless, Bloodless, Painless	
Surgical Procedures and Reconstruction	
Tumors, Ulcerations, and -plasties	

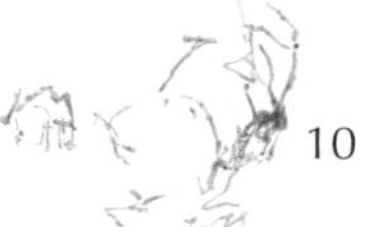

Otologic Concerns

Nursing Process
Otic Structures and Physiology
  Function and Innervation
Pathology
  Otitis, Trauma, and Tumors — Chapter 27
Perianesthesia Priorities
  Bleeding and Spinal Fluid Leaks
  Instructions and Dressings
  Neurologic Weaknesses and Hearing Deficit
  Pain and Position
  Vertigo and Vomiting
Surgical Procedures and Reconstruction
  -ectomies, -otomies, and -plasties

Nasopharyngeal Concerns

Nasal Structures and Physiology
Nursing Process
Pathology
  Mucous, Polyps, Septum, and Sinuses
Perianesthesia Priorities
  Airway, Bleeding, and Emesis — Chapter 27
  Packing, Pain, and Position
Surgical Procedures and Reconstruction
  -ectomies, -otomies, and -plasties
  Fractures, Reconstructions, and Windows

Maxillofacial and Laryngeal Concerns

Nursing Process
Oral and Pharyngeal Structures and Physiology
Pathology
  Adenoids, Tonsils, and Nodules
  Fractures and Tumors
Perianesthesia Priorities
  Airway Patency and Oxygenation — Chapter 27
  Emesis, Hemorrhage, and Mucus
  Endocrine Balance and Nerve Function
  Extubation, Tracheal Tubes, and Jaw Wires
  Position and Communication
  Sepsis, Suction, and Drains
Surgical Procedures and Reconstruction
  -ectomies, -otomies, and -plasties
  -oscopies and Laser Excisions

Issues of Reconstructive Surgery

Coagulation, Healing, and Infection Potential
Nursing Process
Perianesthesia Priorities
  Airway Patency and Oxygenation
  Bleeding, Ecchymosis, and Edema

SET I

Items 10.1-10.37

10.1. Following ocular surgery, stable intraocular pressures are promoted with:

a. prophylactic antiemetics
b. supine bedrest for three hours
c. osmotic diuretics
d. miotic eyedrops

NOTE: Consider scenario and items 10.2-10.3 together.

Mr. E's blood pressure is consistently 180/94 to 200/104 after his left radical neck dissection with tracheostomy, laryngectomy, and partial esophagectomy.

10.2. The PACU nurse closely observes Mr. E for complications and immediately contacts the surgeon to report:

a. laryngospasm and purplish facial color
b. inability to swallow and persistent vomiting
c. emergence delirium and left lower lip palsy
d. severe pain and 90 ml/hour wound drainage

10.3. The nurse titrates a nitroprusside infusion to Mr. E's blood pressure response and anticipates a moderate, dose-related increase in:

a. pulmonary congestion
b. cardiac output
c. PR interval
d. heart rate

10.4. The nurse expects that a patient with ketoacidosis and a serum glucose of 400 mg/dl after retinal reattachment may also have:

a. potassium depletion
b. Biot's respirations
c. septic retinopathy
d. dilutional anemia

10.5. Five minutes after admission of a healthy and drowsy patient to Phase I PACU following a radical antrostomy (Caldwell-Luc operation), the nurse observes rocking respirations and abdominal movement. Prompt intervention includes:

a. an antiemetic per protocol
b. suction of bloody secretions
c. a semi-Fowler's position
d. neck extension

10.6. A 30 year old woman cries inconsolably after her left radical mastectomy and wishes to avoid visitors. When planning nursing care, the nurse recognizes this response may relate to:

a. psychic pain from unexplored sexual abuse
b. hysterical overreaction from fear of pain
c. anticipated rejection from altered body image
d. inappropriate expression of incisional pain

10.7. Damage to the glossopharyngeal nerve (IX) affects patient outcomes by increasing risk of:

a. facial spasm
b. disconjugate eyes
c. aspiration
d. disequilibrium

10.8. Ms S had a left carotid endarterectomy 6 weeks ago and now is in PACU Phase I after a right carotid endarterectomy. The strongest evidence suggesting carotid body dysfunction includes:

a. respiratory rate = 10, pCO_2 = 38 mm Hg, pO_2 = 91 mm Hg

b. systolic BP = 198 mm Hg, disorientation, pCO_2 = 56 mm Hg
c. right eyelid ptosis, ipsilateral tongue deviation
d. hoarseness, heart rate 98, first-degree AV block

10.9. Following left cataract phacoemulsification, the Phase I PACU nurse does *not* position Ms E on her left side, thereby reducing the risk of:

a. increasing ocular pressure
b. vitreous humor leakage
c. triggering oculocephalic reflex
d. postemesis wound infection

10.10. During ethmoidectomy and nasal polypectomy, cocaine may be used to promote:

a. dissociative sedation
b. long-term analgesia
c. localized hemostasis
d. craniofacial relaxation

NOTE: Consider items 10.11-10.12 together.

10.11. Following tympanoplasty, an 8 year old child must learn:

a. ear irrigation with antibiotic solution
b. atraumatic sneezing techniques
c. to cope with altered self image
d. how to insert a hearing device

10.12. During assessment prior to transfer of this child from Phase I PACU, the nurse both documents and contacts the surgeon about discovery of:

a. reoccurring nausea
b. serous rhinorrhea
c. unabated dizziness
d. muffled hearing

10.13. Following cosmetic dermabrasion, rhytidectomy, and blepharoplasty, the patient in Phase I PACU has ptosis of the left eye. The nurse:

a. notifies the surgeon immediately
b. medicates for acute-angle glaucoma
c. consults preoperative documentation
d. applies warm, moist compresses

NOTE: Consider scenario and item 10.14 together.

Ms V had a left scalp, temporofacial and forehead surgery that involved placing full thickness skin grafts. Thirty minutes later, the nurse observes serosanguineous fluid oozing between the sutures at the temporal site and trickling down the left cheek.

10.14. The *most appropriate* nursing intervention for this situation is to observe, notify the surgeon and:

a. apply an occlusive dressing
b. turn Ms V toward her left side
c. place warm compresses on her temple
d. elevate the head of Ms V's stretcher

10.15. The most critical nursing assessments of the postthymectomy patient focus on preventing:

a. autonomic hyperreflexia
b. malignant hyperthermia
c. hypothyroid crisis
d. respiratory muscle failure

10.16. Ms F is admitted to Phase I PACU after abdominal and thigh suction lipectomy. A priority nursing diagnosis specifically related to Ms F's *immediate* postanesthesia care is potential for:

a. wound dehiscence
b. fluid volume deficit
c. systemic hypertension
d. reactive hyperthermia

NOTE: Consider scenario and item 10.17 together.

Ms B is a healthy woman who was NPO for 14 hours preoperatively, partly due to surgical delays. She had an estimated 250 ml blood loss during her elective second-stage breast reconstruction. Her fluid deficit was estimated at 1000 ml. Vital signs are now within 10% of preoperative levels and stable in PACU.

10.17. Initial attempts to restore fluid volume most likely will include:
a. 500 ml hetastarch
b. 1000 ml lactated Ringer's solution
c. 500 ml 5% dextrose in water
d. 1 unit packed red cells

10.18. Ms H, an 87 year old woman, is scheduled for a cataract phacoemulsification with lens implant. Her preexisting medical condition of greatest concern for positive outcome is:
a. digitalis-managed congestive heart failure
b. chronic obstructive pulmonary disease
c. insulin-dependent diabetes mellitus
d. aortic stenosis with LVEDP = 15 mm Hg

NOTE: Consider scenario and items 10.19-10.23 together.

During Mr. J's preanesthesia assessment prior to scheduled parathyroidectomy, the nurse notes that his medical history includes two past episodes of congestive heart failure. These were treated with thiazide diuretics and digitalis medications, which Mr. J still uses daily. Depression is treated with a monoamine oxidase inhibitor.

10.19. His serum calcium of 12.5 mg/dl may increase Mr. J's potential to develop:
a. digitalis tolerance
b. high output heart failure
c. muscle weakness
d. extrapyramidal movements

10.20. One cause of hyperparathyroidism is:
a. chronic renal calculi
b. end-stage renal disease
c. prolonged hypotension
d. thyroid adenoma

10.21. When planning Mr. J's postparathyroidectomy nursing care, the PACU nurse considers the potential for altered neurologic function related to:
a. hypocalcemia, hyperphosphatemia
b. hypercalcemia, hypophosphatemia
c. hypocalcemia, metabolic acidosis
d. hypercalcemia, metabolic alkalosis

10.22. The PACU nurse inflates a blood pressure cuff on Mr. J's upper arm to a pressure above systolic pressure for 3 minutes to determine:
a. capillary filling pressure
b. Chvostek's sign
c. carpopedal spasm
d. tendon hyporeflexia

NOTE: The scenario continues.

Thirty minutes after admission to PACU, Mr. J is aware, oriented, becomes restless and anxious, states dyspnea and develops "crowing" airway sounds. SaO_2 is 92%; respiratory rate is 26 breaths per minute.

10.23. The PACU nurse continues to deliver humidified oxygen at FiO_2 = 0.8, consults with the anesthesiologist and anticipates administering:
a. midazolam 2 mg
b. succinylcholine 1 mg
c. furosemide 20 mg
d. calcium gluconate 1 g

10.24. Signs of the oculocardiac reflex include:
a. decreased blood pressure, pulse and consciousness
b. miosis and widened pulse pressure with anxiety
c. hypertension and tachycardia with hyperthermia
d. vomiting, pulsus paradoxus and mydriasis

10.25. The *most appropriate* intervention when a patient develops severe right eye pain after retinal reattachment is:
a. provide analgesia according to PACU protocol
b. flatten the head and reposition to the left side

c. immediately notify the ophthalmic surgeon
d. transfer the patient to a quiet, dim area of PACU

NOTE: Consider scenario and items 10.26-10.27 together.

Intubation for resection and biopsy of her parotid gland and dissection of adjacent lymph nodes was difficult. During admission assessment to PACU, the nurse notes Ms D is extubated and attempts to sit up, looking about the unit with a wide-eyed and anxious gaze. The nurse observes minimal chest movement, auscultates no breath sounds and feels no air exchange.

10.26. In this situation, the nurse expects that restoring Ms D's airway patency may require:

a. humidified oxygen and nasopharyngeal airway
b. albuterol nebulization and lidocaine
c. oropharyngeal suction and hydrocortisone
d. succinylcholine and assisted ventilation

10.27. Today, Ms D's specific postoperative airway management complication is *least likely* to arise from:

a. challenging endotracheal intubation
b. smoking-related small airway hyperreactivity
c. otolaryngologic surgical manipulation
d. blood-tinged secretions on laryngeal structures

10.28. Potential consequences related to the *most frequently* used intraoperative position include:

a. back pain, alopecia and heel tissue compression
b. corneal abrasion and air embolism
c. neck pain, brachial plexus stretch and knee redness
d. breast ulceration and facial edema

NOTE: Consider items 10.29-10.30 together.

10.29. Intraoperative events that could *most* exacerbate a patient's preexisting congestive heart failure during cataract extraction include:

a. mannitol infusion, flat position
b. nitroprusside infusion, semi-Fowler's position
c. nitroglycerin infusion, flat position
d. enflurane, semi-Fowler's position

10.30. *Initial* medical intervention to treat this patient's congestive heart failure is *most* likely to include:

a. rotating tourniquets
b. phenylephrine
c. nasotracheal intubation
d. morphine sulfate

NOTE: Consider scenario and items 10.31-10.32 together.

Ms B had a right radical mastectomy without breast reconstruction. One wound drain has already removed approximately 30 ml of thin red fluid. The PACU nurse discontinues Ms B's intravenous site after noting redness and tenderness.

10.31. The new IV site is inserted into the left arm *primarily* to minimize potential for:

a. flow of fluid exudate into wound drain
b. muscle immobility after right shoulder disuse
c. altered circulation in right arm tissues
d. physical dependence by limiting dominant arm use

10.32. After 1 hour in PACU, Ms B's nurse is *most* concerned to discover:

a. only 10 ml additional red drainage in the wound drain
b. Ms B's tearful cries of right breast phantom pain
c. stinging pain and sensory deficit in right axilla
d. right inner forearm swelling and numbness

10.33. To minimize damage to an adult's tracheal tissue while assuring adequate protection, the optimal endotracheal cuff pressure is:

a. uninflated
b. near 20 mm Hg
c. fully inflated
d. near 30 mm Hg

10.34. A 46 year old diabetic patient is in Phase I PACU after vitrectomy. Maintaining the position requested by the ophthalmic surgeon is essential to:

a. reduce incidence of postoperative nausea and vomiting
b. maintain a nonvarying intraocular pressure
c. apply pressure by intraocular air bubble against retina
d. prevent paroxysms of pain associated with motion

10.35. Intraocular pressure is decreased by:

a. coughing and hyperventilation
b. hypocarbia and hypovolemia
c. respiratory acidosis and elevated central venous pressure
d. hypoventilation and Valsalva's effect

10.36. Potential for postoperative nausea and vomiting (PONV) is *least* likely to occur after:

a. strabismus repair
b. tympanomastoidectomy
c. laparoscopic ovum retrieval
d. transurethral resection of the prostate

10.37. Following radical mastoidectomy, Ms B is asked to grimace, grin and purse her lips to assess function of:

a. masseter muscles
b. facial nerve
c. temporal lobe
d. cranial nerve VIII

Set I

Answer Key

10.1.	a
10.2.	d
10.3.	d
10.4.	a
10.5.	d
10.6.	c
10.7.	c
10.8.	b
10.9.	a
10.10.	c
10.11.	b
10.12.	b
10.13.	c
10.14.	d
10.15.	d
10.16.	b
10.17.	b
10.18.	a
10.19.	c
10.20.	b
10.21.	a
10.22.	c
10.23.	d
10.24.	a
10.25.	c
10.26.	d
10.27.	b
10.28.	a
10.29.	a
10.30.	d
10.31.	c
10.32.	d
10.33.	b
10.34.	c
10.35.	b
10.36.	d
10.37.	b

SET I

Rationales and References

10.1. Correct Answer: **a**

The incidence of postoperative nausea, retching, and vomiting reportedly reaches up to 50%. When nausea develops after eye surgery, the strain of vomiting increases the risk of elevated intraocular pressure and even hemorrhage while adding to general discomfort. A calm, dimly lit environment and sedative medications effectively promote rest, which then reduces intraocular pressure.

Burden, N: Ambulatory Surgical Nursing. *Philadelphia, Saunders, pp. 459-465, 199; Maes, KS, Britton, T & Bell, B: The Ophthalmic Surgical Patient in* ASPAN's Core Curriculum for Post Anesthesia Nursing Practice, *3rd ed (Litwack, K, Ed). Philadelphia, Saunders, pp. 590-600, 1994.*

10.2. Correct Answer: **d**

After radical neck surgery and laryngectomy, Mr. E's greatest, and dire, potential postoperative complications are hemorrhage, perhaps with carotid artery rupture ("blowout"), and obstruction of his tracheostomy, his only airway. Pain is usually not severe, and wound drainage can be expected to be minimal. The nurse expects to gently suction his mouth because spitting and swallowing are challenges for Mr. E. She also assures a patent nasogastric tube and expects to observe lower face droop from facial nerve dissection. Edema and facial discoloration from venous congestion are also likely. The nurse judiciously sedates Mr. E; she expects he may be restless upon awakening, usually related to anxiety and apprehension, but perhaps to alcohol withdrawal. After laryngectomy, laryngospasm cannot occur.

Silcox, S: The Otorhinolaryngologic and Head and Neck Surgical Patient in ASPAN's Core Curriculum for Post Anesthesia Nursing Practice, *3rd ed (Litwack, K, Ed). Philadelphia, Saunders, pp. 584-586, 1994; Marks, L, Gurwin, A & Farrar, S: Post Anesthesia Care of the Ear, Nose, Throat, Neck, and Maxillofacial Surgical Patient in* The Post Anesthesia Care Unit: A Critical Care Approach to Post Anesthesia Nursing, *3rd ed (Drain, C, Ed). Philadelphia, Saunders, pp. 339-340, 1994.*

10.3. Correct Answer: **d**

Tachycardia is a reflex response when nitroprusside (Nipride) relaxes and dilates vascular (both arterial and venous) smooth muscle. As peripheral vascular resistance decreases, preload, afterload and cardiac work also decrease. Blood pressure can plummet rapidly; continuous blood pressure monitoring and infusing nitroprusside with a volume-controlled pump are required to administer nitroprusside.

Shannon, MT, Wilson, BA & Stang, CL: Govoni & Hayes Drugs and Nursing Implications, *8th ed. Norwalk, CT, Appleton & Lange, pp. 836-837, 1995; Morgan, GE & Mikhail, MS:* Clinical Anesthesiology. *Norwalk, CT, Appleton & Lange, pp. 169-172, 1992.*

10.4. Correct Answer: **a**

This hyperglycemic patient is metabolizing fat, causing diabetic ketoacidosis (DKA). Overall, cellular potassium depletion is associated with DKA, though a serum potassium measure could reflect either hyperkalemia *or* hypokalemia. Acidosis releases intracellular potassium to extracellular fluid, initially producing hyperkalemia. As insulin treatment gradually decreases serum glucose, potassium replacement and close monitoring are necessary. Deep and regular Kussmaul's, not Biot's, respirations correct metabolic acidosis.

Kraft, SA, Mihm, FG, & Feeley, TW: Postoperative Endocrine Problems in Post Anesthesia Care *(Vender, JS & Speiss, BD, Eds). Philadelphia, Saunders, pp. 216-222, 1992; Loriaux,TC & Drass, JA: Endocrine and Diabetic Disorders in* AACN's Clinical Reference For Critical-Care Nursing, *3rd ed (Kinney, MR, Packa, DR & Dunbar, SB, Eds). St. Louis, Mosby, pp. 942-958, 1993.*

10.5. Correct Answer: **d**

Chest and abdominal "rocking" in a sedated patient boldly signals *airway obstruction!* No air passes through this patient's nose because of the surgical procedure and intranasal packing. Repositioning the head; extending the neck; head jaw support; perhaps inserting an artificial oral or nasal airway; or lateral position likely will relieve the obstruction. The relaxed tongue frequently is the source of an obstruction that limits air passage through the mouth.

Burden, N: Ambulatory Surgical Nursing. *Philadelphia, Saunders, pp. 263-265, 1993; Brockmann, DC, Jacobsen, WK & Lobo, DP: Respiratory Management in* Manual of Post Anesthesia Care *(Jacobsen, WK, Ed). Philadelphia, Saunders, p. 84, 1992.*

10.6. Correct Answer: **c**

The woman's beliefs surrounding altered body image are important to consider when supporting a postmastectomy patient. Fear of rejection is common. Postanesthesia patients display varied emotional responses. Some cry easily from relief of anticipatory stress; for others, residual anesthetic sometimes relaxes emotional control, allowing tears to flow.

Burden, N: Ambulatory Surgical Nursing. *Philadelphia, Saunders, pp. 541-542, 1993; Taylor, C, Lillis, C & LeMone, P:* Fundamentals of Nursing: The Art and Science of Nursing, *2nd ed. Philadelphia, Lippincott, pp. 1153-1154, 1993.*

10.7. Correct Answer: **c**

Motor dysfunction of cranial nerve IX affects the airway-protecting gag reflex and the ability to swallow and control secretions. Potential for aspiration increases. Glossopharyngeal motor function is typically assessed with vagus nerve function.

Taylor, C, Lillis, C & LeMone, P: Fundamentals of Nursing: The Art and Science of Nursing Care, *2nd ed. Philadelphia, Lippincott, pp. 465-466, 1993; Stalheim-Smith, A & Fitch, GK:* Understanding Human Anatomy and Physiology. *Minneapolis / St. Paul, West Publishing, pp. 432-440, 1994.*

10.8. Correct Answer: **b**

Headache, confusion and severe hypertension within the first 24 postoperative hours may indicate cerebral edema or intracranial hemorrhage. Carotid endarterectomy impairs carotid body function and expected physiologic responses to changes in blood flow (autoregulation). Cerebral perfusion is affected by the severe hypertension or profound hypotension that results. In addition, Ms S's pCO_2 may be chronically elevated; *bilateral* carotid artery surgery may affect the normal physiologic response to hypoxia and hypercarbia, which is to increase ventilation. Carotid body damage must be weighed with residual anesthetic effect when assessing Ms S's respiratory and vascular status.

Flynn, TC & Laydon, AJ: Postoperative Care of Patients Following Vascular Surgery. Anesth Clin North Am *13(1): 222-224, 1995; Mahla, ME: Carotid Artery Surgery: Anesthesia and Monitoring Update.* Semin Anesth *13(1): 75-85, 1994; Lowdon, JD & Isaacson, IJ: Postoperative Considerations After Major Vascular Surgery in* Post Anesthesia Care *(Vender, JS & Speiss, BD, Eds). Philadelphia, Saunders, pp. 120-124, 1992.*

10.9. Correct Answer: **a**

Position Ms E on her right side, the nonsurgical side, to prevent pressure on the left eye. Nursing interventions after cataract surgery focus on preventing increases in intraocular pressure, hemorrhage, suture stress and infection.

Saleh, KL: Practical Points in the Care of the Patient Undergoing Cataract Surgery. J Post Anesth Nurs *8(2): 113-115, 1993; Zehren, C: Post Anesthesia Care of the Ophthalmic Surgical Patient in* The Post Anesthesia Care Unit: A Critical Care Approach to Post Anesthesia Nursing, *3rd ed (Drain, C, Ed). Philadelphia, Saunders, p. 345-347, 1994.*

10.10. Correct Answer: **c**

Cocaine is a local anesthetic used (legally) in surgery for its strong vasoconstrictive properties. This action contrasts with the dilating actions of other local anesthetics. Cocaine shrinks mucous membranes, reduces bleeding and provides brief, topical anesthesia during intranasal surgery.

Saleh, KL: Practical Points in Understanding Local Anesthetics. J Post Anesth Nurs *7(1): 45-47, 1991.*

10.11. Correct Answer: **b**

Immediately postoperatively, this child must learn to sneeze with the mouth and both nostrils open to prevent pressure increases within the ear. Nose blowing is avoided. Tympanoplasty involves repair of the child's tympanic membrane after tear or damage from middle ear trauma or chronic otitis media. The child may have continued hearing loss and vertigo.

Sands, JK: Clinical Manual of Medical-Surgical Nursing: Concepts and Clinical Practice, *2nd ed. Mosby, St. Louis, pp. 74-76, 1991; Silcox, S: The Otorhinolaryngologic and Head and Neck Surgical Patient in* ASPAN's Core Curriculum for Post Anesthesia Nursing Practice, *3rd ed (Litwack, K, Ed). Philadelphia, Saunders, pp. 568-575, 1994.*

10.12. Correct Answer: **b**

Clear fluid draining from the patient's nose after any ear procedure may herald leak of cerebrospinal fluid. The surgeon must be notified. Severe pain and significant hearing deficit, beyond dressing-related barriers to clear hearing, should also be reported. Sensations of nausea and dizziness, though troublesome to manage, occur regularly; persistent vomiting, despite nursing and pharmacologic intervention, should be reported.

Silcox, S: The Otorhinolaryngologic and Head and Neck Surgical Patient in ASPAN's Core Curriculum for Post Anesthesia Nursing Practice, *3rd ed (Litwack, K, Ed). Philadelphia, Saunders, pp. 568-575, 1994.*

10.13. Correct Answer: **c**

Family members and preoperative documentation are ideal sources to confirm any presurgical neurologic deficits affecting the face or eye, visual acuity, and shape and symmetry of facial structures. The nurse's awareness of ptosis and facial droop from prior trauma, irregularly shaped pupils from prior surgery, or visual deficits avoids unnecessary concern and confusion. Though nerve damage and compression from bleeding are possible, this patient's ptosis may have a preexisting cause totally unrelated to the current surgical procedure. Acute-angle glaucoma is a rare possibility and is indicated by severe pain and unrelenting nausea.

Burden, N: Ambulatory Surgical Nursing. *Philadelphia, Saunders, p. 470, 1993.*

10.14. Correct Answer: **d**

Head elevation helps prevent accumulation of additional fluid beneath the graft and reduces wound swelling. Pools of fluid beneath the graft may interfere with healing at the site. Principles of care after skin grafting generally include minimizing bleeding and infection potential, preventing pressure at the graft site and decreasing edema. Though surgeon preferences widely vary, head or extremity elevation, ice (not heat) to the site, and avoiding graft pressure (no occlusive dressings or lying on graft) are likely interventions.

Mussler, CA: Post Anesthesia Care of the Plastic Surgical Patient in The Post Anesthesia Care Unit: A Critical Care Approach to Post Anesthesia Nursing, *3rd ed (Drain, C, Ed). Philadelphia, Saunders, pp. 492-493, 1994; Fritsch, DE: The Plastic Surgery and Burn Patient in* ASPAN's Core Curriculum for Post Anesthesia Nursing Practice, *3rd ed (Litwack, K, Ed). Philadelphia, Saunders, pp. 608-611, 1994.*

10.15. Correct Answer: **d**

Myasthenia gravis may be treated with surgical removal of the thymus gland (thymectomy). A patent airway, preventing respiratory muscle fatigue, and observing overall muscle strength are important considerations. Anticholinesterase medications continue following thymectomy, perhaps at reduced doses.

Lazear, SE: Neuromuscular Disorders in Critical Care Nursing, *2nd ed (Vazquez, M, Lazear, SE & Larson, EL, Eds). Philadelphia, Saunders, pp. 198-202, 1992; Barash, PG, Cullen, BE & Stoelting, RK:* Handbook of Clinical Anesthesia. *Philadelphia, Lippincott, pp. 157-159, 1991.*

10.16. Correct Answer: **b**

Up to 2500 ml of fat may be removed during liposuction, making fluid volume replacement an essential consideration during the immediate postanesthesia period. Colloid solutions like hetastarch may augment crystalloid volume replacement when large volumes of fat are removed. Blood lost with fat may cause anemia and need for transfusion. Hypothermia, pain and movement difficulty are also likely postlipectomy occurrences.

Burden, N: Ambulatory Surgical Nursing. *Philadelphia, Saunders, pp. 493-495, 1993; Mussler, CA: Post Anesthesia Care of the Plastic Surgical Patient in* The Post Anesthesia Care Unit: A Critical Care Approach to Post Anesthesia Nursing, *3rd ed (Drain, C, Ed). Philadelphia, Saunders, pp. 609-610, 1994.*

10.17. Correct Answer: **b**

Fluid deficits are generally first restored with a plasma-approximating isotonic solution like lactated Ringer's solution. The concept of fluid deficit calculates the patient's preoperative NPO and insensible loss, then considers gastric and urine fluid losses plus intraoperative blood loss. Infused volume varies with evidence of clinical shock, ongoing bleeding, or diuresis. Infusing crystalloid avoids the osmotic diuresis of hetastarch or hypertonic dextrose solutions; lactate absorbs hydrogen ion and can buffer metabolic acids. Hypertonic crystalloids like 5% dextrose in water are sometimes used for volume replacement; however, the 500 ml in this example is probably an insufficient volume. Ms B is healthy and had a relatively small blood loss, so a need for blood transfusion is unlikely.

DeFranco, M: Fluid and Electrolyte Balance in ASPAN's Core Curriculum for Post Anesthesia Nursing Practice, *3rd ed (Litwack, K, Ed). Philadelphia, Saunders, pp. 162 & 170-173, 1994; Ellison, N: Managing Fluids, Electrolytes and Blood Loss in* Dripps/Eckenhoff/Vandam Introduction to Anesthesia, *8th ed (Longnecker, DE & Murphy, FL, Eds). Philadelphia, Saunders, pp. 168-175, 1992.*

10.18. Correct Answer: **a**

Preexisting heart failure is reportedly "the single most important indicator for predicting postoperative mortality." In patients with a history of either congestive heart failure or recent myocardial infarction, the death risk approaches 25%; over 10% of patients can develop life-threatening complications. Both general and regional anesthetic techniques have cardiovascular effects. Profound hypotension or hypertension, fluid imbalances, and supine positioning can contribute to cardiac symptoms.

Burden, N: Ambulatory Surgical Nursing. *Philadelphia, Saunders, p. 397, 1993; Morgan, GE & Mikhail, MS:* Clinical Anesthesiology. *Norwalk, CT, Appleton & Lange, pp. 308-310, 1992.*

10.19. Correct Answer: **c**

Hypercalcemia, a result of parathyroid oversecretion (hyperparathyroidism), decreases both muscle strength and reflex responsiveness. Parathormone (PTH) regulates ionized serum calcium in conjunction with vitamin D and calcitonin. Cardiac muscle is particularly vulnerable to calcium excess. Hypercalcemia also increases sensitivity to digitalis, potentially producing symptoms of digitalis toxicity. Increased risk of fracture due to bone demineralization, hypertension, kidney stones, nausea and lethargy also may occur.

Yucha, CB & Toto, KH: Calcium and Phosphorus Derangements. Crit Care Nurs Clin North Am *6(4): 747-766, 1994; Jacobsen, WK: Endocrine Disorders in* Manual of Post Anesthesia Care *(Jacobsen, WK, Ed). Philadelphia, Saunders, pp. 128-129, 1992.*

10.20. Correct Answer: **b**

Chronic and end-stage renal failure, insufficient vitamin D, osteomalacia, and intestinal malabsorption syndromes decrease serum calcium. Reciprocally, serum phosphorus increases. Chronic hypocalcemia persistently stimulates a compensatory response by the parathyroid glands to produce additional parathormone (PTH). Eventually the parathyroid gland adapts to the increased demand for PTH and enlarges. Parathyroid adenomas, malignancies, and neck radiation are also linked with parathyroid overactivity.

Yucha, CB & Toto, KH: Calcium and Phosphorus Derangements. Crit Care Nurs Clin North Am *6(4): 747-766, 1994; Miller, B & Keane, CB:* Encyclopedia and Dictionary of Medicine, Nursing, and Allied Health, *4th ed. Philadelphia, Saunders, pp. 602-603, 1987.*

10.21. Correct Answer: **a**

Plan to observe for life threatening signs of hypocalcemia (seizure and respiratory failure) in PACU. Parathyroidectomy abruptly "shuts off" parathormone secretion. Calcium then reshifts into bone, rapidly reducing ionized serum calcium. Chemically, decreases in calcium stimulate a reciprocal increase in phosphorus; kidneys retain both phosphorus and bicarbonate, producing hyperphosphatemia and slight metabolic alkalosis.

Stalheim-Smith, A & Fitch, GK: Understanding Human Anatomy and Physiology. *Minneapolis/St. Paul, West Publishing, pp. 561-564, 1994; Taylor, C, Lillis, C & LeMone, P:* Fundamentals of Nursing: The Art and Science of Nursing Care, *2nd ed. Philadelphia, Lippincott, p. 1002, 1993.*

10.22. Correct Answer: **c**

Trousseau's sign, the development of carpal spasm after 3 minutes of circulatory interruption with a tourniquet or blood pressure cuff, and Chvostek's sign, twitching of the upper lip after stimulation, indicate neuromuscular irritability. Hypocalcemia alters acetylcholine release at the synapse. Even minor calcium deficits can produce symptoms of neuromuscular weakness or irritability. Early postoperative cardiac conduction delays may also occur.

Anderson, JL & Lobo, DP: Recovery of the Patient With Head and Neck Surgery in Manual of Post Anesthesia Care *(Jacobsen, WK, Ed). Philadelphia, Saunders, pp. 33-34, 1992; Christoph, SB: Post Anesthesia Care of the Thyroid and Parathyroid Surgical Patient in* The Post Anesthesia Care Unit: A Critical Care Approach to Post Anesthesia Nursing, *3rd ed (Drain, C, Ed). Philadelphia, Saunders, pp. 444-445, 1994.*

10.23. Correct Answer: **d**

Laryngeal stridor may indicate neuromuscular irritability related to hypocalcemia. Intravenous calcium gluconate or calcium carbonate reverses symptoms of neuromuscular irritability. Stridor may also reflect postoperative bleeding, nerve injury or airway edema. Determine serum calcium with a laboratory measure. A diuretic treats hypercalcemia by increasing urinary excretion of calcium; sedation may relax the patient but certainly will not improve ventilation.

Tuman, KJ: Fluid and Electrolyte Abnormalities and Management in Post Anesthesia Care *(Vender, JS & Speiss, BD, Eds). Philadelphia, Saunders, p. 174, 1992; Baer, CL: Fluid and Electrolyte Balance in* AACN's Clinical Reference for Critical-Care Nursing, *3rd ed (Kinney, MR, Packa, DR & Dunbar, SB, Eds). St. Louis, Mosby, pp. 193-194, 1993.*

10.24. Correct Answer: **a**

The oculocardiac reflex is a response to manipulation of eye muscles and tissue. Heart rate, blood pressure and level of consciousness decrease. An oculocardiac reflex can be elicited preoperatively during placement of a retrobulbar block with a local anesthetic. During surgery, direct pressure on the eyeball, traction on eye muscles, a child's strabismus repair, or retinal surgery can also evoke this reflex response. Hypotension and varied intracardiac conduction blocks can continue into the postoperative period.

Maes, KS, Britton, T & Bell, B: The Ophthalmic Surgical Patient in ASPAN's Core Curriculum for Post Anesthesia Nursing Practice, *3rd ed (Litwack, K, Ed). Philadelphia, Saunders, p. 599, 1994; Burden, N:* Ambulatory Surgical Nursing. *Philadelphia, Saunders, pp. 461-464, 1993.*

10.25. Correct Answer: **c**

The surgeon should be immediately informed when a postoperative eye patient develops severe pain. Intense pain may mean hemorrhage or increased intraocular pressure. The cause of pain must be promptly explored to prevent eye damage. Low-grade pain can be anticipated and treated after ocular surgery. Position is generally determined by surgeon-preference, often to achieve pressure on the retina by air or gas injected into the eye.

Litwack, K: Post Anesthesia Care Nursing, *2nd ed. St. Louis, Mosby, pp. 261-262, 1995.*

10.26. Correct Answer: **d**

Ms D's symptoms indicate complete airway obstruction. Relaxing rigid airway structures with succinylcholine and then supporting ventilation with positive pressure and 100% oxygen are likely necessary to open her airway. After such otolaryngologic surgeries as tonsillectomy, adenoidectomy, or parotid gland procedures, the incidence of laryngospasm and complete airway obstruction is high. Anterior displacement of Ms D's mandible and positive pressure ventilation may not "break" a spasm that causes complete obstruction.

Berge, KH & Lanier, WL: Problems After Head, Neck and Maxillofacial Surgery in Post Anesthesia Care *(Vender, JS & Speiss, BD, Eds). Philadelphia, Saunders, pp. 283-285, 1992.*

10.27. Correct Answer: **b**

Ms D's airway complication is laryngeal, not bronchiolar. The nurse should anticipate increased likelihood of airway obstruction for any patient after otolaryngologic surgery. Airway irritants, like vocal cord secretions (especially fresh blood or mucous) near the operative site, can stimulate the vocal cords into spasm. History of smoking, anatomic deviations and intubation trauma may only be contributing causes. One study of nearly 137,000 otolaryngologic surgical patients reported a nearly 1% incidence of partial or complete airway obstruction.

Feinstein, R & Owens, WD: Anesthesia for ENT in Clinical Anesthesia, *2nd ed (Barash, PG, Cullen, BF & Stoelting, RK, Eds). Philadelphia, Lippincott, p. 1525, 1992; Berge, KH & Lanier, WL: Problems After Head, Neck and Maxillofacial Surgery in* Post Anesthesia Care *(Vender, JS & Speiss, BD, Eds). Philadelphia, Saunders, pp. 283-285, 1992.*

10.28. Correct Answer: **a**

The supine position is used for most surgical procedures. This position can be modified in several ways. Postural hypotension, backache, circulatory compromise at bony prominences (i.e., sacrum, heels, or elbows), hair loss from the posterior scalp, and extremity nerve damage are all possible. Anesthesia produces relaxed muscles, inability to move, and no awareness of positions that are painful or that compromise circulation. Tissue ischemia or edema, nerve injury, and joint or muscle pain may become evident in the postanesthesia period. Preexisting medical conditions and surgical procedures of more than 2 hours' duration add to the potential for position-related injury.

Litwack, K: Post Anesthesia Nursing Practice, *2nd ed. St. Louis, Mosby, pp. 480-485, 1995; Walsh, J: Postop Effects of OR Positioning.* RN *56(2): 50-58, 1993.*

10.29. Correct Answer: **a**

Administering large volumes of intraoperative crystalloid fluids or using hyperosmolar solutions like mannitol increases the potential for congestive heart failure in elderly patients. A flat position only compounds this potential. Nitroprusside and nitroglycerin benefit coronary blood flow and contractility.

Florete, OG & Gallagher, TJ: Cardiac Disease: Congestive Heart Failure, Coronary Artery Disease, and Valvular Disease in Manual of Anesthesia and the Medically Compromised Patient *(Cheng, EY & Kay, J, Eds). Philadelphia, Lippincott, pp. 2-20, 1990.*

10.30. Correct Answer: **d**

Morphine sulfate relaxes vascular smooth muscle, producing peripheral vasodilation to decrease both venous return and afterload, and eases anxiety from respiratory distress. The alpha adrenergic effects of phenylephrine vasoconstrict and increase both preload and afterload. Rotating tourniquets, a seldom used form of "bloodless phlebotomy," and intubation are more likely adjuncts after intervention with diuretics, morphine and vasoactive medications.

Benz, J: Heart Failure in Critical Care Nursing: A Holistic Approach, *6th ed (Hudak, CM & Gallo, BM, Eds). Philadelphia, Lippincott, pp. 318-322, 1994; McKenry, SM & Salerno, E:* Mosby's Pharmacology in Nursing, *18th ed. St. Louis, Mosby, pp. 215-216, 1992.*

10.31. Correct Answer: **c**

Blood pressure measures, intravenous lines or venipuncture for serum sampling are avoided in the arm on the surgical side. Such compressive or invasive interventions can impair circulation. Radical mastectomy involves removal of breast tissue, underlying pectoral muscles and fascia and dissection of axillary lymph nodes. The resulting alteration of lymph circulation and drainage from the right (surgical) arm promotes fluid stasis and edema formation.

Saleh, KL: Practical Points in the Care of the Patient Post-Breast Surgery. J Post Anesth Nurs *7(3): 176-178, 1992; Johnson, JR: Caring for the Woman Who's Had a Mastectomy.* Am J Nurs *94(5): 25-32, 1994.*

10.32. Correct Answer: **d**

Report lower arm sensory loss to the surgeon. Swelling, sensory loss on the front of the upper arm or anywhere below the elbow, and strong pain in the lower arm typically do not accompany axillary node dissection. Decreased sensation at the axilla and inner portion of the upper arm and movement difficulty are expected. The nurse positions the right arm on pillows for muscle support, to facilitate venous drainage, and to minimize swelling. Up to 100 ml of red drainage is expected from the incisional area during the first 24 hours, with decreasing amounts thereafter.

Johnson, JR: Caring for the Woman Who's Had a Mastectomy. Am J Nurs *94(5): 25-32, 1994.*

10.33. Correct Answer: **b**

The capillary filling pressure of the tracheal wall is 27-30 mm Hg. Thus to prevent obliteration of blood flow to tracheal tissues, maintaining an endotracheal tube's cuff pressure near 20 mm Hg is recommended. Some cuff inflation is required to prevent air leakage and reduce aspiration risk.

Hudak, CM & Gallo, BM: Critical Care Nursing: A Holistic Approach, *6th ed. Philadelphia, Lippincott, pp. 468-469, 1994; Drain, C:* The Post Anesthesia Care Unit: A Critical Care Approach to Post Anesthesia Nursing, *3rd ed. Philadelphia, Saunders, pp. 308-309, 1994.*

10.34. Correct Answer: **c**

During vitrectomy and retinal surgeries, the surgeon may place a small bubble of air or gas into the eye globe. The purpose of the air is to maintain the retina's position. The surgeon specifies the desired position for each patient. Air rises in solution and will shift with the patient's position.

Litwack, K: Post Anesthesia Care Nursing, *2nd ed. St. Louis, Mosby, pp. 261-262, 1995.*

10.35. Correct Answer: **b**

Normal intraocular pressure (IOP) is 10-20 mm Hg. Hypocarbia (decreased pCO_2 through hyperventilation and respiratory alkalosis) vasoconstricts and reduces aqueous humor production. This decreases IOP. Anesthesia-related events like coughing, Valsalva's maneuvers, straining, or vomiting strongly increase intrathoracic pressure and therefore central venous pressure. These activities increase IOP by as much as 40 mm Hg.

Castro, AD: Management of Anesthesia for Specialty Procedures in

Dripps/Eckenhoff/Vandam Introduction to Anesthesia, *8th ed (Longnecker, DE & Murphy, FL, Eds). Philadelphia, Saunders, pp. 403-406, 1992.*

10.36. Correct Answer: **d**

Controversy surrounds establishing any relationship between specific surgical procedures and the undesired outcome of postoperative nausea and vomiting (PONV). PONV is not specifically linked with uncomplicated transurethral prostate resection. However, ophthalmic surgery may produce significant PONV; up to 85% of children vomit after strabismus repairs. In general, laparoscopic procedures are asssociated with increased nausea; researchers report PONV among approximately 50% of women after laparoscopy to obtain ova. PONV is also often reported after ear procedures.

Burden, N: Ambulatory Surgical Nursing. *Philadelphia, Saunders, pp. 75-76 & 476-478, 1993; Parnass, SM: Problems of Ambulatory Surgery in* Post Anesthesia Care *(Vender, JS & Speiss, BD, Eds). Philadelphia, Saunders, pp. 321-326, 1992.*

10.37. Correct Answer: **b**

The facial nerve lies behind the ear, very near the surgical incision used for mastoidectomy. Mouth drooping, drooling, or facial asymmetry when grinning, grimacing, wrinkling the forehead, or closing the eyes are reportable outcomes. Surgical edema or inflammation or trauma to a specific nerve may compromise muscular function. Branches of the acoustic nerve, cranial nerve VIII, have sensory functions associated with hearing and equilibrium.

Burden, N: Ambulatory Surgical Nursing. *Philadelphia, Saunders, pp. 476-478, 1993; Provenzano, SM: Assessment: Nervous System in* Critical Care Nursing: A Holistic Approach, *6th ed (Hudak, CM & Gallo, BM, Eds). Philadelphia, Lippincott, pp. 657-671, 1994.*

Annotated Bibliography

Run to the medical bookstore...empty the shelves at the biomedical library...browse the book collection of your friends and colleagues...dig into a sampling of excellent resources. Borrow, borrow, borrow!! This bibliography represents but a few of the thousands of texts, journals, and newsletters you could select for your certification review.

- Choosing references from this list can help focus your study plan and steer you toward *other* resources.
- Please note that **this list is neither exhaustive nor exclusive.** You can and will find other equally valuable resources to support your review.
- Expand your literary repertoire. Don't *limit* yourself to anesthesia-focused texts.
  - Keep a basic nursing, pharmacology, and anatomy and physiology text at your side for reference.
  - Explore nursing and medical publications from other specialties that intersect with perianesthesia nursing, particularly those that describe critical care, cardiovascular and pulmonary, neuroscience, orthopedic, nephrologic, urologic, gastrointestinal, and reconstructive nursing.
  - As often as possible, locate **the most current** editions of a journal. While basic anatomy, physiologic and pharmacologic principles and anesthetic concepts don't change, interventions, medications, and philosophies of practice do.

ASPAN-SPONSORED PUBLICATIONS

American Society of Post Anesthesia Nurses: Redi-Ref. *Richmond, VA, 1993. (Available through Slack, Inc., Thorofare, NJ.)*

Provides quick, easy access to essential information needed in daily clinical practice. Set in table and outline format, topics range from laboratory measures to commonly used anesthetic medications to physiologic differences among adults, pregnant women, children, and the elderly.

American Society of Post Anesthesia Nurses: Research Redi-Ref. *Thorofare, NJ, ASPAN, (in press).*

Defines research terms and walks the user through the research process.

American Society of Post Anesthesia Nurses: Standards of Perianesthesia Nusing Practice. *Thorofare, NJ, ASPAN, 71 pages, 1995.*

Designed to slip into a three-ring binder with unit protocols, this resource compiles the perianesthesia scope of practice, national standards for patient care, and several position statements and resources. Latex allergy and educational competencies expand the 1995 edition.

Breathline

Fifteen volumes of ASPAN's bimonthly newsletter chronicle the evolution of perianesthesia nursing. Each issue features clinical content and discusses relevant professional and patient care issues.

Journal of Post Anesthesia Nursing

ASPAN's official Journal, now in its 10th volume year, informs readers who practice in ambulatory surgery and inpatient perianesthesia settings. Each bimonthly issue contains clinical, educational and leadership content the reader can apply to patient care and supplement personal knowledge.

Litwack, K (Ed): ASPAN's Core Curriculum for Post Anesthesia Nursing Practice, *3rd ed. Philadelphia, Saunders, 1994. 680 pages.*

This "must have" text outlines the essential concepts of clinical nursing practice in a perianesthesia setting. Applying a nursing process approach, each chapter outlines critical nursing diagnoses, assessments and interventions related to a specific organ system. Describes relevant nursing priorities related to specific anesthetic and surgical procedures. Review questions end each chapter.

Quinn, D: Ambulatory Post Anesthesia Nursing Outline: Content for Certification. *Richmond, VA, ASPAN, 1994, 245 pages.*

Designated as an overview of ambulatory surgery, the outline format of this text presents anesthetic medications and patient assessment considerations appropriate for the outpatient setting. Approaches the scope of ambulatory surgery practice by applying ASPAN Standards of Nursing Practice and essential patient education. Extensive bibliography.

BOOKS

Perianesthesia Nursing Classics

Burden, N: Ambulatory Surgical Nursing. *Philadelphia, Saunders, 1993, 712 pages.*

Don't let the title fool you. This classic text's in-depth, yet easy reading style spans the spectrum of perianesthesia care. From pharmacology to education to surgical procedures to quality management, the nurse finds pearls of wisdom to plan inpatient *and* outpatient care.

Drain, C (Ed): The Post Anesthesia Care Unit: A Critical Care Approach to Post Anesthesia Care Nursing, *3rd ed. Philadelphia, Saunders, 1994, 594 pages.*

A "household staple" in a PACU library for 15 years, this multi-authored reference delves deeply into organ system anatomy and cellular physiology. Graphs, diagrams, tables and illustrations detail the concepts essential to understanding the effects of anesthetic medications and specific surgical procedures.

Litwack, K: Post Anesthesia Care Nursing, *2nd ed. St. Louis, Mosby, 1995, 558 pages.*

This patient-focused reference overviews broad concepts and techniques of anesthetic pharmacology and physiology. Graphs, tables and drawings illustrate and summarize nursing assessments and interventions. Establishes postsurgical priorities, but focuses on *anesthesia*-related complications.

Anesthesia Focus

American College of Surgeons: Care of the Surgical Patient *(Wilmore, DW, et al, Eds). New York, Scientific American Inc., 1993. 2 Volume set.*

A compendium of general reference articles collected in two 3-ring binders reviews most surgical concerns. Many charts and diagrams illustrate a problem-oriented approach to critical care concerns (Volume 1) and elective procedures (Volume 2).

Barash, PG, Cullen, BF, Stoelting, RK: Handbook of Clinical Anesthesia. *Philadelphia, Lippincott, 1991, 515 pages.*

A comprehensive, handbook style reference in outline format with concise, paragraph-length explanations of anesthesia pharmacology. Peppered with graphs, charts and tables for quick access to information.

Benumof, JL & Saidman, LJ: Anesthesia and Perioperative Complications. *St. Louis, Mosby, 1992, 681 pages.*

Geared for the anesthesia provider, this unique text focuses on physiologic and environmental perianesthesia complications. A comprehensive index leads the reader to rarely described topics ranging from laser fires to managing risk.

Brown, DL: Atlas of Regional Anesthesia. *Philadelphia, Saunders, 1992, 250 pages.*

Full of colorful anatomic illustrations that detail placement of regional blocks. Worth scrutiny to appreciate anatomy, techniques of block placement, and mechanisms of analgesia.

Datta, S: Common Problems in Obstetric Anesthesia, *2nd ed. St. Louis, Mosby, 1995, 527 pages.*

A short patient situation sets a real-life tone for each brief chapter. Topics include postoperative pain relief, postdural puncture headache, nonobstetric surgery during pregnancy, and pregnancy risk issues like diabetes, premature labor, and latex allergy. Provides multiple graphs, charts, and algorithms in a reader-friendly style.

Davidson, JK, Eckhardt, WR & Perese, DA: Clinical Anesthesia Procedures of the Massachusetts General Hospital, *4th ed. Boston, Little, Brown & Co., 1993, 650 pages.*

A pocket-sized reference that describes anesthesia for specific organ systems and medical conditions. Helpful "suggested reading" ends each chapter and directs user to references that provide a wider topical discussion.

Gregory, GA: Pediatric Anesthesia, *3rd ed. New York, Churchill-Livingstone, 1994, approximately 1500 pages.*

A medical text with a focus on specific anatomic and physiologic responses of children during surgery and anesthesia. Includes detailed discussions of pediatric procedures, many subheadings and graphs, and an excellent index.

Longnecker, DE, Murphy, FL: Dripps/Eckenhoff/Vandam Introduction to Anesthesia, *(8th Ed). Philadelphia, Saunders, 1992, 475 pages.*

A medical anesthesia text with wide-ranging scope that carries the reader from preanesthesia evaluation to pharmacologic effects, anesthetic techniques, and surgical positions. Includes a 40 page section on postoperative care, from the medical perspective.

Miller, R: Anesthesia, *4th ed. New York, Churchill-Livingstone, 1994, Vol. 1: 1361 pages; Vol 2: 2696 pages.*

Everything you ever wanted to know about anesthesia is contained in this 2 volume medical text. Hundreds of references. The detailed index and easy reading style with subheadings and diagrams offer a plethora of anesthetic principles from trauma to procedures away from the OR and PACU.

Morgan, GE, Mikhail, MS: Clinical Anesthesiology. *Norwalk, CT, Appleton & Lange, 1992, 719 pages.*

Extraordinarily detailed drawings, comparative tables, and focused descriptions of anesthesia's physiologic effects on organ systems distinguish this clinical text. A case discussion ends each chapter. Relevant for nurses interested in expanding clinical knowledge. A great index and reader friendly too.

Schnider, SM & Levinson, G: Anesthesia for Obstetrics, *3rd ed. Baltimore, Williams & Wilkins, 1993, 720 pages.*

This text's best features for nurses are the pathophysiologic details related to high-risk pregnancy and neonatology. A medical text that focuses on specific obstetric-anesthetic concerns.

Stoelting, RK, Dierdorf, SF: Handbook for Anesthesia and Coexisting Diseases. *New York, Churchill-Livingstone, 1993, 378 pages.*

This outlined text full of tables and charts provides a quick look at pathophysiologic assessments for a wide range of anesthesia/surgical patients. Use this handbook, designed as a pocket companion to a more expansive test of similar title, to increase understanding of potential medical complications.

Summers, S & Ebbert, DW: Ambulatory Surgical Nursing: A Nursing Diagnosis Approach. *Philadelphia, Lippincott, 1992.*

A unique blend of nursing diagnosis and ambulatory surgery concepts. The text is based on case studies and identified patient needs from preanesthesia assessment through postoperative discharge.

Vender, JS & Spiess, BD: Post Anesthesia Care. *Philadelphia, Saunders, 1992, 369 pages.*

A physician-authored text that focuses on medical concerns and complications *after* anesthesia. Useful to expand nursing knowledge for a collaborative postanesthesia practice.

Waugaman, WR, Foster, SC & Rigor, BM: Principles and Practice of Nurse Anesthesia, *2nd ed. Norwalk, CT, Appleton & Lange, 1992, 836 pages.*

A one-of-a-kind multiauthored text written by nurse anesthetists. Provides plenty of content depth and descriptive diagrams. Covers dose calculations, organ system and pharmacologic physiology, and anesthesia for specific surgeries and patient populations.

Zichuhr, MT & Atsberger, DB: Pre- and Postanestheisa Nursing Knowledge Base and Clinical Competencies. *Philadelphia, Saunders, 1995, 158 pages.*

Use this clinical workbook as another atlas of the critical perianesthesia concepts to master. Intended as a guide to educational competencies.

Pharmacology

Baer, CL & Williams, BR: Clinical Pharmacology and Nursing, *2nd ed. Springhouse, PA, Springhouse Corp, 1992, 1325 pages.*

Pharmacology presented in nursing process terms. Offers a clear delineation of assessment, related nursing diagnoses, and implementation for each medication. Technical and detailed information presented in a comfortable reading style. Chapters focus on organ systems or specific diseases altered by the pharmacologic intervention.

Katzung, BG: Basic and Clinical Pharmacology, *6th ed. Norwalk, CT, Appleton & Lange, 1995, 990 pages.*

A general pharmacology paperback full of terrific diagrams and detailed text. Useful discussions for broad classifications of drugs and clearly described pharmacokinetic and pharmacodynamic concepts applied to clinical physiologic changes. A book to pore over, definitely not a quick reference.

Lehne, RA: Pharmcology for Nursing Care, *2nd ed. Philadelphia, Saunders, 1994, 1230 pages.*

An introductory pharmacology text with easy reading style that presents nursing considerations related to the clinical effects of medications. More than a handy reference, this book is written with adequate detail to inform about drug classifications.

Shannon, MT, Wilson, BA & Stang, CL: Govoni & Hayes Drugs and Nursing Implications, *8th ed. Norwalk, CT, Appleton & Lange, 1995, 1196 pages.*

Comprehensive yet nursing focused and filled with need-to-know information. Medications are catalogued in alphabetical order; content provides details not included in many quick-reference nursing texts.

Vallerand, AH & Deglin, JF: Davis's Guide to IV Medications, 2nd ed. *Philadelphia, FA Davis, 1993, 956 pages.*

Alphabetically-sequenced spiral-bound reference for the clinical nurse. Highlights pharmacology essentials and emphasizes incompatibilities, precautions and clinical assessments. Useful study for nonanesthetic medications.

Anatomy and Physiology

Berne, RM & Levy, MN: Physiology, 3rd ed. *St. Louis, Mosby, 1993, 1024 pages.*

Heavily illustrated physiology text that covers neurophysiology to hormones. Best features are the many bi-color diagrams and the topical summary comments that close each chapter.

Copstead, LC: Perspectives in Pathophysiology. *Philadelphia, Saunders, 1165+ pages, 1995.*

Pathophysiology presented in nursing diagnosis terms! Describes normal anatomic and physiologic organ system function, then delves into alterations created by aging and disease. Applies research to nursing care.

Cummins, RO: Textbook of Advanced Cardiac Life Support. *Dallas, American*

Heart Association, 1994, approximately 250 pages.

A compilation of anatomy, physiology, and pharmacology applied to the cardiopulmonary system. Describes airway management, distinguishing features of electrocardiography and life-supporting medications. Many diagrams and algorithms.

Guyton, AC: Textbook of Medical Physiology, *8th ed. Philadelphia, Saunders, 1991 950 pages.*

A classic of cellular fundamentals. Describes normals of organ system function with detail. Colorful and easy reading.

Stalheim-Smith, A & Fitch, GK: Understanding Human Anatomy and Physiology. *Minneapolis/St. Paul, West Publishing, 1994.*

Designed to educate non-medical people, this text clearly explains difficult-to-comprehend physiologic interactions in layman's terms. Visually appealing text with colorful diagrams and charts. Brief clinical capsules in each chapter apply physiology to life.

A Plethora of Specialized Nursing Wisdom

American Association of Critical Care Nurses (AACN): Core Curriculum for Critical Care Nursing, 4th ed; Core Review for Critical Care Nursing; Procedure Manual for Critical Care. *Philadelphia, Saunders, 1991-1993.*

Several society-sponsored publications provide readers with essential critical care content and procedure descriptions. Designed with education and preparation for CCRN certification in mind.

Black, JM & Matassarin-Jacobs, E: Luckmann & Sorensen's Medical-Surgical Nursing: A Psychophysiologic Approach, *4th ed. Philadelphia, Saunders, 1993, 2430 pages.*

A back-to-basics classic that discusses and illustrates general medical-surgical nursing. Considers ethics, education and health concerns from a nursing process approach.

Clochesy, JM, Breu, C, Cardin, S, et al: Critical Care Nursing. *Philadelphia, Saunders, 1993, 1418 pages.*

Focuses on the critically ill adult and describes nursing assessments, techniques and interventions, including pharmacology.

Dossey, BM, Guzzetta, CE, Kenner, CV: Critical Care Nursing: Body-Mind-Spirit *(3rd Ed), Philadelphia, Lippincott, 1992, 980 pages.*

Each chapter combines the essence of nursing—empowerment, healing and independent nursing intervention—with detailed physiology and specialized technical knowledge. Outcome-based care plans describe nursing orders with rationales for specific observations.

Hickey, JV: The Clinical Practice of Neurological and Neurosurgical Nursing, *3rd ed. Philadelphia, Lippincott, 1992, 666 pages.*

Several authors provide detailed discussions of intracranial and spinal neurologic procedures, complications and concepts of patient management. Photographs, diagrams and tables review neuroanatomy and physiology.

Hudak, CM & Gallo, BM: Critical Care Nursing: A Holistic Apporach, *6th ed. Philadelphia, Lippincott, 1994, over 1000 pages.*

A chapter devoted to postanesthesia care rounds out this detailed yet reader friendly text. Includes many diagrams, photographs and tables to illustrate critical care concepts. Written with a nursing process approach.

Kozier, B, Erb, G, Blais, K, et al: Fundamentals of Nursing: Concepts, Process and Practice. *Redwood City, CA, Addison-Wesley. 1995.*

A case management focus in this basic nursing text emphasizes critical pathways and influencing change. The book's novel style invites the reader to think in nursing diagnosis terms, to lead the patient through lifespan changes, and to practice with awareness of outcome-focused criteria.

Lounsbury, P, Frye, SJ: Cardiac Rhythm Disturbances: A Nursing Process Approach, 2nd ed. *St. Louis, Mosby, 1992, 375 pages.*

Discusses and diagrams electrocardiographic principles that underlie the rhythms a nurse monitors each day. Considers the diagnostic features of each monitoring lead. Self-assessment questions end each chapter. Text includes a comprehensive glossary of cardioactive medications.

Maher, AB, Salmond, SW & Pellino, TA: Orthopedic Nursing. *Philadelphia, Saunders, 1994, 978 pages.*

Delve into an in-depth presentation of congenital and acquired orthopedic concerns. Case studies illustrate patient situations, describe assessments, interventions, and education information for specific disorders. Heavily incorporates diagrams to explain chapter content.

Meeker, MR & Rothrock, JC: Alexander's Care of the Patient in Surgery, *10th ed. St. Louis, Mosby, 1995, 1306 pages.*

A descriptive book with the words, photographs and diagrams to explain most surgical procedures and the patient's intraoperative experience. Written with nursing diagnosis and outcome focus in mind, the reader also learns surgical tools to anchor bone or snip and suture organ tissue. Includes a postanesthesia care chapter.

Miller-Keane Encyclopedia & Dictionary of Medicine, Nursing & Allied Health, 5th ed. *Philadelphia, Saunders, 1992, 1810 pages.*

Use this reference full of definitions and concise descriptions to verify spelling and obtain general information about any health care topic.

Phippen, ML & Wells, MP: Perioperative Nursing Practice. *Philadelphia, Suanders, 1994, 1088 pages.*

Graphically describes specific surgical procedures through photographs, lists, and diagrams to portray the intraoperative environment. Appreciate intraoperative issues of patient positioning and sterility.

Roth, MA: AORN's Perioperative Nursing Core Curriculum. *Philadelphia, Saunders, 1995, 450 pages.*

Offers a glimpse into knowledge required for perioperative nursing practice and to certify as a CNOR. Useful for preprocedural assessment information and to become familiar with AORN standards and recommendations.

Taylor, C, Lillis, C, LeMone, P: Fundamentals of Nursing: The Art and Science of Nursing Care, *(2nd Ed). Philadelphia, Saunders, 1993, 1385 pages.*

A colorful, detailed basic nursing text. Good reference to review cardiac physiology, medication calculations, fluid and chemical balance, and procedural techniques and rationales. Chapters end with key point summaries and review questions.

PERIODICALS

Regularly scan medical and nursing journals. Update your literature search for relevant articles. Specialty journals publish review articles, research, and clinical considerations that apply to perianesthesia patients.

AANA: Journal of the American Association of Nurse Anesthetists (bimonthly)

American Journal of Nursing (monthly).

Presents general clinical topics in a brief, colorful format. For fun, test your knowledge with the CE test.

Anesthesia and Analgesia (monthly)

Anesthesiology Clinics of North America (quarterly):

Compiles contributed review-style articles related to each issue's theme. Provides useful overview of a topic.

Anesthesiology (monthly)

ANNA Journal: American Nephrology Nurses Association's publication (bimonthly)

AORN Journal: American Operating Room Nurses official publication (monthly)

Critical Care Nurse (monthly): sponsored by the American Association of Critical Care Nurses

Critical Care Nursing Clinics of North America (quarterly).

More nurse-focused than many textbooks, content of articles in each issue is geared largely for the clinical nurse.

Journal of Neuroscience Nursing (bimonthly).

Minimally Invasive Surgical Nursing (quarterly)

Orthopaedic Nursing (monthly)

Plastic Surgical Nursing (quarterly)

Post Anesthesia and Ambulatory Surgery Nursing Update (bimonthly).

Current information from selected journals presented in abstract form; commentary links information from widely diverse publications to perianesthesia nursing practice.

Seminars in Anesthesia (quarterly).

Assembles easily read yet technical articles related to an issue's theme. Considers diseases from an anesthesia perspective.

Seminars in Perioperative Nursing (quarterly).

Discusses specific patient populations or nursing issues from the perioperative perspective.

Surgical Clinics of North America (quarterly).

Guest-edited theme issues compile articles about a specific surgical topic.

Answer Sheet

1.	a	b	c	d	**26.**	a	b	c	d
2.	a	b	c	d	**27.**	a	b	c	d
3.	a	b	c	d	**28.**	a	b	c	d
4.	a	b	c	d	**29.**	a	b	c	d
5.	a	b	c	d	**30.**	a	b	c	d
6.	a	b	c	d	**31.**	a	b	c	d
7.	a	b	c	d	**32.**	a	b	c	d
8.	a	b	c	d	**33.**	a	b	c	d
9.	a	b	c	d	**34.**	a	b	c	d
10.	a	b	c	d	**35.**	a	b	c	d
11.	a	b	c	d	**36.**	a	b	c	d
12.	a	b	c	d	**37.**	a	b	c	d
13.	a	b	c	d	**38.**	a	b	c	d
14.	a	b	c	d	**39.**	a	b	c	d
15.	a	b	c	d	**40.**	a	b	c	d
16.	a	b	c	d	**41.**	a	b	c	d
17.	a	b	c	d	**42.**	a	b	c	d
18.	a	b	c	d	**43.**	a	b	c	d
19.	a	b	c	d	**44.**	a	b	c	d
20.	a	b	c	d	**45.**	a	b	c	d
21.	a	b	c	d	**46.**	a	b	c	d
22.	a	b	c	d	**47.**	a	b	c	d
23.	a	b	c	d	**48.**	a	b	c	d
24.	a	b	c	d	**49.**	a	b	c	d
25.	a	b	c	d	**50.**	a	b	c	d

Use this generic answer sheet for each set of items in the text. May be reproduced as often as necessary.

Index

In this index, subjects are located by *item* (question) number not by page number. Select a subject from the alphabetized list; the string of item numbers following that subject indicate each subject's location in the text. Each item's level of difficulty appears in parentheses after the item number. For example, item 4.61 (II) is found in chapter 4; its level of difficulty is II. Also refer to the Core Concepts outlined at the beginning of each section in this text; master these key concepts; refer to information contained in the affiliated chapter of *ASPAN's Core Curriculum for Post Anesthesia Nursing Practice, 3rd ed.*

-I-

-J-

-K-

-L-

-M-

-N-

-O-

-P-

-R-

-S-

-T-

-U-

-V-

-W-